CURRENT ISSUES IN HEALTH

THIRD EDITION

CURRENT ISSUES IN HEALTH

THIRD EDITION

Stephen Brown

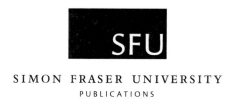

SIMON FRASER UNIVERSITY
PUBLICATIONS

CURRENT ISSUES IN HEALTH
Copyright © 2018 by SFU Publications

Third edition

Library and Archives Canada Cataloguing in Publication

Brown, Stephen (Professor of kinesiology), author
     Current issues in health / Stephen Brown. -- Third edition.

Includes bibliographical references and index.
ISBN 978-1-77287-045-9 (softcover)

     1. Public health--Canada. I. Title.

RA449.B76 2018   362.10971   C2018-903810-1

Printed in Canada by Hignell Book Printing
Cover design and graphics by Greg Holoboff
Book design and typesetting by Robert D. MacNevin
Copy editing by Rebecca Coates

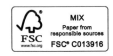

SFU Publications
Simon Fraser University
Faculty of Arts & Social Sciences
8888 University Drive
Burnaby, British Columbia V5A 1S6
Canada

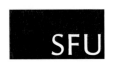

Contents

Preface   x

Acknowledgements   xii

About the Author   xiv

1 The Concept of Health   1
    1   What is Health?   1
    2   Indicators of Health   2
    3   Models of Health   3
    4   How Are We Doing?   14
    5   Conclusion   15

2 Evaluating Health Claims   19
    1   Overview   19
    2   Scientific Evidence   20
    3   Clinical Evidence   28
    4   Personal Experience   29
    5   Anecdotal Evidence   29
    6   Critical Thinking   30
    7   Conclusion   35

3 Infectious Disease   39
    1   Overview   39
    2   Mechanism of Infectious Diseases   40

3   Protection Against Infection   41
4   Transmission of Communicable Diseases   43
5   Colds and Influenza   46
6   Control of Infectious Disease   47
7   Infectious Disease in the Developing Countries   52
8   Conclusion   53

4   Cardiovascular Disease and Diabetes   59
1   The Cardiovascular System   59
2   Prevalence   61
3   Risk Factors for Cardiovascular Disease   62
4   Diabetes Mellitus   69
5   Treatment   73
6   Conclusion   77

5   Cancer   83
1   Overview   83
2   Mechanisms of Cancer   84
3   Major Types of Cancer   90
4   Treating Cancer   100
5   Preventing Cancer   102
6   Conclusion   104

6   Physical Activity   109
1   Overview   109
2   Physical Activity of North Americans   110
3   Activity, Exercise, and Fitness   111
4   Components of Physical Fitness   112
5   Benefits of Exercise   113
6   Nature of the Evidence   115
7   Risks of Exercise/Physical Activity   116
8   How to Develop Aerobic Fitness   118
9   How to Develop Muscular Fitness   120
10   How to Develop Flexibility   123
11   Prevention of Activity-Related Injuries   124
12   Treatment of Activity-Related Injuries   125
13   Conclusion   126

7   Nutrition   **131**

    1   Overview   131

    2   The Main Categories of Nutrients   132

    3   What Is a Healthy Diet?   133

    4   Nature of the Evidence   135

    5   The Modern North American Diet   137

    6   Dietary Recommendations for North Americans   138

    7   How Healthy are Diets of Different Cultures?   144

    8   Vegetarian Diets   145

    9   Organic Foods   148

    10   Genetically Modified Foods   150

    11   Nutritional Concerns of the Developing World   151

    12   Conclusion   152

8   Body Weight and Weight Management   **157**

    1   Overview   157

    2   Definitions of *Overweight, Overfat,* and *Obese*   158

    3   Methods of Determining *Ideal Weight*   158

    4   Prevalence of Obesity   164

    5   Causes of Obesity   164

    6   Social Issues Regarding Obesity   167

    7   Unsound Weight-Loss Dieting   169

    8   Eating Disorders   170

    9   Guidelines for Sound Weight Control   172

    10   Conclusion   177

9   Mental Health   **183**

    1   Overview   183

    2   Mental Health   184

    3   Psychological Disorders   185

    4   Suicide   189

    5   Treatment for Mental Health Problems   191

    6   Stress   192

    7   Sleep   200

    8   Gratitude   203

    9   Conclusion   204

10   Intimate Relationships and Human Sexuality   211

    1   Overview   211

    2   Intimate Relationships   212

    3   What Is *Love?*   215

    4   Human Genital Anatomy   216

    5   Human Sexual Response   221

    6   Variations in Sexual Behaviour   225

    7   Commercial Sex   228

    8   Pornography   230

    9   Sexual Health Promotion   232

    10   Conclusion   233

11   Sexually Transmitted Infections   239

    1   Overview   239

    2   HIV/AIDS   240

    3   Hepatitis   250

    4   Human Papillomavirus   251

    5   Herpes Simplex   253

    6   Other STIs   255

    7   Conclusion   258

12   Fertility Management   265

    1   Overview   265

    2   Choosing a Fertility Management Plan   266

    3   Contraceptive Technology   270

    4   Abortion   285

    5   Pregnancy and Childbirth   290

    6   Conclusion   295

13   Drugs   301

    1   Overview   301

    2   Routes of Administration   302

    3   Common Psychoactive Drugs   304

    4   Why People Take Drugs   322

    5   Models of Drug Abuse   325

    6   Strategies to Address Substance Misuse   326

    7   Conclusion   334

14 Health Care Delivery Systems   **341**

    1   Overview   342

    2. Health Care in Canada   342

    3   Strengths of the Canadian Medical Care System   350

    4   Problems with Health Care in Canada   356

    5   Conclusion   363

15 Environment   **369**

    1   Overview   369

    2   Water   370

    3   Air   372

    4   Land   375

    5   Energy   380

    6   Population   385

    7   Conclusion   390

16 Index   **393**

Preface

This book is the product of many years of teaching a university course called Contemporary Health Issues. It is written for a broad university audience and hopefully will also interest readers from a wide general public who are interested in health. This book introduces readers to the methods by which scientific knowledge develops, and summarizes our current understanding on a variety of health topics. I examine health at both the personal and population levels. In places, I contrast the current Canadian situation with circumstances in other parts of the world or at other times in history.

At times the book presents questions asked by students in my Contemporary Health Issues courses over the years, and attempts to answer these. I pose other questions to stimulate readers to apply a concept, relate it to their own experiences, or reflect on an issue. The text sometimes deals with controversial topics, and it tries to understand and respect different points of view without imposing a particular set of values. There is, however, a common theme of freedom of choice and empowerment of the individual.

Overall, the purpose of this book is to:

- Immerse readers in a way of looking at health that we will call the *holistic view*. This construct considers the inter-relatedness of genetics, physical environment, lifestyle, family status, and other factors as they influence the health of individuals, communities, and nations.
- Demonstrate some principles and methods readers can use to evaluate health information.
- Challenge readers to take greater responsibility for their health (and for the health of their families, communities, and the world) and to make thoughtful, intelligent health decisions.

Acknowledgements

IT TAKES MANY HANDS to produce a textbook. I am especially grateful to:

Dr. Glen Tibbits (former Chair of the Department of Biomedical Physiology and Kinesiology [BPK] at Simon Fraser University), Dr. Charles Krieger (Associate Chair), and Dr. Claire Cupples (Dean, SFU Faculty of Science) for supporting my 2013 study leave, during which the first edition of this book was produced;

Dr. Brooks-Wilson (Chair, BPK), Dr. Krieger, Dr. Cupples, and Van Truong (Manager, BPK) for supporting the 2018 study leave that allowed me to produce this third edition;

Simon Fraser University for its willingness to invest in its employees by providing this type of study leave;

Dr. John Whatley (Managing Editor, SFU Publications) for encouraging me to produce this textbook and for his skillful editorial advice, Greg Holoboff for producing the fine illustrations, Robert MacNevin for the book design, and Rebecca Coates for the copy editing.

Stephen Brown
Victoria, Canada
June 2018

About the Author

Stephen Brown was born in 1951. He obtained BSc and MSc degrees in Kinesiology from Simon Fraser University in British Columbia, Canada. He wrote his Master's degree thesis in the area of exercise and environmental physiology. He has been interested in health and fitness since he was a teenager and has participated in a wide range of sports and activities.

Mr. Brown is a senior lecturer in the Department of Biomedical Physiology and Kinesiology at Simon Fraser University; he has taught there since 1984.

Mr. Brown enjoys the outdoors, yoga, gardening, reading, crossword puzzles, cycling, hiking, travel, warm weather, swimming in the ocean, dogs, ballet, and theatre. He lives in Victoria with his wife, a poet, performer, and retired federal treaty negotiator. Their two daughters (born in 1990 and 1994) live in the Vancouver area.

Contact Information:
Stephen Brown MSc
Department of Biomedical Physiology and Kinesiology
Simon Fraser University
Burnaby, British Columbia v5a 1s6
Canada

CURRENT ISSUES IN HEALTH

THIRD EDITION

1   The Concept of Health

Learning Objectives

By the time you have finished this chapter, you should be able to

- Name the leading causes of human death globally
- State the most common metrics of population health
- List some determinants of health
- Explain what a model is and why models are important
- Describe, compare, and contrast different models of health
- Identify the elements in the holistic model of health
- State the World Health Organization definition of health
- Outline some personal health behaviours that can improve a person's wellness

1 What is Health?

We speak of healthy skin, a healthy bank account, or a healthy lead over a competitor. We say we feel healthy or we're going to get healthy. Health food is presumed to be better than the alternative. These various uses collectively imply something beneficial and associated with soundness, vigour, and happiness. This chapter presents several different views of health, each inherently valid but with different implications for the individual and health professionals.

In this book we will explore health at both the *individual* and the *population* level. ***Populations*** are large groups of people. Sometimes we are interested in populations of whole countries, and other times we study smaller populations, such as prison inmates, elderly women living alone, or people with HIV infection. We will see that an individual's health depends on genetic potential, personal health behaviours, and broader socio-economic and environmental factors. Similarly, a population's health is a composite of the health of the individuals who compose the population, plus broader structural and ideological factors.

2 Indicators of Health

Perhaps the most commonly used indicator of population health is **life expectancy at birth**. Clearly, length of life doesn't give the whole picture. Some people may experience a *long* life but a poor *quality* of life in the later years or even decades. However, life expectancy is much more easily measured than quality of life.

> Imagine *you* were designing a seven-item index of individual quality of life. What items would you include in this index?

A second common metric of population health is ***infant mortality rate (IMR). Mortality*** means death. IMR is calculated as the deaths of infants in the first year of life per 1,000 births. For example, if 1,000 babies were born in Richmond General Hospital in a given year and seven of them died before reaching age one, the IMR equals 7, which is a typical value for Canada and other developed countries. On the other hand, in a country with an IMR of 200, one of every five babies die before its first year of life. Like life expectancy, IMR is commonly used because (a) it is easy to obtain, as even countries that don't keep very good statistics usually record births and deaths; and (b) it hints at living conditions that can lead to death, such as poor nutrition, poor sanitation, overcrowding, violence, and disease.

The World Health Organization (2017) reported the top 10 causes of death worldwide in 2015:

1. Heart disease
2. Stroke (caused by blood vessel problems in the brain)
3. Respiratory infections
4. Chronic obstructive pulmonary disease (a category of lung diseases)
5. Cancer of lung and airways
6. Diabetes
7. Alzheimer's disease and other dementias
8. Diarrhea
9. Tuberculosis (an infectious disease of lung and other tissues)
10. Road traffic injuries

The study noted that annual deaths from dementias more than doubled since 2010. Meanwhile, death rates from diarrheal diseases almost halved. Tuberculosis mortality rates were also down, as was HIV/AIDS mortality (the latter dropped off the "top 10" list).

Worldwide, average life expectancy at birth continues to increase, but at a much slower pace than in the 1950s and 1960s. Not surprisingly, the biggest recent gains have occurred in countries with the shortest life expectancies; these countries had the most room for improvement, while life expectancy in high-income countries approaches a biological upper limit. In 2015 global life expectancy averaged 71.4 years (WHO, 2015). Grouping all countries together, infant mortality rate declined from about 65 deaths per 1,000 live births in 1990 to 30 in 2016 (WHO, 2016). Despite this overall decrease, IMR was still more than six times higher in Africa than in Europe.

As lower-income countries continue to develop economically, their health problems increasingly resemble those of high-income countries: fewer deaths from infectious diseases, and more chronic conditions such as heart disease, cancer, and diabetes. Tobacco use—blamed for almost six million deaths annually—is a rising threat, especially in the developing world. Diabetes (strongly associated with too much body weight and not enough physical activity) is also spreading quickly.

3 Models of Health

Scientists often use *models* to study and think about problems. A model means a representation. A model airplane is not a real airplane but is a representation of an airplane. A fashion model shows how clothes might look on a person's body. A mouse model allows a researcher to follow the life history of a disease such as diabetes at reduced scales of time and size.

This chapter discusses several models of health. Models are important because the framework a person uses and the perspective she adopts influence her interpretations, decisions, and behaviours.

For example, *prevalence* of and mortality from tuberculosis (TB) vary widely around the globe, being much higher in developing than industrial countries. TB is strongly associated with overcrowding, poorly ventilated housing, and poor nutrition. Diabetes and HIV infection increase risk for active TB infection. TB impacts specific subgroups of Canadians disproportionately. For example, "in 2012, Indigenous peoples, who comprised approximately 4% of the population of Canada, accounted for 23% of reported cases of active TB disease in Canada" (PHAC, 2014).

How should we think about tuberculosis in Canada? How is housing different from nutrition as a health issue? Is poverty a health issue? What special measures could address TB among Indigenous Canadians?

Let's look at several different views of health. See if you can deduce how each approach would handle the problem of TB in Canada differently.

3.1 Health through treatment of illness

The **illness model** views health as the absence of disease (Figure 1.1). When one develops *signs* (which means things one can see, such as spots on the skin) or *symptoms* (which means things one feels, such as fever or nausea) of disease, doctors and/or other practitioners begin treatment to try to cure the disease. If the disease is not cured, disability and perhaps even premature death can ensue. When the individual returns to the neutral position (the point where there are no signs or symptoms), the intervention stops.

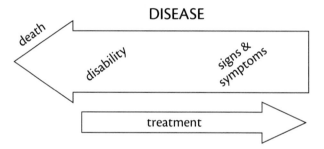

Figure 1.1. The illness model.

The **medical model** refers to a scientific empirical[1] approach that attempts to form a specific diagnosis based on the symptoms of a disorder (Bhate, 1990). The empirical tradition in Western thought began with Greek thinkers such as Pythagoras and Hippocrates (around 500 BCE) and Aristotle (around 350 BCE). "In the 17th century [CE] the natural sciences moved forward on a broad front. There were attempts to grapple with the nature of science, as expressed in the works of thinkers like Francis Bacon, [René] Descartes, and [Isaac] Newton" (Thomson, 2014). A **mechanistic** view, which saw nature as an intricate system or machine, like a very complex clock, increasingly replaced non-scientific thinking. By extension, these thinkers began trying to understand and treat human disease through a detailed understanding of human structure and function.

---

1   *Empirical* means originating in, or based on, observation or experience; relying on experience or observation alone, often without due regard for system and theory; capable of being verified or disproved by observation or experiment (Merriam-Webster, 2014).

The medical model produced many important advances in the 19th and 20th centuries, including, for example, knowledge that tiny living organisms could directly cause certain diseases and infection of wounds, and that washing hands before delivering babies led to dramatic decreases in maternal mortality; this was also the period when researchers discovered insulin (1921), penicillin (1928), and a polio vaccine (1954) (Thomson, 2014).

The medical model is mechanistic. Sachs (2010) describes the medical model in psychiatry as a specific and narrow **_discipline_**. Neuroscientists increasingly understand mental illness as the result of abnormal brain structure or function, with treatment (e.g., drugs) directed at correcting neurochemical imbalance. Brain-imaging technology has shown differences between brains of psychopaths and alcoholics, for example, compared with subjects who do not have these disorders.

Psychiatrist R. D. Laing (1971) used the term "medical model" in a more negative sense. He argued that since diagnosis of mental illness was based on the individual's behaviour rather than on physical pathology, the medical model wasn't really appropriate. Laing believed the feelings patients expressed were valid descriptions of the patient's life as he experienced it, rather than just symptoms of some separate disorder.

Another feature of the classic medical model is that it positioned the physician as the expert. The practitioner prescribed treatment and gave advice, and patients were expected to comply. Perhaps as a result of the "human potential movement" and the humanistic psychotherapies that became popular in the 1960s and early 1970s, medical practice has become more patient centred.

A third aspect of the traditional medical model is focus on the disorder rather than the person. An orthopedic surgeon might mention how many "knees he did" in a given day, rather than how many people with knee problems he treated. In recent years, public health experts have increasingly recognized the importance of psychosocial and environmental **determinants of health**. This more holistic view is now part of medical school education, and modern medical practice tends to use a broader approach than seen in the traditional medical model.

How about *you*?

What kind of relationship do you have with your doctor or other health care provider?

Do you feel intimidated when you are in your doctor's office?

Do you feel that you are a "lesser" person being told what to do?

Or, do you feel like your doctor is a partner in the process of helping you to become healthier?

3.2 *Health through* **prevention** *of illness*

Population data use statistics to show how *morbidity* (illness) and *mortality* correlated with various **risk factors**, such as age, sex, family health history, tobacco use, seat belt use, family income, and occupation. The 1974 report from the Canadian federal health minister, titled *A New Perspective on the Health of Canadians,* pointed out that the main causes of mortality in Canada at that time (which remain the same today) derived from a number of known risk factors (Lalonde, 1974). For example, drinking alcohol is a risk factor for motor vehicle accidents, suicide, and liver disease. Cigarette smoking is a risk factor for lung cancer. A high-fat diet and lack of exercise are risk factors for heart disease.

Such risk-factor inventories cannot predict with certainty if a particular individual will or will not get a given disease. However, the **risk-factor model** is useful in three ways:

- At the **community or population** level, health promoters can identify high-risk groups and target prevention or early detection efforts (e.g., blood pressure screening) toward them.
- At the **individual** level, high-risk individuals can decide to change health behaviours to reduce their own risks.
- At the **health care provider** level, physicians and other practitioners can act as resource people to raise awareness and impart knowledge to individuals and communities.

> What do *you* know about your health risk factors?
> Are certain diseases more common in your family?
> What factors in your personal medical history or your current health behaviours increase your risk of specific disorders or early death?

3.3 *Health viewed holistically*

A **holistic** view of health goes further still (Figure 1.2), viewing health as more than the intersection of a person's health behaviours and the health care provided to him. The holistic model is broadly consistent with an **ecological** perspective, in which we can best understand an individual or species in the context of its environment. In human health, this means not just the physical environment (air, water, food, shelter, etc.) but also the social, psychological, economic, and even political environments. Researchers have developed **ecological models** to better understand interactions among individual, family, community, and societal factors for a number of health issues, including family violence (American Academy of Pediatrics, 2014), child obesity (Davison & Birch, 2001), and children with special health needs (Newacheck, Rising & Kim, 2006).

Let's take a look at various elements in the holistic view of health.

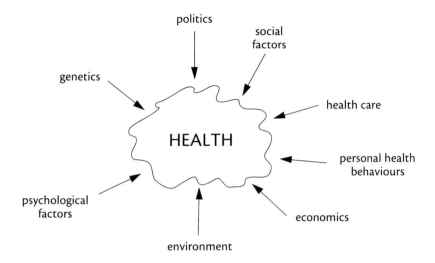

Figure 1.2. From a holistic perspective, many things contribute to health.

3.3.1 Genetics

Each person has a different set of genes, which come from a combination of material from the mother and the father at the moment of conception, when the father's sperm penetrates the mother's ovum, or egg. The genes comprise a long set of "instructions" that tell cells what to do, including manufacturing the proteins and other molecules that make up our bodies.

Some disorders clearly result from genetic defects. Down syndrome is a genetic disorder that results in developmental delays, heart defects, and certain characteristics of facial appearance, among other things. Genes damaged by things like chemicals or radiation can cause cancer (uncontrolled cell multiplication). Other disorders that are not so directly caused by faulty genes are still related or linked to genetic factors. For example, genes determine whether one is male or female: males have one X and one Y chromosome, while females have two X chromosomes. One impact this has on health is that, on average, females have a longer life expectancy than males do.

Why do women live longer than men?

This is not completely understood. It's an interesting question at this point in the book, as it leads us to consider several factors.

Lifestyle: Traditionally, women have followed healthier and safer lifestyles than men: women typically smoke less and drink less alcohol; women are less likely to drive after drinking or to drive aggressively; women are less likely to work in dangerous occupations, such as fishing, mining, and forestry; they are less likely to participate in risky recreational activities, such as automobile racing, scuba diving, or mountain climbing; and they are less likely to experience combat in the armed forces.

However, the gap between female and male life expectancy is decreasing. While life expectancy is increasing for both females and males, it is increasing more rapidly in males. This may be related to increasing similarity between female and male lifestyles; for example, contemporary females are more likely to work in dangerous jobs and more likely to drive automobiles than they were a generation ago. There has been a steady decrease since the 1960s in the number of females and males in Canada who smoke cigarettes regularly, but this trend is more dramatic among men, such that the difference between males and females is shrinking (Reid et al., 2012).

Biology: Research in humans and in mice suggests females' immune systems age more slowly than males'; in fact, the aging process *in general* may be slower in females than males (Briggs, 2013). Females have higher blood levels of the hormone estrogen, which appears to have a protective effect on the heart (Deschamps, Murphy, and Sun, 2010). Kirkwood (2010) notes that in most species females live longer than males, and explains that at the biological level aging results from the gradual accumulation of many small faults, such as damage to genetic material; we will explore this concept further in Chapter 5: Cancer. Briefly, cellular damage occurs every day, and the body detects and repairs much, but not all, of the damage. Animal species with longer lifespans generally have better maintenance and repair systems than animals with shorter lifespans. Rodent studies provide evidence that cells in a female body repair damage better than cells in a male body, and that surgically removing the ovaries[2] eliminates this difference. Conversely, surgically removing the testicles[3] seems to prolong the lives of males in domestic cats and dogs, and "... in one study of several hundred men at an unnamed institution in Kansas,

---

2   The ovaries are two walnut-sized structures in the female lower abdomen. Ovaries store and develop *ova* (eggs), and secrete the female hormones estrogen and progesterone.

3   The male *testes* (testicles) produce sperm and the male hormone testosterone. See Chapter 10: Intimate Relationships and Human Sexuality for more discussion of human genital anatomy.

the castrated men were found to live on average 14 years longer than their uncastrated fellows" (Kirkwood, 2010).

3.3.2 *Health care*
Health care comprises a continuum from public health promotion (e.g., vaccination against common childhood diseases) to primary care by family physicians, to the more intensive care hospitals and medical specialists provide. Later in this text we will see how health care has reduced the burden of infectious disease, heart disease, and some types of cancer. We will also see that other disorders, such as obesity, diabetes, other types of cancer, mental health disorders, and suicide, continue to trouble Canadians despite our sophisticated and expensive health care system.

3.3.3 *Psychological factors*
How we feel mentally also has an impact on our health. The prevalence of illness from colds or "the flu" increases in university students around exam time. Accountants tend to experience a rise in blood pressure at the end of the calendar year and as income-tax deadlines approach, the two times when their workload increases. We will see more extreme examples of the impacts of psychological factors on health when we examine mood disorders, such as depression, in Chapter 9: Mental Health.

3.3.4 *The physical environment*
Mortality rates from melanoma of the skin (a type of skin cancer) among white males in the USA are higher in the southern states, because the sun's cancer-causing ultraviolet rays are more intense closer to the equator. A similar pattern presents among females and to a lesser extent in darker-skinned people. The quality of the water we drink and the air we breathe, our exposure to noise, and other environmental factors also affect health; we will explore this more in Chapter 15: Environment. Life expectancy varies regionally as well as globally.

Where are the highest and lowest life expectancies in Canada?

Statistics Canada (2015) data show people in British Columbia have the highest life expectancy (84.6 and 80.5 years for women and men, respectively) while life expectancy is lowest in Nunavut (73.9 and 69.2 years).

An article from the popular magazine *Canadian Living* claimed that at 83.4 years overall, Richmond residents have a higher life expectancy than residents of any other Canadian city (Beun-Chown, 2007).

> What do *you* think about these figures?
>
> Why do you think British Columbia, and especially Richmond, is home to people with the longest life expectancy in Canada?

3.3.5 Social factors

The 2010 report by British Columbia's Provincial Health Officer (Kendall, 2010), titled *Investing in Prevention,* lists "early childhood development" and "poverty reduction" as two of the five broad policy areas in which government should invest to promote health and prevent disease. Social factors in health, which are sometimes referred to as **social determinants of health,** include the following:

Employment status (full-time, part-time, unemployed) and occupation: Employment is obviously a source of income (see below). More subtly, work can provide a sense of satisfaction and meaning, an opportunity to express and develop one's talents, and a social group within which to find a sense of belonging and status. One of the first questions people often ask a new acquaintance is "What do you do?" by which they mean, "What kind of work do you do?" Unemployment, even if it's voluntary retirement, often reduces self-esteem. "Unemployment increases the likelihood of turning to unhealthy coping behaviours such as tobacco use and problem drinking" (Mikkonen & Raphael, 2010, p. 17). On the other hand, overwork, irregular work hours, and work perceived as lacking meaning or satisfaction can also undermine health. In addition, certain occupations expose workers to increased risk of disease or injury.

Education:
There are various pathways by which education leads to better health. First, level of education is highly correlated with other social determinants of health such as the level of income, employment security, and working conditions. Viewed in this light, education helps people to move up the socioeconomic ladder and provides better access to other societal and economic resources. Second, higher education makes it easier to enact larger changes in the Canadian employment market. Better educated citizens have more opportunities to benefit from new training opportunities if their employment situation suddenly changes. Furthermore, education facilitates citizens' possibilities for civic activities and engagement in the political process. In other words, people attain better understanding of the world and they become more able to see and influence societal factors that shape their own

health. Finally, education increases overall literacy and understanding of how one can promote one's own health through individual action. (Mikkonen & Raphael, 2010, p. 15)

Income: This presents as a determinant of health in various ways. For example, those who live in the wealthiest 20% of neighbourhoods in Canada live longer than those who live in the poorest 20% of neighbour-hoods—four years longer for males and two years longer for females (Mikkonen & Raphael, 2010, p. 12). Low-income Canadians suffer much higher rates of suicide, adult-onset diabetes, and heart attacks than their high-income counterparts (Mikkonen & Raphael, 2010, p. 12).

Marital status: Married people live longer. This may also be true for people who are *cohabitating* (living together) in long-term relationships, but I haven't seen data on this.

Housing:
Overcrowding allows for transmission of respiratory and other ill-nesses. Some Canadian homes, especially on Aboriginal reserves, lack even clean water and basic sanitation—a fundamental public health risk. Housing provides a platform for self-expression and identity. High housing costs reduce the resources available to support other social determinants of health. Living in poor housing creates stress and unhealthy means of coping such as substance abuse." (Mikkonen & Raphael, 2010, p. 30)

Ethnicity: This probably has both genetic and social components. For example, South Asian people (e.g., those from India, Pakistan, Sri Lanka, and Bangladesh) living in Canada have higher rates of hypertension (high blood pressure), diabetes, and heart disease than other Canadians of the same age, income, and similar factors. Some of the difference may be due to lifestyle (e.g., high-fat diet and low levels of physical activity), while some may result from genetic differences in physiology.

Community engagement: People who participate actively in their com-munities through volunteering, voting, donating blood, and so on, tend to be healthier overall.

Religion: The impact of religion on health appears to result from a com-plex mix of spirituality, health-related behaviours (e.g., some religions prohibit drinking alcohol, smoking, or eating meat), and the social, psychological, and material support provided by a community of those who attend a particular place of worship, whether it's a church, temple, synagogue, or mosque.

3.3.6 Personal health behaviours

A group of researchers at the University of Cambridge Institute of Public Health in England studied over 20,000 men and women aged 45 to 79 (Tufts, 2008). During the follow-up period, about 10% of the participants died. Lifespan was an average of 14 years longer for those with four simple health habits:

1. Not smoking
2. Drinking moderately (one to 14 drinks per week)
3. Keeping physically active
4. Eating five servings of fruits and vegetables per day

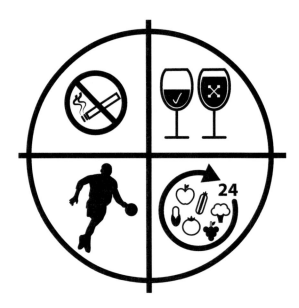

Figure 1.3. Four health habits associated with longevity (Tufts, 2008).

The authors noted these health-promoting behaviours are not extreme, but very simple and do-able.

Another study (Tufts, 2008), called *The Physicians Health Study*, looked at longevity over a 22- to 25-year period in over 2,000 healthy men with an average age of 72. During the study period, a total of 970 men lived to the age of 90 or older. Participants who smoked, had diabetes, were obese, or had high blood pressure were significantly less likely to live to age 90 than those without these risk factors. On the other hand, regular vigorous exercise substantially improved their chances of a long life.

> Think about *your* situation in a holistic way.
>   What factors are most influential on your health?
>   What could *you* do to bring more wellness into your life?

3.3.7 Political factors

We can define politics as the use of power to achieve certain results. Several examples show how political factors influence health:

- The USA has a powerful right-to-firearms lobby, a high rate of gun violence, and a huge prison population.
- In Canada, mortality from violent death is much higher among Indigenous people than among other Canadians. There is a similar pattern for suicide. These rates are probably *not* caused by genetic differences. While many of these deaths are alcohol-related, alcohol alone cannot explain the differences. The roots of these phenomena may lie in the systematic discrimination and abuse of Indigenous Canadians, which leaves many feeling alienated from the Canadian dream, disenfranchised from the political process, and experiencing feelings of anger, frustration, hopelessness, or despair.
- Wars in various parts of the world break out sometimes for ideological reasons and sometimes to gain control of territory or resources. People living in war-torn regions don't need aerobic fitness classes or low-fat diets to improve their health status; they need peace and security.

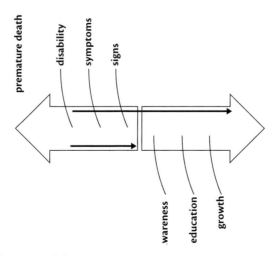

Figure 1.4. Wellness model.

3.4 *Health as* wellness

The World Health Organization (WHO) developed a definition of health that is widely used and completely consistent with the wellness model. The WHO states that "health is the complete state of physical, mental, and social well-being, and not merely the absence of disease or infirmity" (*infirmity* means disorder or frailty).

The **wellness model** (Figure 1.4, above) recognizes the importance of disease treatment. However, it goes much further. The neutral position—the absence of signs and symptoms of illness—is not considered the optimal state of health. Rather, the individual should strive to achieve a high level of wellness by becoming aware of the role she can play in her health, becoming educated about the consequences of different lifestyle choices, and growing as a person, mentally, physically, and spiritually. A high level of wellness is not a state or a place, but rather a *process* or a way of living.

The University of California at Riverside (2012) lists "seven dimensions of wellness":

1. Social
2. Emotional
3. Spiritual
4. Environmental
5. Occupational
6. Intellectual
7. Physical

The 1986 *Ottawa Charter for Health Promotion* presents a view of **health as a resource for everyday life,** not the objective of living.

> Health is created and lived by people within the settings of their everyday life; where they learn, work, play and love. Health is created by caring for oneself and others, by being able to take decisions and have control over one's life circumstances, and by ensuring that the society one lives in creates conditions that allow the attainment of health by all its members. Caring, holism and ecology are essential issues in developing strategies for health promotion. (WHO, 2014)

4 How Are We Doing?

By many measures, Canada is a wealthy and healthy country (WHO, 2013):

- Our gross national income of $40,000 per capita is almost four times the global average.

- Our life expectancy at birth averages 82 years (males and females combined), compared with a global average of 70.
- Only 12 of every 100,000 women in Canada die as a consequence of childbirth, compared with a global maternal mortality ratio of 210 per 100,000.
- The Canadian under-five mortality rate of six per 1,000 live births is much better than the global average of 51.
- Fewer than six of every 100,000 people have the lung disease tuberculosis, compared with a global figure of 170 per 100,000.
- We have excellent access to clean drinking water.
- Our childhood immunization rates are relatively high.
- Our health care is relatively well funded, with the equivalent of over $5,000 (USD) spent per capita per year, which is almost twice the spending of other countries in the Americas.

Mercer, a human resources consultancy, annually ranks 223 world cities based on data from its *Quality of Living Survey*. "Canadian cities dominate North America's top-five list. Ranking fifth globally, Vancouver tops the regional list, followed by Ottawa (14), Toronto (15), Montreal (23), and San Francisco (27)" (Mercer, 2014).

However, this overall positive picture hides substantial disparities within Canada. The gap between the richest and poorest segments of society is growing. Disadvantaged groups include people with disabilities, street-involved youth, older women living alone, Indigenous Canadians, single women with children, and people of colour.

5 Conclusion

We may view health as merely the absence of disease or as a broader but vaguer sense of wellness. We can discuss health status as captured at the individual level by measures such as blood pressure and body weight, or at the population level by indicators such as longevity and infant mortality rate. We can think of health as simply one's physical soundness, or include mental, emotional, social, spiritual, and environmental balance. We can view health as a process, as the goal of continuing adaptation and growth in response to stressors and challenges from the environment.

Regardless of how we think of it, health is precious. Our personal health significantly influences not only how long we live but our enjoyment of and satisfaction with our lives, and the achievements and contributions we can realize. The health of families, neighbourhoods, societies, and nation-states rests on the health of the individuals they comprise, and on systems that optimize collaboration among individuals.

We have just started our examination of health. The next chapter presents some methods and criteria to evaluate the credibility of health claims. The subsequent three chapters discuss major causes of death and disability in Canada and other parts of the world. Then a series of chapters considers health behaviours: physical activity, nutrition, weight management, and mental health. Later chapters deal with some controversial issues around sex and sexuality, sexually transmitted diseases, conception and contraception, and substance use. The final chapters address health care delivery systems and the physical environment of our planet.

Study Questions

1. What do we mean by "model" when we say "models of health"?
2. What two common indicators of population health does this chapter introduce?
3. Name five of the 10 leading causes of death globally (you don't have to list them in the correct order).
4a. What does it mean to say "the medical model takes a mechanistic view of health"?
4b. What are the three keys features of the medical model?
5. What is the difference between morbidity and mortality?
6. From a health-promotion point of view, in what three ways is the risk-factor approach to health useful?
7. State the World Health Organization's definition of health.
8. What are the seven dimensions of wellness proposed by University of California at Riverside? Explain each of these components briefly in your own words.
9. What four simple health habits could add an average of 14 years to longevity?
10. List at least three factors other than personal health behaviours that affect health.
11. State at least four social determinants of health.
12. Give two different examples of how political factors affect health.
13. Is a strong correlation with mortality a good indication of health? Explain.

Glossary

discipline—a particular area of study, usually with a specific vocabulary and way of thinking and acting

infant mortality rate—deaths of infants in the first year of life per 1,000 births

infirmity—frailty or disorder

model—a representation, or way of looking at things

morbidity—illness

mortality—death

populations—groups of people

prevalence—how common a condition is, usually expressed as a rate (e.g., number of cases per 100,000 population)

signs—things that can be observed or measured (e.g., swelling, redness, hotness)

symptoms—feelings that cannot be observed or measured (e.g., nausea, headache, fatigue, pain)

Additional Resources

Public Health Agency of Canada

http://www.who.int/gho/countries/can.pdf?ua=1

Simon Fraser University, Health and Counselling Services

http://students.sfu.ca/health.html

Provides a range of services for SFU students and employees, including in-person health and medical services, vaccination, sexual health services, counselling, physiotherapy and chiropractic services, and a number of online resources.

World Health Organization

http://www.who.int/countries/en/

References

American Academy of Pediatrics. (n.d.). *Preventing sexual violence: An educational toolkit for health care professionals.* Retrieved January 21, 2014 from http://www2.aap.org/pubserv/PSVpreview/pages/preventsv.html

Beun-Chown, J. (2007). Canada's healthiest city. *Canadian Living.* Retrieved January 12, 2013 from http://www.canadianliving.com/health/prevention/canadas_healthiest_city.ph

Bhate, S. (1990). Medical model. *British Medical Journal.* 301(6746), 299.

Briggs, H. (May 15, 2013). Biological clue to why women live longer than men. *BBC News.* Retrieved May 10, 2014 from http://www.bbc.com/news/health-22528388

Davison, K. K., Birch, L. L. (2001). Childhood overweight: A contextual model and recommendations for future research. *Obesity Reviews* 2(3), 159–171.

Deschamps, A. M., Murphy, E., Sun, J. (2010). Estrogen receptor activation and cardioprotection in ischemia reperfusion injury. *Trends in Cardiovascular Medicine.* 20(3), 73–78.

Empirical. (n.d.). In *Merriam-Webster online.* Retrieved May 10, 2014 from http://www.merriam-webster.com/dictionary/empirical

History of medicine. (n.d.). In *Encyclopedia Britannica online.* Retrieved May 10, 2014 from http://www.britannica.com/EBchecked/topic/372460/history-of-medicine

Kendall, P. R. W. (September, 2010). *Investing in prevention: Improving health and creating sustainability: The provincial health officer's special report.* British Columbia: Office of the Provincial Health Officer. Retrieved July 24, 2014 from http://www.health.gov.bc.ca/library/publications/year/2010/Investing_in_prevention_improving_health_and_creating_sustainability.pdf

Kirkwood, T. (October 1, 2010). Why women live longer. *National Geographic*. Retrieved May 10, 2014 from http://www.scientificamerican.com/article/why-women-live-longer/

Laing, R. D. (1971). *The politics of the family and other essays*. London: Tavistock Publications, pp. 23 and 39–42.

Lalonde, M. (April 1974). *A new perspective on the health of Canadians*. Ottawa, ON: Minister of National Health and Welfare.

Mercer. (February 18, 2014). *Quality of living city rankings*. Retrieved April 20, 2014 from http://www.mercer.com/qualityofliving

Mikkonen, J., Raphael, D. (2010). *Social determinants of health: The Canadian facts*. Toronto: York University School of Health Policy and Management. Retrieved July 24, 2014 from http://www.thecanadianfacts.org/

Newacheck, P. W., Rising, J. P., Kim, S. E. (2006). Children at risk for special health care needs. *Pediatrics*. 118(1), 334–42.

PHAC. (2014). *Tuberculosis prevention and control in Canada: A federal framework for action*. Ottawa: Public Health Agency of Canada. Retrieved July 1, 2014 from http://www.phac-aspc.gc.ca/tbpc-latb/pubs/tpc-pct/assets/pdf/tpc-pcta-eng.pdf

Reid, J. L., Hammon, D., Burkhalter, R., Ahmed, R. (2012). *Tobacco use in Canada: Patterns and trends, 2012 Edition*. Waterloo, Ontario: Propel Centre for Population Health Impact, University of Waterloo. p. 14. Retrieved December 16, 2012 from http://www.tobaccoreport.ca/2012/adtu_sic_ht.cfm

Sachs, D. M. (2010). Beyond the medical model. *Psychoanalysis and the Human Sciences* 67(4), 597–600.

Statistics Canada. (2015). *Deaths and causes of death, 2015*. Retrieved May 1, 2018 from http://www.statcan.gc.ca/daily-quotidien/180223/dq180223c-eng.htm

Tufts University. (2008). Four simple habits add 14 years to life. *Tufts University Health & Nutrition Letter*, April 2008, 26(2), 1–2.

University of California, Riverside. (September 27, 2012). *Seven dimensions of wellness*. Retrieved April 16, 2014 from http://wellness.ucr.edu/seven_dimensions.html

WHO. (1986). Ottawa Charter for Health Promotion: First International Conference on Health Promotion, Ottawa, 21 November 1986. Geneva: World Health Organization, Health Promotion. (WHO/HPR/HEP/95.1). Retrieved June 20, 2006 from http://www.who.int/healthpromotion/conferences/previous/ottawa/en/. Retrieved July 1, 2014 from http://www.who.int/healthpromotion/conferences/previous/ottawa/en/index1.html

WHO. (May, 2013). Canada: General health statistical profile. *Global Health Observatory, Country Profiles*. Retrieved April 16, 2014 from http://www.who.int/gho/countries/can.pdf?ua=1

WHO (2015). Global Health Observatory data. Life expectancy. Retrieved May 7, 2018 from http://www.who.int/gho/mortality_burden_disease/life_tables/en/

WHO (2016). Global Health Observatory data. Infant mortality. Retrieved May 7, 2018 from http://www.who.int/gho/child_health/mortality/neonatal_infant_text/en/

WHO (January 12, 2017). The top 10 causes of death. Retrieved May 1, 2018 from http://www.who.int/en/news-room/fact-sheets/detail/the-top-10-causes-of-death

2   Evaluating Health Claims

Learning Objectives

By the time you have finished this chapter you should be able to

- Describe the scientific method
- State the limitations of human experiments and suggest alternative solutions
- Explain how epidemiology works
- Pinpoint the weakness of epidemiological evidence
- Discuss how to determine whether an association between two things implies that one causes the other
- Identify whether a particular example represents experimental, epidemiological, clinical, or anecdotal evidence

1 Overview

We are exposed to many different health claims. But not everything circulated in print or by other media is true. How do you know what to believe? Here's a question one of my students asked:

> *How can you determine which products on the market provide options for healthy eating and good nutrition?*

This is an important question. In this chapter we will examine several different types of evidence and suggest some criteria you can use to evaluate the credibility of health claims.

2 Scientific Evidence

Early, pre-scientific people tended to explain events in terms we now consider superstitious. For example, they thought a mentally ill person was full of evil spirits. They believed a disease such as measles was a curse sent by the gods as punishment for failing to observe a religious ritual. Then the Egyptians, Persians, Greeks, and others began making systematic observations of the world. This scientific view became increasingly prevalent (which means "common") in Europe of the 18th and 19th centuries. Scientists attempted to explain things in **mechanistic** terms—that is, in terms of cause-and-effect mechanisms. For example, astronomers discovered that the reason the sun rises every morning and sets every evening is that the earth revolves, or spins, on its axis, making one complete revolution every day.

Much of the information presented in this text is based on scientific evidence. Scientists are trained to follow a certain method in conducting scientific experiments. The **scientific method** is a way of testing ideas under controlled conditions before accepting them as true.

2.1 Experimental evidence

A scientist starts with a *hypothesis*, which is a statement phrased in a way that can be tested. Scientists base hypotheses on existing knowledge, with a good dose of logic, intuition, and educated guessing. For example, in coronary artery disease (we will study this more in Chapter 4: Cardiovascular Disease and Diabetes) the blood vessels are clogged with fat. So, a reasonable hypothesis is that "reducing dietary fat intake will decrease the prevalence (percentage of the population who have this condition) of coronary artery disease (CAD)."

The scientist then tests the hypothesis. One way to test this hypothesis would be to establish the prevalence of CAD, then change the level of fat in the diet and re-measure CAD levels in your sample. Many things besides diet also affect the incidence of CAD. These factors need to be controlled. For example, CAD is also more common among smokers, among older individuals, and among those exposed to excessive stress. The scientist will need to be sure, for example, that the reduced CAD is due to the reduced fat in the diet and not because the subjects also stopped smoking.

One way to control for the effect of other factors in a scientific study is to use a *control group*. A sample of subjects can be separated into two groups (Figure 2.1.):

- Half of the subjects make up the *experimental group*. This group would get the experimental *treatment*—in this case, the low-fat diet.

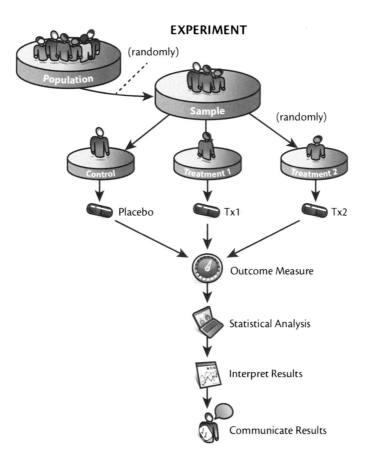

Figure 2.1. Design for a controlled scientific experiment with a control group and two experimental groups.

- The other half make up the control group. The control group should ideally be identical to the experimental group in all respects except for the experimental treatment. That is, individuals in the control group should live in the same area, work in the same types of occupations, be the same age and sex, have the same percentage of smokers, and so on as the subjects in the experimental group. Also, the control group should continue practising all the same health habits as the experimental group except for the low-fat diet.

If the scientist observes that after the experimental group has been on the low-fat diet for some time, CAD is lower in the experimental group than in the control group, this is evidence that a lower fat diet reduces incidence of CAD.

However, individuals can vary greatly in how their bodies respond to the same situation. You probably know some people who can eat almost anything they choose and never gain weight. Scientists call this **individual variability**. Individual variability is another factor to consider in a good scientific experiment. If a study has one person as a control and one person as the experimental subject, how valid do you think the results will be? Maybe the person in the control group will have less heart disease than the experimental person who eats the low-fat diet, but it could be because the control person is less susceptible to heart disease. Good scientific studies usually have a **large sample size**; that is, they use a large number of subjects. Larger samples even out the effect of individual variability. Thus, if a study had 500 people in a control group, it is highly unlikely that the control group differed from the experimental group in its susceptibility to heart disease.

Scientists use a couple of other methods to help produce valid results. One of these is the *placebo*. A placebo is something that has no effect on the variable being tested and that the subject cannot tell is different from the experimental treatment. For example, suppose a scientist wants to test the effect of alcohol consumption on automobile driving performance. He may give the experimental group a solution of alcohol and lemonade and give the control group plain lemonade. In this case, if the **subjects** (those participating in the experiment) cannot tell (from the taste or smell, for example) whether they are drinking plain lemonade or lemonade with alcohol, the plain lemonade is an effective placebo. Sometimes an experiment using a placebo is said to be a *blind experiment*, because the subjects are "blind" to whether they are receiving a placebo or the real treatment. Placebos may have powerful effects. If the subjects know the purpose of the study is to examine the effect of alcohol on driving, some of the subjects who receive the placebo may behave as if they are intoxicated and may actually feel they are intoxicated.

Another method that helps produce valid results is a *double-blind experiment*. In this type of experiment, neither the *subjects* nor the *experimenter* know who received the placebo and who received the real treatment. In a study on alcohol and automobile driving with a double-blind experimental design, the solutions would be mixed by a laboratory assistant and placed in bottles labelled with a code number. The assistant would note on a code sheet which solutions contained alcohol and which did not. Then the experimenter would give a bottle to each subject, the subjects would drink the solutions, and the experimenter would record the driving test results. Only after all of the driving test results were recorded would the experimenter look at the code sheet to see which subjects received the placebo.

The purpose of the double-blind method is to minimize the effects of the experimenter's **bias** on the results. That is, if the experimenter has hypothesized that alcohol ingestion will affect driving performance adversely, and he knows which subjects drank the alcohol, he may unconsciously grade the driving tests of those who drank alcohol more harshly, and that unconscious judgment would reflect his bias.

> Have *you* ever been a subject in a scientific experiment?
> Did that experiment have a control group?
> Were you in the control group or in the experimental group?

2.1.1 *Problems with experiments*

Time can pose a problem in testing some hypotheses. For example, some types of cancer have a long *latent period* (the time from exposure to the cancer-causing agent to the appearance of signs or symptoms of cancer). The latent period for lung cancer in humans is 30 years or so. In this case, a researcher could spend her entire career waiting for the results of a treatment that might cure the cancer. In the meantime, millions of people would have died needlessly. Also, research-granting agencies may be reluctant to fund a study for 30 years with no interim results. And publishing papers—often several or more a year—is important for the career progress of scientists. We need a way to speed up the process of getting results.

There are also **ethical considerations** in scientific research. It is usually considered unethical to expose human subjects to procedures that increase risk of disease. For example, suppose a scientist wanted to see if tobacco smoking increases risk of lung cancer. One logical approach to this problem would be to gather a number of volunteers who have never smoked and divide them into an experimental and a control group. The scientist would then tell the control group to remain non-smokers, while telling the experimental group to smoke 20 cigarettes per day. This proposed experiment would be ethically unacceptable. Even if the scientist could find subjects to volunteer, he could not justify exposing subjects to a suspected (or known) health risk.

Scientists have some options for avoiding the long timelines and ethical problems they might encounter with human subjects. One option is **animal experimentation**. Researchers often use mice and rats as subjects because these animals are small, they are relatively easy and inexpensive to handle and keep, they reproduce readily, they have a relatively short life span (which means an experimenter can see in weeks or months effects that might take decades to appear in humans), and they respond a lot like humans physiologically. A scientist might expose a group of mice to tobacco smoke for six months and then compare the amount of lung cancer in this group to the amount in a control group not exposed to tobacco.

The issue of animal experimentation has become increasingly controversial. Some people feel it is unethical to use animals as experimental subjects. You have probably heard of "animal rights activists." Pressure from this vocal and growing group has made scientists more sensitive to how they treat animal subjects and whether they can ethically justify a particular animal experiment they might propose.

> How do *you* feel about the use of animals in scientific experiments?
> Does it depend on what type of animal is used?
>> For example, is it okay to experiment with ants but not with dogs?
> Does it depend on the purpose of the experiment?
>> For example, is it okay if the purpose is to find a cure for breast cancer but not to find a shampoo that makes hair shinier?

Another option is **tissue cultures**. For example, subjects may be asked to rub a toothbrush over their tongue and the inside of their mouth. Scientists can take the skin cells that come off on the toothbrush and grow the cells in little covered glass dishes. Later, they can expose the cells to a cancer-causing material and then treat half the cells with a cancer-fighting chemical. After a while, they can look at the cells under a microscope to see if the cancer-fighting chemical worked.

Computer modelling is another way to avoid problems with time and ethics in human experiments. If a scientist knows how different variables in a system behave, she can describe it mathematically. Computers can then simulate the effect of different manipulations. For example, we understand the human circulatory system well enough to simulate what would happen to blood pressure if a person were to lose a litre of blood. The limiting factor in computer models is that systems are often complex and incompletely understood, so predictions can be quite inaccurate.

2.2 Epidemiological evidence

Another option a scientist may exercise to avoid the possible ethical problems of exposing human subjects to experimental procedures is *epidemiology*. You can think of epidemiology as medical detective work. Let me illustrate with three real examples:

Example A: In London, England, in the 1850s, thousands of people began dying of a strange new illness. The victims all experienced similar symptoms, so doctors concluded they all had the same illness, but none of the doctors knew what the illness was or how to treat it. One clever doctor had an idea. He posted a large map of the city of London on his office wall. When a new patient arrived with the symptoms of the unknown illness, he asked the patient where he lived and placed a pin in this location on the map. Soon he noticed a pattern. A definite cluster of pins surrounded a particular pub (Frerichs, 2018).

Still not knowing how the pub was connected with the illness, he convinced city authorities to close the pub. The number of new cases of the mysterious illness in the area of the pub dropped sharply. We now know this mysterious illness as cholera, caused by a type of bacteria that lives in contaminated water. How was the pub related to cholera? In those days, people got their drinking water from wells. The pub's well was contaminated, and all the people who drank this water were exposed to the cholera-causing bacteria.

Example B: Since 1948, scientists have examined more than 5,000 residents of the small town of Framingham, Massachusetts, (near Boston) at yearly intervals. Investigators have recorded blood pressure, serum cholesterol levels, smoking habits, body weight, drinking habits, exercise habits, and a number of other traits for each of the participants in this study. Over the years, many of the original subjects have died. The cause of death and the age of the subjects at the time of death have been noted. As is typical of epidemiological studies, no attempt has been made to modify the lifestyle of the subjects; they have just been studied. The Framingham Study has revealed correlations between certain traits and cardiovascular disease. These traits are known as **risk factors** (Figure 2.2).

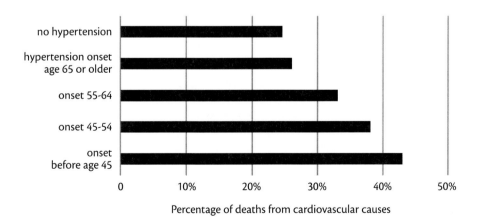

Percentage of deaths from cardiovascular causes

Figure 2.2. Risk of dying from cardiovascular disease increases with earlier onset of hypertension (high blood pressure) (Niiranen et al., 2017).

Example C: In 1980, physicians in the United States became aware of a strange new disease. Patients, often in their 20s and 30s and otherwise in good health, showed symptoms of a rare type of lung disease and a type of skin cancer normally only seen in older people. The usual medical tests revealed nothing, yet the patients often died in a matter of months.

Medical researchers took an epidemiological approach. They asked patients all sorts of questions, without really knowing what they were looking for. Soon, a peculiar pattern emerged. Most of the patients were young male homosexuals who lived in urban areas. Another smaller group were not gay but were drug users who used needles to inject the drug intravenously. An even smaller minority were hemophiliacs. We now know the disease as AIDS, or acquired immune deficiency syndrome. The initial epidemiological findings made it possible to identify the virus that causes AIDS. Subsequent research showed that this virus can be spread through semen or blood.

The weakness of epidemiological evidence is that just because two things are associated does not mean one *causes* the other. For example, I wake in the morning and 10 minutes later the sun rises. Did my waking cause the sun to rise? If I slept in, would the sun wait? Did the sun cause me to wake? Or is it a coincidence, with the sun and my waking not connected in a **causal**, or cause-effect, relationship?

You can read an interesting exchange in two letters to the editor of the British journal *Addiction*. First, Bell and Britton (2013) seem to criticize another author, Fekjaer, for stating that observational epidemiology produces "second-class" evidence compared with experimental studies. Then Fekjaer (2013) replies,

> However, I did not characterize observational epidemiology as a second-class *science*, but only stated that observational studies are second-class *evidence for causality* … My paper summarized findings from observational studies showing that light or moderate drinking apparently prevents no fewer than 24 diseases and health problems. … When such studies are published in scientific journals the conclusion is often carefully formulated, such as "moderate drinking is *associated with* better health." However, we all know that time and again, the association is misinterpreted as an evidence of causality. Therefore, it seems important to issue a reminder that observational studies alone, or even combined with possible biological mechanisms, remain second-class evidence for causality [emphasis in original].

2.2.1 Factors that can allow one to consider an association to be causal

An association can be considered causal if it meets enough of the following criteria. It is not possible to generalize and say, for example, that it must meet four of the six criteria; such a judgment depends upon the total weight of the evidence. We'll look at each criterion using the example of cigarette smoking and lung cancer.

- **Strength of the association:** In 1951, two Oxford professors collected data on 35,000 male physicians in Britain. (The study did not include females because there were few female physicians at the time.) The professors followed this sample for 20 years, by which time 441 of the group had died of lung cancer. The lung cancer mortality rate for smokers in the sample was 14 times that of non-smokers. This is a very strong association and makes it likely that smoking caused the lung cancer.

- **Dose-response:** As the amount smoked per day increases, the mortality ratio increases. "Mortality ratio" in this case is the mortality rate among smokers divided by the mortality rate among non-smokers; that is, a mortality ratio of 20 means a 20-fold increase in risk relative to non-smokers (Figure 2.3). This makes it likely that smoking is the cause of death. If the lung cancer mortality ratio were lower for heavy smokers than for light smokers, it would suggest smoking was not the *cause* but might in fact be the *cure*.

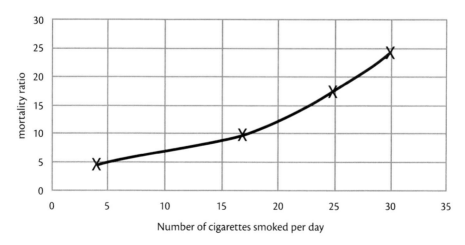

Figure 2.3. Dose-response curve for lung cancer mortality and cigarette smoking (Law et al., 1997).

- **Consistency:** Many studies show lung cancer mortality rates among smokers are 10 to 20 times those of non-smokers. None have observed the opposite effect. This is persuasive evidence.
- **Temporally correct:** In Latin, *tempus* means "time." When we refer to the "tempo" of music, we mean the pace or speed at which it is played. If people got lung cancer the day they started smoking, this would be puzzling. (It probably would also be a powerful motivation for others not to smoke.) It would be puzzling because we know normal cells become cancerous in a number of stages, and in most cancers this takes a long time. But the fact that lung cancer develops decades after people have started smoking is temporally correct, and further points to smoking as a cause of lung cancer.
- **Specificity:** If the association between smoking and lung cancer were 100%, every person who smoked would get lung cancer, and no non-smokers would get lung cancer. This is not true, and it is the only weak point in the evidence proving smoking causes lung cancer. Only 15% of those who smoke get lung cancer—although smokers also die from other forms of lung disease and from heart disease. Apparently, most people have cellular repair mechanisms that correct the damage caused by cigarette smoke before it can progress to cancer. But 80% of those with lung cancer are or were smokers, and this suggests smoking *does* cause lung cancer.
- **Biological plausibility:** Is there a reasonable mechanism that explains how smoking might cause lung cancer? Yes, there is. You can make a machine suck air through lit cigarettes, collect the smoke, and concentrate the "tar" from the smoke. If you rub the tar into the skin of mice, the mice will develop skin cancer. We know there are cancer-causing agents in cigarette smoke, and we know that when humans smoke, they inhale the smoke into their lungs. So it is logical that smoking exposes the cells of the lungs to cancer-causing agents, and likely this smoke is a cause of lung cancer.

3 Clinical Evidence

Clinical evidence comes from the experience of clinicians—people such as physicians, dentists, chiropractors, psychologists, athletic trainers, and so on. In other words, clinical evidence reflects what is seen in a clinic. For example, an athletic therapist may notice that when a newly sprained ankle is put into a hot tub, it swells badly. By contrast, when the therapist treats a similar sprain with rest, ice, compression, and elevation, it heals faster.

Often clinical evidence is consistent with scientific evidence. However, many clinical procedures have not been tested scientifically. For example, when a drug company introduced a drug called Valium (diazepam) in the 1950s, doctors hailed it as a "miracle drug" to relieve anxiety. Later, it became known that it had a strong potential to cause drug dependence.

Medicine, physiotherapy, and many other health care practices are grounded in basic sciences, such as biology, chemistry, and physics. However, doctors, physiotherapists, and others are *not scientists*; they are primarily *healers* who focus on trying to improve the patient's well-being. The best health care comes from clinicians and scientists working together, learning which treatments are most effective.

4 Personal Experience

Information acquired through personal experience is *not valid scientific evidence*, because the conditions are not controlled. Nevertheless, personal experience is a powerful source of health information. We tend to remember things that have happened to us, or to friends, more easily than things we read in scientific articles or hear on television.

Generalizations derived from personal experience are sometimes consistent with scientific evidence. For example, if you start running several times a week, you may, over a period of months, notice your endurance improves markedly. This personal experience is consistent with evidence from numerous scientific studies. On the other hand, conclusions based on your personal experience may contradict scientific evidence. For example, you may rub olive oil into your scalp and notice your memory seems to improve, even though no scientific evidence supports this.

> Have *you* had a powerful personal experience that has altered your health beliefs and behaviours?

5 Anecdotal Evidence

An "anecdote" is a story. Imagine a friend tells you, "My grandmother smoked a cigar every day of her adult life and she's still in good health at age 90." Of course, this will be a memorable story. But is it evidence that cigar smoking helps people live to old age? Perhaps if she had not smoked, she would be in better health. Maybe the average longevity of 100 female cigar smokers is less than the non-smokers, and your grandmother is an exception. In this way, anecdotal evidence is as **unscientific** as personal experience.

However, anecdotal evidence can have the same powerful impact as personal experience. A student approached me after a lecture on heart disease and described how his father's middle-aged friend had been over on the weekend to help move a refrigerator. The friend was overweight and smoked cigarettes. While moving the heavy refrigerator, the friend collapsed on the kitchen floor, where he died from a heart attack. This is a very powerful story, and in this case the point of the story *does* line up with scientific evidence on heart disease.

6 Critical Thinking

How can you sift through the mass of health "information" available in order to separate scientific *evidence* from personal *opinion?* Here are some guidelines to help you make better decisions when evaluating the credibility of health claims.

6.1 Source

Where did the information originate? Was it a television documentary? A radio interview? Was it a pamphlet produced by an organization such as the Canadian Cancer Society, Mothers Against Drunk Driving, the Canadian Dairy Council, or the Pro-Life Society? Did the information come from articles published in your local newspaper, the *New York Times,* the *Canadian Medical Association Journal,* the *Canadian Journal of Public Health, Runner's World, Shape,* or *Cosmopolitan* magazines? Knowing the source tells you something about the credibility of the information and may also alert you to bias.

6.1.1 Scientific journals

For a couple of hundred years, scientists have communicated their findings by publishing them in periodicals called **journals**. Some journals have a new issue every week, some publish monthly, and others publish once every three months. Journals are like popular magazines in that they are usually soft-covered and are about the size of magazines. However, popular magazines tend to have a lot of colourful photographs and lots of advertisements (medical journals also have lots of advertisements, most commonly for pharmaceutical products, also known as "drugs"). By contrast, scientific journals have a more serious appearance and tone, few photographs, and many figures (graphs and other images) and tables of numbers.

Virtually all scientific journals now publish digital editions in addition to, or instead of, print issues, and some researchers post summaries of their work as short videos on sites such as YouTube.

6.1.2 Peer review

Scholars prefer journals that are **peer reviewed**. This means the articles have gone through a "quality control" process. Peers are people like oneself. My peers are university teachers. The peer-reviewed journal *Cardiology* is aimed at heart doctors and heart scientists. It publishes articles that have been reviewed by other heart doctors and scientists.

6.1.3 *Impact factors*

An organization called ICI calculates **impact factors,** which measure how frequently authors cite a particular journal. Journals that are frequently cited by other authors tend to be the more important journals in that field. It is likely that journals that contain more articles in each issue will be cited more often than those with fewer articles. Thus, the impact factor is calculated as the number of citations to that journal divided by the number of articles published in that journal. High impact scores are considered better. The prestigious journal *Nature* has an impact factor of over 40, while *Scientific American*'s impact factor is less than 2.

There is growing concern regarding the intricate system behind peer-reviewed journals. David Eisner (2017) of the University of Manchester claims that "… despite the peer review of both the grants that fund the work and the papers in which it is published, serious errors are being published." There can be tremendous pressure on academics to publish, and to publish in the "best" journals. Publishing in journals with high impact factors can be key to career advancement, research funding, and in some cases, large cash payments. Eisner urges the reader to judge researchers on the merit of their work per se, and not by the journals in which they publish.

> A major reason that people take note of bibliometric factors such as the Impact Factor is that they are very convenient measures to use when assessing others for jobs, promotion etc. They are not a substitute for the only real test of a scientific paper; that its results stand over time and influence the work of others. (Eisner, 2017)

6.2 Date

Knowledge changes over time. It is likely that some of today's commonly accepted wisdom regarding diet or exercise will, in the future, be discredited. Newer information is usually preferred. However, in cases where other investigators have replicated original research, the original studies are often interesting and important to read.

6.3 Author experience or qualifications

Does the article say where the author works? Does the author have a university degree or other specialized training or experience? For example, is the author a person "with 20 years' experience as a tree planter, who has since served as a consultant to government and industry on the effects of clear-cut logging on water drainage"? Is the author described as "a freelance journalist specializing in environmental issues"? Often you will have to do some digging to determine the author's experience or qualifications. A little healthy skepticism is also useful. Remember, periodicals publish a mountain of articles every year. Just because a person's writing is in print or they speak on the air does not mean they have an informed point of view. This has become especially true with the explosion of self-publishing through new media, such as Internet blogs and YouTube videos.

6.4 Evidence

Determine what evidence the author has presented to support the main idea. To a lawyer, "evidence" refers to facts that connect the accused to the crime: fingerprints, blood, hairs, and so on. As a reader, you can allow yourself to be entertained, impressed, or shocked, but you should also be skeptical. The author should convince you. An article on the Amazon rainforest might include statements that "we lose 50,000 hectares of forest every minute," "satellite photographs taken in 1970 and again in 1990 show a 40% increase in the amount of deforested land in the Amazon basin," or "according to Brazilian government census data, 200,000 settlers relocated to the provinces in the northeast last year." Statements such as "we must protect the rainforest for the benefit of all mankind" are not evidence. They are opinions or conclusions, although they may be supported by the evidence provided.

6.5 Bias

Does the author seem to present both sides of the issue fairly, or do her personal opinions distort the evidence? Does the author have a personal reason for persuading you to agree with her? For example, is she encouraging you to "send $19.95 plus $3.00 for shipping and handling for your copper bracelet to use as protection against tennis elbow"? Does the author have a connection that might make you suspect bias? For example, the conclusions of a study showing that drinking milk regularly lowers risk of heart disease might be less convincing if the report were written by the senior scientist on the staff of the Canadian Milk Producers Council than if the author were an employee of Health and Welfare Canada.

6.6 Logic

Finally, look for examples of faulty reasoning. The evidence may be extensive and well documented, but the conclusions drawn from the evidence might be faulty. Consider the following hypothetical example:

- The Maasai people of Africa have a low incidence of heart disease despite a high consumption of meat. Therefore, North Americans would be advised to eat more meat as a protection against heart disease.

This argument has several flaws.

- First, the low incidence of heart disease might be the result of other factors (such as lower level of urban stress, higher degree of social cohesion, or lower rate of cigarette smoking) than the meat consumption.
- Second, the findings might not be transferable to North America. It would be more convincing to learn that Canadians who eat large amounts of meat have lower rates of heart disease than their counterparts (of similar age, gender, and lifestyle) who eat less meat.
- The argument is also flawed by lack of detail, although this is not "faulty reasoning." It would be helpful to have meat consumption specified in kilograms per person per year, and for heart disease incidence to be reported in deaths per 1,000 people per year.

Consider another example of faulty reasoning:

- Of the 1,800 persons arrested last year in Vancouver for possession of heroin, 89% reported they had been habitual marijuana smokers (defined as use at least once per day) before first using heroin. This demonstrates that smoking marijuana can lead to addiction to heavier drugs.

> Can *you* see the flaw in the reasoning?

What if this researcher had questioned these marijuana smokers regarding milk consumption? Probably most of them were milk drinkers before they were heroin users. Would this suggest milk leads to heroin addiction? No, because only heroin users were questioned. If the researcher questioned a group of habitual marijuana users, probably much less than 89% of them would report ever using heroin.

6.7 Additional guidelines

A website produced by the US Food and Drug Administration gives some additional guidelines to help readers evaluate material they find on the Internet (FDA Staff, 2005):

- Discuss the information you find with your health care professional.

- Determine the purpose of the website. Most fundamentally, is the purpose to provide objective information or to sell a product or service?
- Determine who runs the website (e.g., from the "About Us" link).
- Look for sites with URLs ending in .gov, .edu, or .org. These are sponsored by government, universities or medical schools, and not-for-profit organizations, respectively.
- Be aware that sites ending in .com are often selling something.
- Be cautious about chat rooms or discussion groups, because what people say there may or may not be true, is usually not checked or verified by anyone, and may be posted as a way to promote a product for financial gain. It is a good idea to follow a discussion and feel comfortable with it before you join in.
- Try to ascertain the original source of the information. Many websites compile information that was originally published elsewhere. Be cautious with sites that don't share the original source of the information.
- Note whether the website distinguishes between what parts of its content are opinion and what parts are based on evidence.
- Be cautious about any website that does not share a way to contact its owners (e.g., a "Contact Us" link).
- Check some of the links on the site. Lots of broken links suggest the owners may not keep the website current.
- Try to find out whether the website has a policy regarding linking to other sites (check the "About This Web Site" link). Some websites link to any other site that asks, or that pays for a link, while others only link to sites that meet certain criteria.
- Be careful about sites that ask for your personal information. Check the "Privacy Statement" link to see what the site will do with this information.

So, let's get back to that student question posed at the beginning of this chapter:

> *How can you determine which products on the market provide options for healthy eating and good nutrition?*

Here are some questions you can ask to guide your evaluation of the evidence:

- **Is the website making a claim that seems too good to be true?** If it seems too good to be true, it probably isn't true. For example, I wouldn't believe a claim that a product "melts body fat from thighs" because I know from my study of body weight and weight loss that fat is not lost preferentially from any area of the body. You can reduce the total amount of fat you have, but you can't direct your fat loss to any particular area of the body, even if that part has more fat than other parts.

- **What is the source of the claim and how credible (believable) is that source?** I would be more suspicious of claims made by people with a financial interest in the product, such as a salesperson in a nutritional supplement store, an advertisement, or a special interest group (e.g., the Canadian Milk Producers Association) than I would of claims made by researchers at a university, a government agency, or a not-for-profit organization (such as the BC Heart Association) who usually provide unbiased, objective information.

- **Where was the claim published?** Peer-reviewed scientific journals and websites of universities, government agencies, and not-for-profit organizations are, in general, more reliable sources than popular magazines such as *Shape* or *Muscle and Fitness*. Almost anybody can put up a website. So, if you are reading something on the Internet, look at the "About Us" and "Contact Us" links to learn more about who is behind the website and what their motivation is.

- **How consistent is the claim with what you already know?** In most cases, knowledge develops in small steps rather than amazing new discoveries overnight. For example, I have read in many places over many years that losing one pound of body fat is associated with a negative caloric balance of 3,500 kilocalories (kcal). Similarly, I know that the average daily caloric requirements for average adult females and males are about 2,400 and 2,800 kcal, respectively. A day of bed rest consumes about 1,200 kcal. Very active people may need 4,000 kcal per day. So, I wouldn't believe a promise that I will lose a pound of fat a day every day for a week. I would need to eat *nothing* and be *very* active every day for this to happen.

7 Conclusion

By now you should have a better understanding of the way in which scientists (experimenters and epidemiologists) and clinicians behave. You should be better able to decide for yourself whether or not to believe a particular health claim. Hopefully, you will want to know what evidence supports a headline or news story, and you will be in a better position to weigh the evidence.

Study Questions

1a. Define "placebo."
1b. Give a couple of examples of placebos other than the ones given in the book.
2a. Explain what is meant by a "blind" study.
2b. How is a "double-blind" study different from a "blind" study?
3.   Explain the term "latent period" in relation to disease.
4.   What alternatives do researchers have to address the potential problems of time and ethics in experimental research on human health?
5.   Explain the difference between an experimental study and an epidemiological study.
6a. List the six criteria given for determining whether an association or correlation between two variables means that one causes the other.
6b. Pick an example (real or hypothetical) other than the one given in the book and use it to illustrate these criteria.
7.   Consider the hypothesis "sweating in a sauna helps prevent colds." Give a hypothetical example of each of the following types of evidence in relation to this hypothesis:
     • Anecdotal
     • Experimental
     • Epidemiological
     • Clinical
8a. How can you tell the difference between a scientific journal and a popular magazine?
8b. Explain briefly the terms "peer review" and "impact factor."
9a. Give six guidelines you could use to evaluate printed material (e.g., material in a newspaper or magazine).
9b. Give six additional guidelines you could use to evaluate material found on the Internet.

Glossary

blind experiment—an experiment in which the subjects know the purpose of the experiment, but they do not know whether they are in the control group or in one of the experimental groups

control group—a group of experimental subjects intended to be the same as the experimental group (see below) except for the factor to which the experimental group is exposed (see *treatment*)

double-blind experiment—an experiment in which the subjects are blind (see *blind experiment*), and in addition the experimenters do not know which subjects are in the control group and which are in the experimental group until the end of the experiment

epidemiology—the branch of health science concerned with the distribution and determinants of disease

experimental group—a group of experimental subjects who receive the experimental treatment or manipulation

hypothesis—an idea, phrased in a way that can be tested

latent period—the time from exposure to something (in this context, a disease-causing agent) and the appearance of results (in this context, the development of signs or symptoms of a disease)

placebo—something that has no physiological effect but that subjects in an experiment cannot distinguish from the real treatment or manipulation

treatment—in this context, the thing that is done to the experimental group (i.e., the experimental manipulation)

Additional Resources

Centre for Science in the Public Interest (CSPI)

http://www.cspinet.org/

This website says, "CSPI carved out a niche as the organized voice of the American public on nutrition, food safety, health and other issues during a boom of consumer and environmental protection awareness in the early 1970s."

Health Fraud Scams (video)

US Food and Drug Administration

http://www.fda.gov/ForConsumers/ProtectYourself/HealthFraud/default.htm.

Health-Related Web Site Evaluation Form

http://www.sph.emory.edu/WELLNESS/instrument.html

Rollins School of Public Health, Emory University, Georgia, USA

This is an "instrument" (a numerical rating sheet) to help readers evaluate websites.

National Council Against Health Fraud (NCAHF)

http://www.ncahf.org/

This website says, "The NCAHF is a USA voluntary health agency that focuses its attention upon health fraud, misinformation and quackery as public health problems."

Quackwatch

http://www.quackwatch.com/

This website provides a guide to quackery and health fraud, with tips on how to make intelligent health decisions.

The website says it is operated by Stephen Barrett, who describes himself as "a retired psychiatrist who resides near Chapel Hill, North Carolina, has achieved national renown as an author, editor, and consumer advocate."

Solving the Diet-Cancer Mystery: Scientific Studies Provide Clues
  American Institute for Cancer Research
  http://www.pacificcancer.org/pacp-resources/food-nutrition-physical-
  activity/solving-the-diet-cancer-mystery.pdf

References

Bell, S., Britton, A. (2013). A second-class science? A defence of observational epidemiology to make causal inferences (letter to the editor). *Addiction.* 109, 163–164.

Eisner, D. A. (2017). Reproducibility of science: Fraud, impact factors and careless-
  ness. *Journal of Molecular and Cellular Cardiology.* http://dx.doi.org/10.1016/j.
  yjmcc.2017.10.009

Frerichs, R. (2018). John Snow. *Encyclopedia Britannica.* Retrieved May 8, 2018 from
  https://www.britannica.com/biography/John-Snow-British-physician

FDA Staff. (December 2005). How to evaluate health information on the internet. US
  Food and Drug Administration. Retrieved July 5, 2012 from http://www.fda.gov/
  Drugs/ResourcesForYou/Consumers/BuyingUsingMedicineSafely/BuyingMedi-
  cinesOvertheInternet/ucm202863.htm

Fekjaer, H. O. (2013). Second-class evidence for causality, not second-class science
  (letter to the editor) *Addiction.* 109,164–165.

Law, M. R., Morris, J. K., Watt, H. C., Wald, N. J. (1997). The dose-response relationship between cigarette consumption, biochemical markers and risk of lung cancer.
  British Journal of Cancer. 75(11):1690-1693.

Niiranen, T. J., McCabe, E. L., Larson, M. G., Henglin, M., Lakdawala, N. K., Vasan,
  R. S., Cheng, S. (May 17, 2017). Heritability and risks associated with early onset
  hypertension: multigenerational, prospective analysis in the Framingham Heart
  Study. *British Medical Journal.* 357: j1949 DOI: 10.1136/bmj.j1949

3 Infectious Disease

Learning Objectives

By the time you have finished this chapter you should be able to

- Explain the basic biology of infection
- Outline the links in the chain of infection and illustrate with examples of specific infectious diseases
- Describe the body's defences against infection
- Describe the trends in mortality from infectious diseases in developed and developing countries and explain the reasons for these trends.
- Describe what you can do to decrease your risk of contracting and transmitting infectious diseases.

1 Overview

In this chapter we look at infectious diseases, a leading cause of disability and death throughout human history. Most infectious diseases are *communicable*, which means they can be passed from person to person. In the following two chapters, we study heart disease, stroke, diabetes, and cancer. These are non-communicable. If a person on the bus sneezes in your face, you might "catch" a communicable disease such as a cold or the flu, but you won't catch heart disease or cancer.

Incidence of and mortality from infectious diseases has dropped dramatically in Canada and other developed countries in the last 100 years. "Incidence" refers to the number of *new* cases of a condition per year; unless otherwise stated, it is expressed as a rate (e.g., per 100,000 people). Progress has also been made in much of the developing world. For example, in 2010 there were 130,000 deaths globally from measles, compared with 630,000 deaths in 1990. Tetanus deaths decreased from 270,000 to 60,000 (Lozano et al., 2012).

However, these diseases remain one of the major public health challenges in *developing* countries. For example, there were 52.8 million deaths globally in 2010. Tuberculosis and malaria were responsible for 1.2 and 1.17 million of these deaths, respectively. The same year, 1.5 million died from AIDS (Lozano et al., 2012).

Infectious diseases also remain a major cause of death in North Americans with poorer immune system function, including infants, the elderly, and those weakened by malnutrition, alcohol abuse, or other illness. Furthermore, *acute* (short-term, sudden, temporary) respiratory infections (such as influenza and colds) are the main cause of acute **morbidity** (sickness) and lost time from school or work.

In this chapter we will examine the mechanisms of infectious disease, study reasons for the decline in infectious disease rates in industrial countries, and observe that the same progress has not been made in less-developed countries. Then we will look at what you can do to decrease your risk of contracting an infectious disease or transmitting it to someone else.

2 Mechanism of Infectious Diseases

Infectious diseases are characterized by *infection*, which means the invasion by and multiplication of microorganisms in body tissue, usually accompanied by local cellular injury. The *latent period,* or *incubation period* (the time from entry of the pathogen until the appearance of symptoms), usually ranges from a day to a few weeks for most infectious diseases. However, with cholera it is only a few hours, and with HIV it appears to usually be several years

There are many different types of infectious diseases, each caused by a specific *pathogen* (infectious disease-causing agent) or "germ." Most pathogens are tiny and can only be seen with a microscope. Bacteria, viruses, fungi, and protozoa can all act as pathogens for specific diseases.

> Have *you* ever looked through a microscope at a drop of pond water?
> What did you see?

All pathogens have proteins called *antigens* on their surface. Different pathogens have antigens of different shapes. The immune system recognizes and responds to specific pathogens by their specific antigens.

3 Protection Against Infection

Bacteria, viruses, and other **microbes (micro-organisms)** surround us in the air, in the water, on the ground, on our hands, in our bedding—virtually everywhere. It's surprising we don't get infected more often. But not all microbes are harmful to humans. Also, most people normally have layers of natural protection against infection.

Hundreds of species of *bacteria* and trillions of individual bacteria live in our "gut," or gastrointestinal tract (GI tract, i.e., stomach, intestines, etc.), where they help us digest food. These "good" bacteria also help by competing with and excluding harmful microbes such as *Clostridium difficile* (*C. difficile*) bacteria. In addition, gut microbes help the immune system of the gut and the whole body. At birth the gut of the newborn has no or few microbes. Microbes from the environment colonize the gut, and the newborn develops tolerance to these early colonizing species. That is, it treats them as "friends," while it reacts against microbial species encountered later in life as "foreign."

Broad-spectrum **anti-microbial agents** taken to fight an infection kill many of the good bacteria in the gut and can decrease ability to digest food, sometimes resulting in diarrhea. **Probiotics** are microbes people deliberately ingest in food (e.g., yogurt) or as supplements. There is some evidence for the beneficial effects of probiotics, for example, in some types of bowel disease and in treatment of diarrhea in infants and children. "Probiotics are generally considered safe—they're already present in a normal digestive system—although there's a theoretical risk for people with impaired immune function" (Harvard Medical School Family Health Guide, 2005).

3.1 Natural defences against infection

In addition to maintaining bacterial balance in the GI tract, our bodies have several other methods of protecting us against infection in the course of daily life:

- **Intact skin** provides an excellent barrier against pathogens. However, pathogens can enter through cuts or sores, when the skin is pierced (e.g., with needles), or through body openings such as the mouth.
- **Cilia** are small, hair-like structures that protrude from cell surfaces. They sweep up pathogens and other particles that enter the airways and sweep them out.
- **The mucous coat** that covers tissues in the mouth, lungs, digestive tract, vagina, and urethra provides another physical barrier against infection.
- **The fever** (elevated body temperature) that accompanies many infections impairs pathogens' metabolism.

- **The immune system** provides a complex cellular and chemical response to infection. Various types of white blood cells will
    - Surround and "eat" foreign material, including pathogens.
    - Destroy infected cells.
    - Produce and release large numbers of ***antibodies***. Antibodies are proteins with particular shapes that fit the shape of the antigens on pathogens (Figure 3.1). The antibodies then stick to the pathogens, making it harder for the pathogens to enter cells and causing them to clump together so they can be more easily "eaten" by one type of white blood cells.
    - Create a cellular "memory" for specific pathogens. If the same pathogen enters the body again, these cells quickly recognize and neutralize it, often before it can cause an infection. In this way, the body acquires immunity to pathogens.

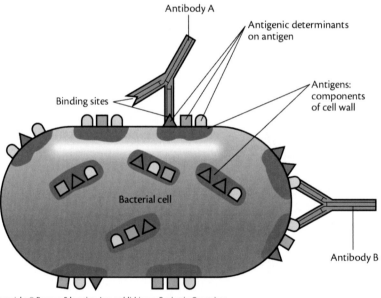

Figure 3.1. Antibodies match the shape of specific binding sites on the surface of other cells.

3.2 Immunity

There are four different ways in which you can develop ***immunity***, a state in which your body can be exposed to a particular pathogen without becoming infected:

- The fetus gets antibodies from its mother through the placenta while in the uterus (I explain placenta in Chapter 12: Fertility). Breastfed infants get antibodies through breast milk.
- You can get an injection of antibodies.
- You can be exposed to the pathogen and develop immunity to subsequent infections.
- You can be vaccinated. I explain this below.

The first two methods are temporary because the antibodies wear out over a period of months. The last two methods are long lasting because they stimulate your body to make its own antibodies.

3.3 Vaccination

Vaccination (or *immunization,* which is essentially the same thing) involves deliberately exposing a person to a weakened form of a pathogen, usually as an injection or "shot," although sometimes orally or with a nasal spray. The vaccine contains the antigen parts of the pathogen, which triggers the immune system of the person receiving the vaccination. The person's immune system keeps a memory of the antigens for that pathogen and uses that memory to make antibodies later when it encounters that antigen on a pathogen.

This immunity is usually specific; that is, the vaccinated person is only immune to that specific form of the pathogen. This is fine for most pathogens, but the influenza (flu) virus mutates quite rapidly, so every year there are several major new strains or varieties of it.

> What immunizations have *you* had:
>   a) as a child?
>   b) more recently?

4 Transmission of Communicable Diseases
4.1 Modes of transmission

Communicable diseases can be transmitted in several ways:

- The pathogen can be transmitted through **direct contact**, such as a touch, a kiss, sexual intercourse, or blood transfusion.
- The pathogen can be transmitted through **indirect contact**, when it is deposited on an object (such as eating utensils, toys, towels, bedding, or hypodermic needles) and then picked up when another person handles the object.
- Pathogens can be carried through **airborne transfer** (e.g., sneezing).

- **Contaminated water** carries pathogens for many communicable diseases; people become sick when they drink it.
- In *vector* **transmission,** an animal is an intermediate carrier of the disease. For example, dogs and rodents are vectors for the rabies virus. The bubonic plague ("black death") is transmitted to humans chiefly by fleas from infected rats. Certain species of mosquitoes are the vector for the parasite that is the pathogen for malaria.

As you can see, sexual contact (kissing, intercourse, etc.) is one transmission mode for communicable disease. We will study this more in Chapter 11: Sexually Transmitted Infections.

4.2 The chain of infection
Infectious diseases travel through the human population through a **chain of infection** (Figure 3.2), which involves the following steps:

- Pathogen
- Human reservoir
- Portal (door) of exit
- Transmission
- Portal of entry
- Establishment of disease in a new host

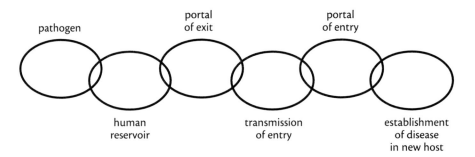

Figure 3.2. The chain of infection.

Let's look at several examples of the chain of infection in action:

- **Example A:** The **influenza** virus (pathogen) infects person A and multiplies in her upper respiratory tract. Then when person A sneezes, the pathogen leaves the mouth (portal of exit) in water droplets (transmission). Person B inhales it through the nose (portal of entry) and it multiplies in her body (establishment of disease in a new host).

- **Example B:** The bacteria that are the pathogens for **cholera** multiply in person A, leave through the anus in his feces, and may enter food or drinking water (for example, if he defecates in a stream or near a well, or prepares food without washing his hands). If person B consumes this contaminated food or water, the pathogen enters through the mouth and he can become infected.
- **Example C:** The **hepatitis** virus leaves person A's body on a contaminated hypodermic needle. If person B uses this needle without sterilizing it (killing the pathogens), the pathogens enter the body through the skin.
- **Example D:** The **gonococcus** bacteria (the pathogen for gonorrhea) can leave person A through the penis during sexual intercourse. The pathogen travels in the semen and infects person B through his or her mouth, vagina, or anus.
- **Example E:** The protozoan that is the pathogen for **malaria** lives in a particular species of mosquito (the vector), which breeds in warm, swampy areas. When the mosquito bites a person, the malaria pathogen can enter the person's body through the skin.

4.3 *Non-communicable infectious disease*

Not all infectious diseases are communicable. For example, a person infected with **tetanus** cannot pass it to another person. The tetanus pathogen is a bacterium that produces endospores, typically when the bacteria run out of nutrients. The endospores represent a reduced form of the bacteria that allows the bacteria to remain dormant. The endospores, which are found worldwide, get into the body through a puncture wound, such as might be caused by stepping on a rusty nail. The endospores then germinate inside the body, and the resulting bacteria multiply and release toxins.

Another example is **food poisoning. Botulism** is a type of food poisoning. Like tetanus, botulism spores produce toxins that humans take in when they eat contaminated food. Food poisoning is very common. According to one source, up to 13 million Canadians suffer from food-borne illnesses yearly (*The Ottawa Citizen*, 2013).

Modern society has become very complex, integrated, and interdependent. Consumers often live far from the sources of the food they eat. We depend upon producers, shippers, distributors, retailers, and government agencies that set and enforce standards for safety and quality. We can take some measures, such as proper refrigeration and cooking, to protect ourselves from food-borne pathogens at the individual level. As individuals, we can also do more to source food locally or even grow it ourselves, an issue we pursue in Chapter 7: Nutrition and Chapter 15: Environment.

5 Colds and Influenza

Colds and influenza are both **respiratory illnesses** but are caused by different *viruses* (CDC, 2013c). Influenza and the common cold have some similar symptoms, so it can be hard to tell whether you have one or the other. Flu symptoms, such as fever, body aches, extreme tiredness, and dry cough, are more common and intense. Conversely, colds are more likely to cause a runny or stuffy nose (CDC, 2013c).

Colds usually last a few days, while the flu can last for 7 to 10 days (CHICA, 2013). Generally, colds don't cause serious health problems. Flus are worse and can lead to pneumonia (a serious lung condition), bacterial infections, or hospitalizations (CDC, 2010). According to the Public Health Agency of Canada, 2,000–8,000 Canadians die of influenza and its complications annually, depending on the severity of the season (PHAC, 2012). The mortality estimates of the Community and Hospital Infection Control Association of Canada are more conservative: 500 to 1,500 per year (CHICA, 2013).

Influenza is highly infectious. **Transmission** occurs through droplets (e.g., saliva, sneezing) and by touching objects and surfaces contaminated with the virus (e.g., doorknobs, cell phones). The influenza virus may persist for hours in dried mucus and be transmitted by direct contact (CHICA, 2013). The *incubation period* for influenza is 24 to 72 hours. Adults with influenza remain infectious for three to five days after onset of symptoms, while children may remain infectious for up to a week (CHICA, 2013).

5.1 Vaccination for the flu and colds

The influenza virus **mutates** rather rapidly, exposing people to many different strains of the virus during their lives. "Even though the virus changes, their previous bouts of influenza may offer some protection against infection caused by a similar strain of the virus. However, three to four times each century, for unknown reasons, a radical change takes place in the influenza virus causing a new strain to emerge" (PHAC, 2012).

Influenza tends to be **seasonal,** with peak infection rates in January or February most years (CDC, 2013a). Vaccination does not become maximally effective right away (CDC, 2013a), so it's best to be vaccinated in the fall, before "flu season" starts. However, even if you wait until later, the vaccine can still help, as flu season can last until May (CDC, 2013a).

Because it takes months for pharmaceutical (drug) companies to manufacture the millions of doses of flu vaccine given each year in Canada, they have to start work before the actual flu season. So, the vaccine manufacturers make an educated guess about which strain(s) of flu virus this year's vaccine should combat.

What about a vaccine against the common cold? There is no such vaccine. Because so many different viruses can cause symptoms, there probably never will be a vaccine for it.

> Do *you* usually get an influenza vaccine each year?
>   Why or why not?
>   How does that work for you? Do you usually "catch" the flu or not?

5.2 "Stomach flu"

Viral gastroenteritis, also known as "stomach flu," is *not* influenza. A different virus, the norovirus, causes this stomach problem. Symptoms typically consist of abdominal pain, vomiting, diarrhea, nausea, low-grade fever, chills, body aches, and joint stiffness. The infected person generally feels better in a day or two (Vaesa, 2013).

Norovirus infection symptoms are very similar to food poisoning, although food poisoning symptoms can be more intense. If you ate with a group of people in the hours before you started feeling sick, ask them if they also got sick. If they have symptoms such as yours, you probably all got food poisoning. If not, you probably have a norovirus infection (Vaesa, 2013).

> Have you ever had food poisoning?
>   If so, what did you eat that made you sick?

6 Control of Infectious Disease

6.1 At the personal level

There is much you can do to minimize your risk of contracting or transmitting disease. You can **minimize exposure** to yourself and others if you

- Wash your hands before and after going to the bathroom, especially if you are going to prepare food, before eating, after working outside in the soil, after shaking hands with others, or after handling objects which may have been handled by others. Hand washing doesn't kill the pathogens; it removes them from your skin.
- Promptly clean any cuts or abrasions you sustain.
- Don't bite your fingernails.
- Avoid rubbing your eyes.
- If you sneeze, cover your mouth with a tissue or handkerchief, or sneeze into the crook of your elbow.

- Dispose of used tissues and handkerchiefs.
- Don't spit on the street.
- Avoid contact with those who have a communicable disease, and isolate yourself from others if you are sick.
- Avoid crowded places, especially if they are poorly ventilated.
- Limit the number of people whom you kiss on the mouth. Kissing on the cheek or shaking hands is more hygienic. The custom of bowing in greeting is even better.
- Avoid close contact with people who have active cold sores (herpes simplex virus, or HSV). Many people are permanently infected with HSV by age five; it is common for children to put their fingers and toys in their mouths and their friends' mouths.
- Limit your number of sexual partners, avoid sexual contact with those who may have a large number of sexual partners, and practise safer sex (e.g., by using a condom during sexual intercourse).
- Don't share personal articles such as your toothbrush, eating utensils, soap, face cloths and towels, or underwear. Don't drink out of the same glass or bottle as anyone else.
- Protect yourself from insect bites with repellants, clothing, and screens on windows.
- Control rodents by picking up garbage, putting lids on garbage cans, and repairing cracks and holes in walls of buildings.
- Wash all vegetables and fruits thoroughly.
- Avoid food poisoning (e.g., botulism, salmonella) by keeping cold foods cold and hot foods hot. If food is at a temperature between 4 and 60 °C (40 and 140 °F), bacteria will grow rapidly. These bacteria produce toxins that cause food poisoning. Most food poisoning is temperature-related. Meat is the food most commonly involved in food poisoning.

What other strategies do *you* know for avoiding food poisoning in your home kitchen?

- **Maintain your resistance** to infection with good health habits: sleep, rest, proper nutrition, regular moderate physical activity, and fresh air.
- Get **medical advice** for the following symptoms of a possible infection: sore throat, high fever, skin rash, frequent coughing and sneezing, swollen lymph nodes or glands, repeated diarrhea, or repeated vomiting.

6.2 At the community level
A number of strategies have proved useful in controlling the spread of infectious disease at the community level.

- **Pasteurization:** This refers to the heat-treating of fluids such as milk, orange juice, and beer to kill microorganisms.
- **Antimicrobial agents:** These are a large variety of chemicals that kill microbes or prevent their development, including antiseptics, disinfectants, and *antibiotic* drugs such as penicillin and streptomycin.

  There is growing concern among health experts regarding **antimicrobial resistance** (AMR), which develops when a microbe (microorganism) no longer responds to the drug to which it was originally sensitive. AMR results from a combination of random mutation and natural selection. Mutations occur all the time. Environmental challenges to living organisms result in "the survival of the fittest." This means that if a mutation gives an organism an advantage, then that organism may survive and thrive, passing on this trait to its offspring. The World Health Organization (2014b) reports "very high rates of resistance have been observed in all WHO regions in common bacteria," and states "antimicrobial resistance (AMR) is an increasingly serious threat to global public health ... The problem is so serious that it threatens the achievements of modern medicine. A post-antibiotic era—in which common infections and minor injuries can kill—is a very real possibility for the 21st century."

- **Adequate housing:** Overcrowded, cold, damp, and drafty accommodation increases exposure to pathogens and decreases resistance to infection by these pathogens.
- **Nutrition:** In modern developed countries, we are able to afford and obtain a wide variety of food year-round. Modern food-processing techniques minimize the risk of infection by botulism and other microorganisms in food.
- **Public sanitation:** Today when we turn on the tap, clean water flows. We flush the toilet, and human waste disappears. We put our garbage in the lane, and the garbage collector removes it. But 200 years ago, sewage and garbage were thrown into the streets to rot, be washed away by the rain, or be eaten by rats, dogs, and other vectors of infectious disease.
- **Surveillance:** Developed countries such as Canada have sophisticated systems of reporting and tracking trends in infectious disease. Most emerging infectious diseases (EIDs) come from latitudes closer to the equator, where reporting tends to be low. So unfortunately, "the majority of the scientific and surveillance effort [is] focused on countries from where the next important EID is least likely to originate" (Jones et al., 2008).
- **Vaccination:** Table 3.1 shows how effective vaccination can be in eradicating common infectious diseases.

Table 3.1

The Effectiveness of Vaccination Against Selected Infectious Diseases in Canada.

Disease	Cases per year pre-vaccine*	Year**	cases per year post-vaccine***
Diphtheria	206,939	1921	5
Measles	894,132	1941	135
Mumps	152,209	1968	612
Pertussis	265,269	1934	5,519
Polio (wild)	21,269	1952	0

*   Number of cases of the disease in Canada in the year at which there was the peak number of cases, before the start of immunization for a specific disease.
**   Year in which immunization started.
*** Number of cases in Canada in the year 1997 (University of Ottawa, 2011).

New immigrants to Canada are screened and are offered any immuniza-tions they may be missing. However, individuals are *not required* to get these immunizations in order to enter Canada or attend school (although if there is an outbreak of, e.g., measles, un-immunized children will not be allowed to attend). Therefore, it's possible that polio, which was eliminated from North America by the early 1990s, could be re-introduced from other countries where it is still widespread.

6.3 Relative risk

"Relative risk" compares the risk of taking one action with the risk of taking a different action ... or taking no action. For example, is vaccination safe? If by "safe," you mean absolutely, positively guaranteed to have no adverse effects, the answer is that probably *nothing* is safe. The question could be better posed as "what is the *relative risk* of vaccination?" That is, what is the risk of something bad happening if I get vaccinated compared to the risk of something bad hap-pening if I don't get vaccinated?

Consider **measles**, a highly contagious respiratory viral infection. Most people who contract measles suffer a bad skin rash and then recover in about a week. However, complications (such as blindness, swelling of the brain, and a lung disease called pneumonia) can occur and can be fatal (WHO, 2014a). Complications from measles are more common in very young children and in adults. In developed countries, one or two of 1,000 people infected with measles die (fatality rate = 0.1% to 0.2%). Fatality rates are higher in developing countries with poor nutrition and low access to health care (PHAC, 2014). "Every year, globally, thousands of people die of measles" (Maki, 2014, p. A8).

Measles is transmitted only by human-to-human contact and is *completely preventable* with vaccination. A measles vaccine has been available for over 50 years (WHO, 2014a). On rare occasions, individuals experience adverse side effects from the measles vaccine, for example, swelling, fever (elevated body temperature), and allergic reactions. However, getting the *vaccine* is much safer than getting *measles* (Centres for Disease Control and Prevention, 2017). That is, the risk of getting the vaccine is not zero, but the relative risk is low. In other words, the risk of vaccination is low relative to the benefit, giving a favourable **risk-benefit ratio**.

Spiegelhalter (2012) provides an interesting discussion of this issue. He notes, for example, that in England and Wales in 1940 there were over 400,000 cases of measles, with a fatality rate of 0.2% (i.e., 1 in 500 people who got measles died). Vaccination for measles started in the 1960s. In the year 1990, there were only 13,000 measles cases and one fatality. Since 1992, there have been no childhood deaths from measles in the UK; there have only been problems in adults who get infected with measles because they were *not* vaccinated. On the other side of the equation, the risks of health complications from vaccination are very low—much lower than 1 in 500. These rare instances, however, tend to get a lot of media attention, causing the public to overestimate the real risk of vaccination. Ignorance or complacency can result in re-emergence of disease. For example, after Britain stopped vaccinating against **pertussis** (whooping cough), an outbreak of the disease occurred.

Compliance with vaccine recommendations is reportedly facilitated when health care providers take a directive approach. Opel et al. (2013) analyzed videotape of 111 discussions about vaccines between health care providers and parents of young children. The investigators reported that most providers used *presumptive* ("Well, we have to do some shots") rather than *participatory* ("What do you want to do about shots?") language. Parents were much less likely to resist vaccine recommendations with the presumptive approach. Among parents who initially resisted the recommendation, when the provider pursued the original recommendation ("He really needs these shots"), almost half the resistant parents relented.

6.4 Herd immunity

If you were the only human being on the planet, there would be no need for or benefit from immunization against human-transmitted diseases such as measles. But there are billions of us humans, the vast majority living and interacting in dense human societies. For vaccination to be effective at controlling communicable diseases, community immunization rates of about 90% or higher are needed (Plans-Rubio, 2012).

This is the concept of "herd immunity," which compares human communities to a group or herd of cows. Compliance rates (i.e., the percentage of those who comply with, or follow, the recommendation to get immunized) don't need to be 100%, because some members of the "herd" have already developed immunity as the result of prior infection. In 2013, fewer than 70% of two-year-olds in British Columbia had received all the recommended immunizations (BCCDF, 2014). This isn't high enough to provide herd immunity.

An important issue here is the balance between **individual** and **community** interests.

If I think only of myself, I will encourage *everyone else* to get immunized so that they won't get infected. Then I don't need to get *myself* immunized (avoiding the small risk of adverse reaction to the vaccine), because nobody in my community will get infected, so nobody will infect me. This is somewhat like being at a sports event where somebody stands up so she can get a better view. Then people behind her stand, causing people behind them to stand, and so on. You can observe similar behaviour at airports, where people often stand close to the baggage claim carousel so they can see their bags arrive. If everyone stood back several metres, then everyone could see the luggage come down the chute; when you see your bag, you step forward and claim it. We will see this theme emerge again in Chapter 15: Environment.

7 Infectious Disease in the Developing Countries

In the developing world, public-health agencies have mounted major campaigns against infectious disease, with the financial, technical, and logistical assistance of such international agencies as the World Health Organization. Significant advances have been made in immunizing the global population against major infectious diseases.

- **Smallpox** has been completely eliminated worldwide.
- Most of the world is also free from **polio**, a disease that can cripple and paralyze children. When the Global Polio Eradication Initiative began in 1988, polio paralyzed more than 350,000 children yearly in a total of more than 125 *endemic* countries. In 2009, the disease paralyzed fewer than 1,600 children in 24 countries, and was endemic in only four countries (WHO, June 2010). In 2017, only 5 new cases of polio were reported globally: 3 from Pakistan and 2 from Afghanistan (Global Polio Eradication Initiative, 2018). However, unless these vaccination efforts continue until polio is eradicated globally, the pathogen can spread from remaining human reservoirs and infect unvaccinated people in areas where the disease had been eliminated.

- **Measles** is a major cause of child death worldwide. In developed countries, where children are generally healthy and well nourished, measles is rarely fatal. Significant progress has been made in vaccinating children in developing countries, and global measles deaths fell from about 733,000 in 2000 to 164,000 in 2008 (WHO, 2009).
- **Malaria** has been controlled in some parts of the world by killing the mosquito vector with insecticides and removing the stagnant water that provides breeding grounds for the mosquito, for example by draining swamps and discarding old automobile tires lying in back yards collecting rainwater. However, malaria remains a major problem in much of the tropical developing world. In some areas, success has been achieved in ensuring reliable supplies of clean drinking water and introducing basic principles of public hygiene.

However, general economic and social development in some regions still lags far behind conditions in industrial countries. Malnutrition weakens the body and makes it more susceptible to infection. Hard physical labour worsens the problem. Inadequate housing further erodes resistance to infection. Overcrowding allows disease to spread quickly through the population. Animal and insect vectors thrive. Primitive food-storage methods allow the nutritional content of food to deteriorate and harmful microorganisms to flourish. Illiteracy, unemployment, and poverty perpetuate the cycle of ignorance, despair, and disease.

8 Conclusion

Infectious diseases are caused by invasion of specific pathogens, or germs, and the multiplication of these microorganisms in the body. The body has considerable natural defences against infection. Immunization bolsters these natural defences. The risk of contracting and transmitting infectious disease can be minimized by observing a number of good personal and public health practices. Many major infectious diseases have been eradicated or controlled in North America. However, infectious diseases remain one of the biggest health problems in the developing world, where improving public health conditions and raising the standard of living seem central to success.

Study Questions

1. What does it mean when a disease is "communicable"?
2. Define the following terms:
   - Infection
   - Antibiotic

- Pathogen
- Antibody
- Antigen
- Incubation period/latent period
- Vaccine

3. Outline the natural defences against infection.
4. Explain briefly four different ways that a person may become immune to a specific infectious disease.
5. Explain four different ways in which infectious disease can be transmitted.
6a. Draw and label the "chain of infection" model.
6b. State at which place in the chain each of the following actions works:
   - Covering your mouth when you sneeze
   - Getting sufficient rest
   - Wearing a condom when you are having intercourse with an infected person
   - Washing your hands often
   - Treating infected people with antibiotics
   - Covering food so that flies can't land on it
7. Give an example of a non-communicable infectious disease.
8a. Contrast the flu with the common cold.
8b. Describe briefly transmission of influenza.
8c. What is the "stomach flu"?
9. List 10 things you could do (i.e., at the personal level) to decrease your risk of contracting (not transmitting) an infectious disease.
10. Explain the concept of herd immunity, including a discussion of relative risk and the balance of individual and community interests.
11a. How has mortality from infectious disease changed globally in the last 100 years?
11b. What accounts for this?

Glossary

acute—sudden, short-term (as opposed to chronic)

antibiotics—drugs (such as penicillin) that are effective against some pathogens (e.g., bacteria and fungi)

antibodies—proteins with a particular shape that matches the shape of antigens; antibodies interfere with infection caused by pathogens by binding to the pathogens, which makes it harder for them to enter cells and makes it easier for certain types of white blood cells to consume them

antigen—a protein (e.g., on the surface of a pathogen) that stimulates the body to produce antibodies

bacterium (plural = bacteria)—one of many types of small (typically several micrometres long) single-celled organisms that lack a cell nucleus

communicable—capable of being passed from one person (or animal) to another

endemic—regularly found among particular people or in a certain area

immunity—the state in which a person can be exposed to a particular pathogen without becoming infected

immunization—the process of conferring or giving a person immunity; vaccination is one type of immunization

incidence—the number of new cases of a condition per year, often expressed as a rate (e.g., per 100,000 population)

incubation period—the time from entry of the pathogen until the appearance of symptoms

infection—the invasion of the body by, and the multiplication in the body of, a pathogen

latent period—in this context, the same as *incubation period*

pasteurization—the heat-treating of fluids such as milk, orange juice, and beer to kill microorganisms

pathogen—an infectious disease-causing agent

vaccination—the process of deliberately exposing a person to an altered form of a pathogen in order to stimulate the production of antibodies to that pathogen, thus giving the person immunity against future infection by the real pathogen

vector—an animal carrier of a pathogen

virus—a simple microbe that consists of a small amount of nuclear material surrounded by a protein coat; smaller than a bacterium, a virus cannot grow or reproduce apart from a living cell but invades living cells and uses their chemical machinery to keep itself alive and to replicate

References

Aleccia, J. (October 22, 2010). Winter Olympics gave Canada medals—and measles. *NBC News.* Retrieved April 13, 2014 from http://www.nbcnews.com/id/39768249/ns/health-infectious_diseases/t/winter-olympics-gave-canada-medals-measles/#.UotZLaWCbwI

BCCDF. (February 17, 2014). *Percent of two-year olds with up-to-date immunizations British Columbia, 2009–2013.* Vancouver, BC: BC Centres for Disease Control. Retrieved April 13, 2014 from http://www.bccdc.ca/NR/rdonlyres/B8FB94AC-A216-4AEF-B88A-5C3C539F2575/0/2_Year_Old_Coverage_2010_Cohort.pdf

CDC. (2013a; January 10, 2013). *Misconceptions about seasonal influenza and influenza vaccines.* Atlanta, GA: Centers for Disease Control and Prevention. Retrieved March 4, 2013 from http://www.cdc.gov/flu/about/qa/misconceptions.htm

CDC. (2013b; February 13, 2013) Measles elimination efforts and 2008–2011 outbreak, France. *Perspective.* 19(3). ISSN 1080–6059. Retrieved March 4, 2013 http://wwwnc. cdc.gov/eid/article/19/3/12-1360_article.htm

CDC. (2013c; September 19, 2013). *Cold versus flu: Questions & answers.* Atlanta, GA: Centers for Disease Control and Prevention. Retrieved April 13, 2014 from http:// www.cdc.gov/flu/about/qa/coldflu.htm

CHICA. (March 4, 2013). *Influenza, avian influenza and pandemic influenza.* Winnipeg, MB: Infection Prevention and Control Canada (formerly CHICA: Community and Hospital Infection Control Association). Originally retrieved March 4, 2013 from http://www.chica.org/links_flu.php. Retrieved July 23, 2014 from http://www.ipac-canada.org/links_flu.php

Global Polio Eradication Initiative. (April 10, 2018). World Health Organization. Retrieved April 17, 2018 from http://polioeradication.org/polio-today/polio-now/ this-week/

Harvard Medical School Family Health Guide. (September 2005). *Health benefits of taking probiotics.* Retrieved May 11, 2014 from http://www.health.harvard.edu/fhg/ updates/update0905c.shtml

Jones, K. E., Patel, N. G., Levy, M. A., Storegard, A., Balk, D., Gittleman, J. L., Daszak, P. (2008). Global trends in emerging infectious diseases. *Nature.* 451(7181), 990–993.

Lozano, R., et al. (December 15, 2012). Global and regional mortality from 235 causes of death for 20 age groups in 1990 and 2010: A systematic analysis for the Global Burden of Disease Study 2010. *The Lancet.* 380(9859), 2095–2128.

Maki, A. (April 8, 2014). Measles in Canada: How it got to this. *The Globe and Mail.* pp. A8–A9.

Opel, D. J., Heritage, J., Taylor, J. A., Mangione-Smith, R., Salas, H. S., DeVere, V., Zhou, C., Robinson, J. D. (2013). Provider-parent vaccine discussions. *Pediatrics.* 132(6), 1037–1046.

PHAC. (September 24, 2012). *Influenza.* Ottawa, ON: Public Health Agency of Canada. Retrieved March 4, 2014 from http://www.phac-aspc.gc.ca/influenza/index-eng.php

PHAC. (April 7, 2014). *Measles.* Ottawa, ON: Public Health Agency of Canada. Retrieved April 13, 2014 from http://www.phac-aspc.gc.ca/im/vpd-mev/measles-rougeole-eng. php

Plans-Rubio P. (March, 2012). The vaccination coverage required to establish herd immunity against influenza viruses. *Preventive Medicine.* 55:72-77.

Spiegelhalter, D., (May 23, 2012). Vaccines: risks and benefits. *BBC News.* Retrieved May 11, 2014 http://www.bbc.com/future/story/20120523-vaccines-the-numbers

The Ottawa Citizen. (May 26, 2008). *More Canadians suffer food poisoning.* Retrieved March 4, 2013 from http://www.canada.com/topics/news/national/story. html?id=ee66451e-aa59-4bf1-90d7-7ecd7985f582

University of Ottawa. (November 8, 2011). The impact of childhood immunizations. *Society, the Individual, and Medicine.* Retrieved March 4, 2013 from http://www. med.uottawa.ca/sim/data/Immunization_e.htm

Vaesa, J. (2013). *Norovirus symptoms: 2013 stomach flu bug going around.* Retrieved July 24, 2014 from http://www.decodedscience.com/norovirus-symptoms-2013-stomach-flu-bug-going-around/25151

WHO. (June 17, 2010). *Global polio eradication initiative launches 2010–2012 strategic plan for interrupting polio worldwide.* (News release). Geneva: World Health Organization. Retrieved January 31, 2013 from http://www.who.int/mediacentre/news/releases/2010/polio_eradication_20100616/en/index.html

WHO. (December 3, 2009). *Global measles deaths drop by 78%, but resurgence likely.* (News release). Geneva: World Health Organization. Retrieved January 31, 2013 from http://www.who.int/entity/mediacentre/news/releases/2009/measles_mdg_20091203/en/index.html

WHO. (February 2014a). *Measles (Fact sheet N°286)* Geneva: World Health Organization. Retrieved April 13, 2014 from http://www.who.int/mediacentre/factsheets/fs286/en/

WHO. (April 2014b) *Antimicrobial Resistance: Global Report on Surveillance 2014.* Geneva: World Health Organization. Retrieved July 24, 2014 from http://www.who.int/drugresistance/documents/surveillancereport/en/

4 Cardiovascular Disease and Diabetes

Learning Objectives

By the time you have finished this chapter you should be able to

- Explain the basic anatomy of the cardiovascular system
- Describe the stages in the development of atherosclerosis
- Identify the risk factors for cardiovascular disease (CVD)
- Describe the trend in CVD mortality in North America and the personal and societal changes that have contributed to this trend
- Explain the basic physiology of diabetes
- Summarize the prevention and treatment of CVD and diabetes, noting the difference between primary and secondary prevention

1 The Cardiovascular System

Cardiovascular disease (CVD) refers to diseases of the heart (cardio) and blood vessels (vascular). The heart is a muscular pump about the size of your fist, located a bit to the left of middle in the chest (Figure 4.1). Blood is pumped from the heart to body tissues via blood vessels called *arteries.* Arteries divide like branches of a tree into smaller and smaller vessels, ultimately becoming tiny **capillaries.** In the capillaries, oxygen and other nutrients move from the blood into body cells, and carbon dioxide and other waste products move out of the cells into the blood. The blood returns to the heart via **veins.** The heart pumps steadily throughout life, at about 70 beats per minute at rest and up to 200 or more beats per minute in maximal exercise. The arteries that supply blood to the heart muscle itself are called the *coronary arteries.*

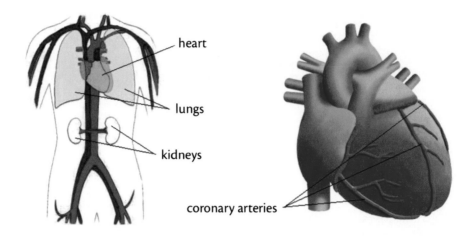

Figure 4.1. The human cardiovascular system. Major arteries are shown in red, with major veins in blue.

Atherosclerosis, a progressive narrowing of the arteries caused by deposits of fat and other material, is a major form of CVD. Atherosclerosis of the coronary arteries is known as *coronary artery disease* (CAD) or *coronary heart disease* (CHD). Atherosclerosis starts with a *lesion* (injury) to the inner wall of the artery (Figure 4.2). This presumably happens thousands of times a day, throughout the body, and starting in early life. A number of things have been blamed for causing the lesions. High blood pressure can cause the artery to overstretch and tear. Various chemicals, including nicotine, cholesterol, and **free radicals,** can injure the artery wall. Free radicals are molecules that are highly reactive chemically.

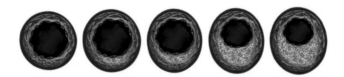

Figure 4.2. Stages in atherosclerosis. The artery progressively narrows as deposits accumulate in the artery wall.

Once the lesion has formed, *cholesterol* begins to deposit between the layers in the artery wall. This seems to happen in young adulthood or earlier. At this stage, the disease seems to be reversible. Over a period of months, calcium and other deposits gradually replace the soft cholesterol, forming a type of hard scar tissue. This is probably not reversible. Once these deposits form, the walls of the artery become stiff and the artery does not adapt well to changes in blood pressure. This is why atherosclerosis often leads to ***arteriosclerosis***, also known as "hardening of the arteries." The deposits in the walls of the artery cause a bulge to protrude into the inside of the artery. This bulge reduces the space through which blood can flow and causes a relative deficiency of blood flow, which reduces the rate at which oxygen is supplied and waste products are removed. The terms "atherosclerosis" and "arteriosclerosis" are often used interchangeably, which can lead to confusion about which is which. The key difference is that atherosclerosis is reversible, while arteriosclerosis is not.

Temporary lack of oxygen in the heart muscle causes pain in the chest, which may also radiate into the arms and neck. In the brain, temporary oxygen deprivation may cause headache, dizziness, loss of consciousness, or temporary inability to speak or move part of the body. More seriously, a clot may form in the region of the lesion. The clot can close off the vessel or break loose and get stuck downstream in a smaller vessel. Cells that do not get oxygen will die. When this occurs in the heart, it is called a **heart attack**. In the brain, this condition is known as a ***stroke***. If the region of the brain or heart that dies is large, the person may die. On the other hand, a blockage in a small blood vessel may not even cause any symptoms.

> Think about *your* family: parents, uncles and aunts, grandparents, siblings:
> a) Which of them has/had cardiovascular disease?
> b) What type of cardiovascular disease is/was this?

2 Prevalence

Heart disease and stroke are two of the three leading causes of death in Canada (Statistics Canada, 2017). Remember that ***prevalence*** refers to the number of people with a particular disease or condition as a portion of the total population (i.e., as a rate or a percentage). According to the Public Health Association of Canada,

- In 2014, 7% of Canadian men and 5% of women reported living with cardiovascular disease (PHAC, 2016a). About 2.4 million Canadians age 20+ live with diagnosed heart disease (PHAC, 2016b).
- Prevalence increases with age. Only about 1% of those aged 20 to 34 reported having CVD. This increased to 8% of those 50 to 64 and 18% of those 65 and older (PHAC, 2016a).

- Heart disease is more common than stroke. Among Canadians of all ages, prevalence of heart disease was about 5%, and for stroke about 1% (PHAC, 2009).

There is some good news. Compared with 2001, in 2013 the number of Canadian adults newly diagnosed with heart disease declined from 221,800 to 158,700. The number of *new cases* of a disorder in a given time period is called *incidence*.[1] Over the same period, the death rate among those with known heart disease decreased by 23% (PHAC, 2016b).

Prevalence based on self-report probably underestimates true prevalence, as heart disease is often asymptomatic. This underscores the value of *primary prevention*, which includes modifying diet and activity level to prevent the disease from starting.

3 Risk Factors for Cardiovascular Disease

Prevention, especially of diseases that have a lengthy, usually "silent" (i.e., asymptomatic) onset, is based on identification and modification of risk factors for the disease. *Epidemiological studies* are used for such identification.

> Do *you* remember from Chapter 2: Evaluating Health Claims what epidemiological studies are?
> Do you remember the example of the Framingham study?

The **Framingham Heart Study** is a great example. This study examined more than 5,000 residents of the town of Framingham, Massachusetts, at yearly intervals. Over time, patterns emerged. Individuals with certain characteristics were more likely to contract and die from cardiovascular disease. Dr. William Kannel, who led the Framingham Study from 1966 to 1979, coined the term "**risk factors**" for these characteristics. This important study has generated over 1,200 scientific research papers (Miller & Wood, 2011).

3.1 Unchangeable risk factors for cardiovascular disease
3.1.1 Age
Risk of CVD increases with age. Atherosclerosis and arteriosclerosis progress over many years. Also, mechanisms that repair damage to arteries and other tissues appear to become less effective as one ages.

3.1.2 Sex
Cardiovascular disease (CVD) used to affect more Canadian males than females, but the picture has changed. The current number of deaths from CVD is virtually

---

1   Incidence is similar to prevalence, except that prevalence focuses on those who *have* the disorder, while incidence considers only *new cases*.

the same for Canadian women and men (The Heart & Stroke Foundation, 2008). The situation in the USA is essentially the same as in Canada. In 2010, CVD mortality rates in the USA for both males and females were 236 deaths per 100,000. In that year, CVD caused the deaths of 387,318 males and of 400,332 females (American Heart Association, 2014).

> Can *you* reconcile the apparent contradiction in the preceding two sentences?

3.1.3 Heredity
If you have had cardiovascular disease already, or if a close relative (e.g., parent or sibling) has had cardiovascular disease, you are more likely to experience cardiovascular disease in the future.

3.1.4 Ethnicity
Canadians of African, Hispanic, and South Asian heritage are at higher risk of CVD than other people in Canada. This is partly due to higher rates of obesity and diabetes in these subgroups. Indigenous people living in Canada are also at a high risk of CVD. Among those living on reserves in Canada,

- About 20% had diabetes (PHAC, 2009, p. 58)
- Over half of adults smoke (PHAC, 2009, p. 56)
- Almost 75% of adults, 42% of youths age 12 to 17, and 58% of children age 0 to 11 are overweight or obese (PHAC, 2009, p. 57)

Half of the Indigenous population are under age 25 (PHAC, 2009, p. 55). It is likely that as these young people age, they will experience CVD at rates higher than those of the overall Canadian population.

3.2 Changeable risk factors for cardiovascular disease
The major modifiable risk factors include (PHAC, 2011)

- Smoking
- Lack of exercise
- Unhealthy eating
- High cholesterol
- Hypertension
- High sodium intake
- Stress
- Diabetes

- Overweight (although this risk factor was not on the PHAC 2011 list, it is widely recognized as a risk factor; see Section 3.2.9 below)

3.2.1 Tobacco smoking

Risk of cardiovascular disease increases with the number of cigarettes smoked. Smoking tobacco in pipes or cigars also increases risk of CVD, though not as much as cigarette smoking does, presumably because cigarette smokers inhale more deeply, which allows more of the substances in cigarette smoke to enter the blood. Cigarette smoke contains dozens of potentially hazardous chemical compounds. Some of these substances are **carcinogenic** (they cause cancer). Others increase the risk of CVD. The two substances in cigarette smoke that have been blamed for CVD are carbon monoxide and nicotine. These chemicals can cause lesions in artery walls. In addition, carbon monoxide may impair the body's natural repair mechanisms by reducing oxygen supply to tissues.

3.2.2 Physical inactivity

Regular, moderate-intensity exercise has beneficial effects on a number of CVD risk factors: it lowers blood pressure, increases HDL cholesterol[2] and decreases LDL cholesterol, reduces stress, controls body weight, and helps with control of certain types of diabetes. Regular exercise has also been associated with improved nutritional habits and better quality of sleep, and it seems to benefit those who wish to quit smoking. Lower intensity activities, such as walking and gardening, may not be vigorous enough to develop aerobic fitness but are nevertheless also associated with decreased risk of cardiovascular disease.

3.2.3 Unhealthy eating

Several nutritional problems can contribute to cardiovascular disease:

- Eating too many calories and the associated problem of accumulating excess body weight.
- Eating too much fat, especially *saturated fat.* Saturated fats become solid at room temperature. They include
  - Meat, especially the visible white fat that can be trimmed before cooking or before eating; when this fat is separated from the meat it is called "lard." Many fried foods (such as French fries, potato chips, donuts, and fried chicken) are fried in lard.

---

2   Cholesterol in blood occurs in combination with proteins, in a molecular structure called lipoproteins. These can be either high density (lots of protein relative to the cholesterol) or low density (less protein relative to the cholesterol). High-density lipoprotein and low-density lipoprotein are abbreviated as HDL and LDL, respectively.

- Milk, cheese, cream, and ice cream.
- Nuts, such as peanuts.
- "Tropical oils," such as cocoa butter and palm oil.
- Not eating enough omega-3 fatty acids. Eating cold-water fish (mackerel, tuna, salmon, herring, and lake trout) reduces risk of CVD, and the omega-3 fatty acids in these fish are believed to be the protective ingredient. There is a health concern with eating too much of certain kinds of fish because they may contain high levels of mercury (a heavy metal that damages the nervous system) and toxins (poisons). Generally, the larger, older, and higher on the food chain the animal is, the more contaminants tend to concentrate in its tissues. For example, mercury levels in tuna are several times higher than in salmon or herring.
- Not eating enough fruits and vegetables. Five to ten servings a day are recommended. They contain fibre and antioxidants, both of which reduce risk of CVD.
- Drinking too much alcohol.

We'll look at food in greater depth in Chapter 7: Nutrition, and discuss alcohol in Chapter 13: Drugs.

3.2.4 *High blood cholesterol*
Cholesterol is a type of fat, or lipid, that occurs normally in various parts of the body, including the blood. Cholesterol is an important component of cell walls and certain hormones. In fact, the body manufactures cholesterol. However, excessive levels of cholesterol in the blood may increase the amount of cholesterol deposited around lesions in artery walls.

It's important to differentiate between *dietary* cholesterol and *blood* cholesterol. The public has become increasingly aware of the dangers of too much cholesterol. For example, you may know that cholesterol is found only in animal products and is especially abundant in eggs, organ meats (liver, kidney, heart), and shellfish (shrimp, crab, oysters).

Elevated blood cholesterol is the big risk factor for CVD. A minority of the population is cholesterol sensitive. For this group, increasing or decreasing dietary cholesterol can increase or decrease blood cholesterol. But most people are not cholesterol sensitive. For cholesterol-insensitive people, large changes in dietary cholesterol are associated with only small changes in blood cholesterol. Health professionals often advise North Americans to reduce their dietary cholesterol intake. There is probably no harm in this recommendation, and it should help a minority of the population reduce their risk of cardiovascular disease. However, most people will not experience much reduction in blood cholesterol levels by following this advice.

Cholesterol is carried in the blood in *lipoproteins*. Cholesterol carried by *low-density lipoproteins* (LDL) can easily move from the blood into the artery wall. Thus, high LDL levels increase risk of CVD. On the other hand, *high-density lipoprotein* (HDL) cholesterol appears to stay in the blood and may even promote the reabsorption of cholesterol from the artery walls back into the blood. The higher the proportion of total blood cholesterol that is present as HDL cholesterol, the lower the risk of CVD (Mayo Clinic, 2012).

> How are *you* doing so far?
> When you think about the preceding four changeable risk factors, do you think your current lifestyle puts you at lower, higher, or average risk for cardiovascular disease compared with other Canadians of your age, sex, and ethnicity?

3.2.5 High blood pressure (hypertension)

> **What can high blood pressure lead to?**

> Blood travels from the heart to the other parts of the body in blood vessels, which are like hoses or tubes, called arteries. When the pressure increases, the walls of the tubes will stretch a bit. Beyond that, they will tear. Even slightly elevated blood pressure increases risk of CVD.
>
> Tearing of the arteries in the kidneys, lungs, heart, brain, eyes, and so on will damage these organs. Thus, high blood pressure is a risk factor not just for heart disease but also for other disorders such as stroke (brain damage), kidney failure, and blindness.

Prevalence of *hypertension* among Canadian adults is over 22%, representing about 7.5 million Canadians (Hypertension Canada, 2016). Hypertension is more common among older adults, with prevalence increasing from less than 10% among those age 20–44 to more than 70% in those over 80. The good news is that Canada has the world's highest rate of hypertension awareness, treatment, and control. In Canada, young males with hypertension are less likely to know they have this condition, so are less likely to have it treated or controlled.

It is probably useful to have your blood pressure measured regularly (Figure 4.3). Blood pressure readings should be interpreted cautiously, since many things can influence them. Exercise, anxiety, lack of sleep, caffeine and

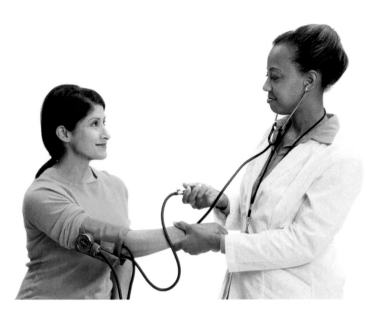

Figure 4.3. A clinician measures a person's blood pressure.

other drugs, food, cold, pain, and many other factors can cause temporary increases in blood pressure. A single measurement, or even several measurements of blood pressure on any given day, is usually insufficient.

The cause of most cases of hypertension remains unknown. However, some lifestyle **risk factors** are known. High dietary sodium (salt) intake and obesity each account for about 32% of lifestyle contribution to hypertension. Low dietary potassium and low physical activity each contribute another 17%. High alcohol intake adds another 3% (Hypertension Canada, 2016).

Drugs are often prescribed to treat hypertension. Although these drugs are effective at reducing hypertension and thus in reducing the health risks of hypertension, they often cause side effects such as dizziness, nausea, or impotence. Remember, hypertension itself often presents no symptoms. Consequently, it is sometimes difficult to convince patients to continue taking anti-hypertensive medication regularly.

3.2.6 High sodium (salt) diet

Sodium is an essential mineral in the body and is present in many foods. In contemporary Western society, we take in most sodium in the form of sodium chloride, which is common table salt. The saltshaker on the table is an obvious source, but many packaged, canned, and dried foods have salt added as a seasoning and preservative.

3.2.7 Stress

The mechanisms connecting stress and the cardiovascular disease process are somewhat speculative. Part of the typical stress response involves increased blood pressure, which is a known risk factor for CVD. Stress also increases blood-clotting rate, which may increase the chance of narrowed arteries becoming blocked. Furthermore, blood cholesterol levels are known to rise during stressful periods. Decreased blood flow to the liver during stress may impair the liver's ability to break down and excrete cholesterol, thus allowing blood levels of cholesterol to rise. Also, people under prolonged stress often sleep less, eat poorly and irregularly, and may smoke more (cigarette smoking seems to have a relaxing effect on the individual who has become dependent on nicotine).

3.2.8 Diabetes mellitus

"Adults with diabetes are two to four times more likely to have heart disease or a stroke than adults without diabetes" (American Heart Association, 2013). Heart disease and stroke are the main causes of death (over 65% of all deaths) and disability for people with Type II diabetes. Diabetes causes elevated blood glucose levels. Normalizing blood glucose levels does not appear to reduce the diabetic's risk of CVD (American Heart Association, 2013). Diabetes is discussed at more length later in this chapter.

3.2.9 Obesity and overweight

Many Canadians are overweight. **Obesity** (defined as being 20% or more above one's ideal weight) is strongly associated with hypertension, poor blood lipid profile (high cholesterol, low HDL, etc.), and diabetes (American Heart Association, 2012a) and "is probably an independent risk factor for atherosclerosis and CHD events" (Lavie, Milani, and Ventura, 2009).

Paradoxically, many studies have suggested that obese patients with CVD had a *better* prognosis than non-obese patients with the same cardiovascular disease. For example, one study reported that, compared with individuals without elevated BMI,[3] overweight and obese heart-failure patients had reductions in CV mortality (–19% and –40%, respectively) and all-cause mortality (–16% and –33%, respectively) (Lavie, Milani, and Ventura, 2009).

Discussion of the paradox includes the validity of BMI as a measure of fat versus muscle, blood levels of **leptin** (see Chapter 8: Body Weight and Weight Management), and inflammatory factors, but most of these concepts are beyond the scope of this book.

---

3   BMI = body mass index; we will discuss BMI and other measures of ideal body weight in Chapter 8: Body Weight and Weight Management.

More to the point, should the clinician advise an overweight or obese patient with CVD to lose weight or not? Lavie, Milani, and Ventura (2009) conclude the balance of evidence supports "purposeful weight reduction in the prevention and treatment of CV diseases."

> Think again about *your* family members with cardiovascular disease. What factors may have been responsible for their disease(s)?

4 Diabetes Mellitus
4.1 *Physiology of diabetes*
Diabetes is a medical condition that involves the hormone **insulin**, which is produced by special cells in the pancreas (Figure 4.4.). Insulin helps glucose (the most basic form of "sugar" in the body) move from the blood into cells.

There are several types of diabetes. In **Type 1 diabetes** (also known as **insulin-dependent** or **juvenile-onset diabetes**), the main problem is that the pancreas does not produce enough insulin (Figure 4.5.). Symptoms usually start in child-hood or young adulthood.

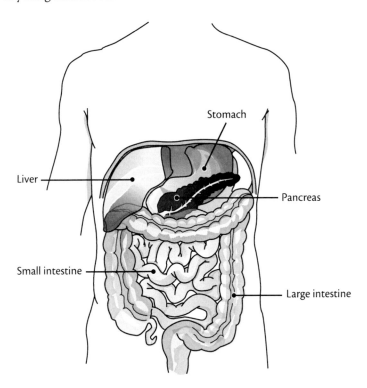

Figure 4.4. The pancreas is an organ that is located near the stomach and intes-tines.

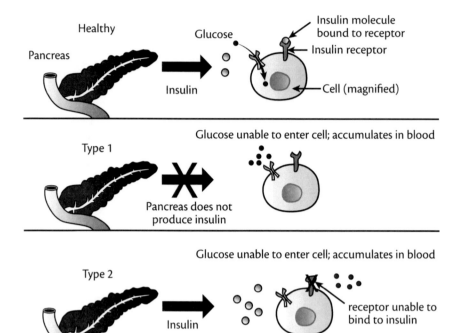

Figure 4.5. Diabetes interferes with the normal movement of glucose from blood to cells.

In **Type II diabetes** (**insulin-independent** or **adult-onset diabetes**), the pancreas produces enough insulin, but the cells lose their sensitivity to insulin, a problem called **insulin resistance.** Type II diabetes is strongly correlated with excess body weight. In perhaps 80% of cases, a combination of physical activity and weight loss can cure Type II diabetes.

People with either type of diabetes can, and some do, lead essentially normal lives, compete at high levels in sports, and live a normal lifespan. However, those who are unable to control blood glucose level within a reasonably normal range are at increased risk of a number of disorders, including

- Blindness
- Peripheral neuropathy (damage to the nerves in the arms and legs, which can result in loss of sensation to those areas)
- Sores and infections, especially of the feet
- Limb amputation
- Cardiovascular disease

4.2 Prevalence of diabetes mellitus

Diabetes was the sixth-leading cause of death in Canada in 2013, after cancer, heart disease, stroke, chronic lower respiratory infections, and accidents (Statistics Canada, 2017). Compared with people without diabetes, those with diabetes are

- Over three times more likely to be hospitalized with CVD.
- Twelve times more likely to be hospitalized with end-stage renal (kidney) disease. Diabetes was the primary cause of 34% of new cases of end-stage renal disease in 2009; people with this disease will die without either regular dialysis or a kidney transplant.
- Almost 20 times more likely to be hospitalized with non-traumatic (i.e., not caused by accidents) lower limb amputations (PHAC, 2011b, p. 4).

According to Diabetes Canada (2016) 9.3% of Canadians have diabetes. The Public Health Agency of Canada estimated that about 20% of people with diabetes do not know they have it (PHAC, 2011b, p. 4). Prevalence of diabetes in Canada is increasing. This could result from any one of several factors, or a combination of factors:

- A decline in mortality (deaths) from diabetes
- An increased prevalence of overweight and obesity, which is an important risk factor for diabetes
- Broader diagnostic criteria, which could have increased the number of cases identified
- A growing awareness by physicians and the public, which could have led to increased detection

Diabetes is more common among males (7.2%) than females (6.4%) (PHAC, 2011b, p. 4). This pattern differs for Indigenous peoples in Canada, where females are more likely to have diabetes than males, perhaps because Indigenous females also have higher rates of obesity and glucose intolerance than their male counterparts (PHAC, 2011b, p. 94).

Diabetes becomes more prevalent with advancing age. The Public Health Agency of Canada estimates that about one in five Canadians over age 65 had diabetes (PHAC, 2009, p. 47). Compare that with a 2010 Statistics Canada survey noting that fewer than one in 200 people aged 12 to 24 report having diabetes (Statistics Canada, 2010).

4.3 Risk factors for diabetes mellitus

- **Ethnicity:** Indigenous peoples or those of Hispanic, Asian, South Asian, or African descent are at increased risk of diabetes (Canadian Diabetes Association, 2012). A majority of Canadian children with Type II diabetes (75%) belong to a high-risk ethnic group (PHAC, 2011b, p. 83). Age-standardized prevalence rates for people age 12 and older show Indigenous people are at two to three times higher risk for diabetes than non-Indigenous people in Canada (PHAC, 2011b, p. 92).
- **Weight:** A 2012 report of the Canadian Diabetes Association shows being overweight or obese are risk factors for diabetes. The 2011 report of the Public Health Agency of Canada notes that just under half of new cases of diabetes were diagnosed in individuals aged 45 to 64 years old, an age range in which over 47% of individuals with diabetes were also obese; by comparison, only about 19% of individuals of the same age without diabetes were obese (PHAC, 2011b, p. 4).
- **Physical activity:** Many studies show physical inactivity increases risk of diabetes.
- **Family history:** The 2012 report of the Canadian Diabetes Association also shows that having a parent or sibling with diabetes increased risk. This may indicate a genetic predisposition and shared behaviours that could lead to diabetes, but it could also suggest that family history increases awareness and leads individuals to seek testing for diabetes (Statistics Canada, 2010).
- **Gestational diabetes:** If a woman develops diabetes during pregnancy, or gives birth to a baby that weighs over 4 kg (9 lb), she may be at risk for diabetes later in life (CDA, 2012).

The Canadian Diabetes Association (CDA) also lists hypertension and high cholesterol levels as risk factors for diabetes. I can't think of how either of these would cause diabetes. Since cardiovascular disease is a major complication of diabetes, I assume the CDA means "if you have diabetes, you should also be concerned about hypertension and blood cholesterol levels, as these would add to your risk for CVD."

Other the other hand, the CDA doesn't list age as a risk factor, yet the prevalence of diabetes certainly increases with age. Maybe age isn't considered a risk factor because Type I (and increasingly Type II) diabetes can start in children.

> A Canadian diabetes campaign once ran with the tag line of "Diabetes. Chances are one in five you've got it."
> What is your reaction to this statement?

5 Treatment
5.1 Treatment of cardiovascular disease
In Western countries, CVD mortality rates peaked in the 1960s and have declined substantially since then (Figures 4.6a and 4.6b). This is partly the result of primary prevention efforts, including reduced rates of smoking and physical inactivity and increased consumption of vegetables and fruits. According to the Heart and Stroke Foundation, "since 1952, the cardiovascular death rate in Canada has declined by more than 75 per cent—and nearly 40 per cent in the last decade—largely due to research advances in surgical procedures, drug therapies and prevention efforts" (Statistics Canada, 2011).

Deaths per 100,000 population

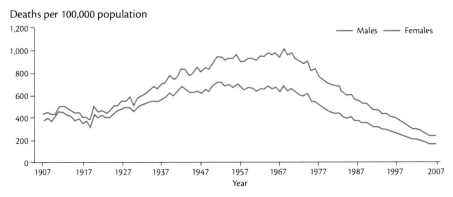

Figure 4.6a. Decline in cardiovascular disease in Australia (from Australian Institute of Health and Welfare, 2011, p. 62).

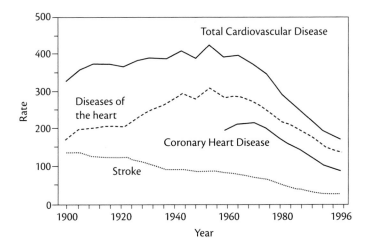

Figure 4.6b. Decline in cardiovascular disease in the USA. Lines show age-adjusted death rates (from Tulchinsky & Varavikova, 2010).

The decline in CVD mortality over the last 50 years is also partly the result of *secondary prevention* efforts—interventions to try to minimize the effects of the disease once it has appeared. These include better diagnosis and treatment of high blood pressure and blood lipids (e.g., cholesterol) and better management of people with CVD, which has increased survival rates (PHAC, 2009 p. 5).

- Improvements in ambulance service and emergency room care have reduced death from heart attacks. Cardiac rehabilitation programs, in which individuals who have suffered a recent heart attack participate in moderate, progressive exercise under medical supervision, have reduced the incidence of recurrent heart attacks.

- A wide range of drugs have been proven effective in reducing blood pressure, reducing blood cholesterol levels, opening blood vessels, and stabilizing the rhythm and strength of the heartbeat.

- Aspirin is effective in primary and secondary prevention of CVD. Aspirin decreases the tendency of blood to clot. However, there are harmful and potentially fatal side effects of aspirin therapy, and people should not start taking aspirin on a regular basis without first consulting their doctors (American Heart Association, 2012b).

- Improved treatment includes new devices (e.g., artificial hearts and implanted electronic pacemakers to keep the heart beating regularly) and surgical procedures such as heart transplants, *coronary artery bypass grafts* (Figure 4.7), and *angioplasty* (Figure 4.8).

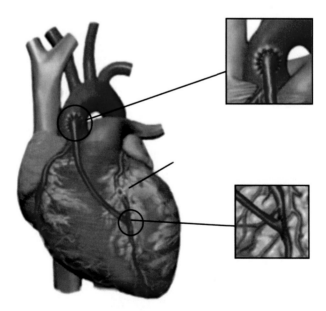

Figure 4.7. A coronary artery bypass graft (CABG) replaces blocked or narrowed blood vessels with sections of healthier blood vessels.

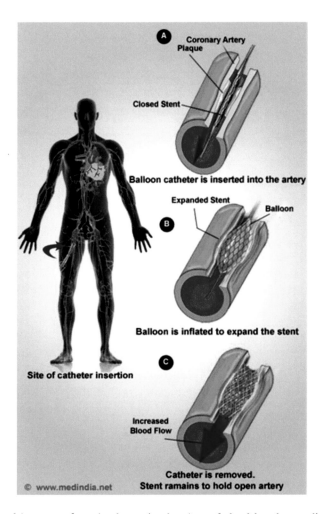

Figure 4.8. In this type of angioplasty (reshaping of the blood vessel), a small balloon is inserted into a narrowed artery. The balloon is inflated to enlarge the opening inside the artery and then withdrawn from the body.

Although CVD mortality has fallen dramatically in the last 50 years, this progress could reverse.

> Nine out of ten individuals over the age of 20 years have at least one of the following risk factors: smoking, physical inactivity during leisure time, less than recommended daily consumption of vegetables and fruit, stress, overweight or obesity, high blood pressure, or diabetes. Two in five have three or more of these risk factors. (PHAC, 2009, p. 6)

5.2 Treatment of diabetes

At present, there is no *cure* for diabetes. *Treatment* typically consists of

- **Insulin:** Regular injections of insulin and/or medication to control blood glucose levels.
- **Diet:** Balancing carbohydrate intake (which makes blood glucose go up) with physical activity and insulin, each of which makes blood glucose go down (Figure 4.9). Physical activity also reduces the risk of developing diabetes and inhibits disease progression by increasing insulin sensitivity.

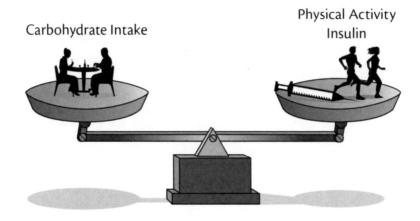

Figure 4.9. Management of blood glucose levels in diabetes by adjusting insulin dose according to carbohydrate intake and energy expenditure.

- **Fibre:** Those at risk of diabetes should meet the USDA recommendation of 14 g fibre per 1,000 kcal and eat at least half of their grains as whole grains.
- **Protein:** Opinions in this area have changed with recent research. The American Diabetes Association (ADA) 2008 nutritional recommendations advised people with diabetes to reduce protein intake, especially for those in the later stages of chronic kidney disease (Bantle JP et al., 2008). The ADA 2013 recommendations (Evert et al., 2013) take a different position, advising that (a) for people with diabetes and no evidence of diabetic kidney disease, protein-intake goals should be individualized; (b) for people with diabetes and diabetic kidney disease, reducing protein below the usual intake is not recommended; and (c) carbohydrate sources high in protein should not be used to treat or prevent hypoglycemia (low blood "sugar" level).
- **Weight loss:** In overweight and obese insulin-resistant individuals, modest weight loss has been shown to improve insulin resistance. Thus, weight loss is recommended for all such individuals who have or are at risk for diabetes.

- **Blood pressure:** People with diabetes should monitor blood pressure and manage hypertension as necessary (Canadian Diabetes Association, 2012).

> What do *you* think?
>
> Having read this chapter, what lifestyle changes could you make that would decrease your risk of getting—or developing complications from—cardiovascular disease and diabetes?

6 Conclusion

The Heart and Stroke Foundation's 2010 Annual Report on Canadians' Health is titled *A Perfect Storm of Heart Disease Looming on Our Horizon*. The report expresses satisfaction overall with the low rates of smoking among Canadians and acknowledges that Canadians are a bit more physically active than they used to be. However, the report also notes the increase in the percentage of Canadians who say they are overweight, have high blood pressure, and/or have diabetes, particularly among younger age groups that have traditionally been less affected by these conditions. The report also notes Canada's population is aging and certain ethno-cultural groups (Indigenous, South Asian, and Afro-Caribbean) who tend to experience higher rates of CVD are growing. Collectively, these trends point to a future increase in heart disease in Canada and threaten to reverse the gains made in the last 50 years.

Study Questions

1. Describe the stages in the progression of atherosclerosis.
2a. What causes a heart attack or stroke?
2b. What is the difference between a heart attack and a stroke?
3a. What is the difference between prevalence and incidence?
3b. Compare the prevalence in Canada of heart disease to living with effects of stroke.
3c. How do prevalence of the two conditions mentioned in Part (b) change with age?
4a. Name the study that created the concept of "risk factors" for cardiovascular disease.
4b. What are the major unchangeable risk factors for CVD?
4c. What are the major changeable risk factors for CVD?
4d. Explain, in a paragraph each, how each of the items in Part (c) affects CVD.
5a. What are lipoproteins?
5b. Differentiate between high- and low-density lipoproteins.

6a. Summarize the physiology of diabetes, differentiating insulin-dependent from non-insulin dependent forms of diabetes.

6b. How prevalent is diabetes in Canada?

6c. Outline the risk factors for diabetes.

7a. Discuss treatment for cardiovascular disease.

7b. Discuss management of diabetes.

8a. What is the trend for mortality from cardiovascular disease in North America?

8b. Explain the reasons for this trend.

9. Identify six lifestyle factors that an individual can change to reduce risk of CVD.

10a. What is the difference between primary prevention and secondary prevention?

10b. Give three different examples of secondary prevention in cardiovascular disease.

Glossary

angioplasty—a procedure in which a narrowed blood vessel is reopened by inserting a small flattened balloon, inflating it several times, then withdrawing it

arteriosclerosis—progressive narrowing of arteries due to an accumulation of fat, cholesterol, and other material, and a hardening of the arteries due to mineral deposits

atherosclerosis—progressive narrowing of arteries due to an accumulation of fatty material

artery—muscular-walled blood vessel that carries blood away from the heart

cardiopulmonary resuscitation (CPR)—an emergency first-aid procedure in which external compressions of the chest and artificial ventilation of the lungs sustain the flow of oxygenated blood necessary for life

cholesterol—a fatty substance produced by the body and also found in food from animal sources, which can accumulate as fatty deposits in the walls of arteries

coronary arteries—blood vessels that supply the heart muscle itself with blood

coronary artery disease—atherosclerosis of the coronary arteries

coronary artery bypass graft—a procedure in which sections of healthier blood vessels are sewn or grafted onto a diseased artery to create an alternate route for blood flow around a narrowed or blocked portion of the artery

coronary heart disease—essentially synonymous with *coronary artery disease*

epidemiological study—an observational study of a population, which observes, but does not manipulate, correlations between disease outcomes and various risk factors

high-density lipoproteins (HDL)—lipoproteins that have lots of protein and little fat, are less likely than *LDL* to deposit fat in artery walls, and may even absorb some cholesterol out of artery walls and into blood

hypertension—high blood pressure

incidence—the number of new cases of a disorder in a specified time period (typically a year), usually expressed as a rate by dividing the number of cases by the population

lesion—injury or damage

lipoproteins—the form in which lipids (fats and oils, including cholesterol) are carried in the blood

low-density lipoproteins (LDL)—lipoproteins that have lots of fat relative to protein and can move easily from blood into artery walls

prevalence—proportion of a population with a particular condition or disease (i.e., how common it is)

primary prevention—modification of risk factors to prevent the disease from starting

saturated fat—fats that have the property of being solid at room temperature

secondary prevention—secondary prevention of CVD means reducing mortality and morbidity once the disease process has started

stroke—sudden loss of brain function resulting from interference with the blood supply to a part of the brain

Additional Resources

American Heart Association
  Risk factor assessments for diabetes, heart attack, and high blood pressure are available at http://www.heart.org/HEARTORG/Conditions/More/Tools-ForYourHeartHealth/Heart-Health-Risk-Assessments-from-the-American-Heart-Association_UCM_306929_Article.jsp

References

American Heart Association. (2012a; September 13, 2012). *Obesity information.* Retrieved February 14, 2013 from http://www.heart.org/HEARTORG/GettingHealthy/WeightManagement/Obesity/Obesity-Information_UCM_307908_Article.jsp

American Heart Association. (2012b; December 11, 2012). *Aspirin and heart disease* Retrieved January 30, 2013 from http://www.heart.org/HEARTORG/Conditions/HeartAttack/PreventionTreatmentofHeartAttack/Aspirin-and-Heart-Disease_UCM_321714_Article.jsp

American Heart Association. (January 31, 2013). *Cardiovascular disease and diabetes.* Retrieved April 15, 2014 from http://www.heart.org/HEARTORG/Conditions/Diabetes/WhyDiabetesMatters/Cardiovascular-Disease-Diabetes_UCM_313865_Article.jsp

American Heart Association. (2014). *Heart disease and stroke statistics—2014 update.* Retrieved April 15, 2014 from http://www.heart.org/HEARTORG/General/Heart-and-Stroke-Association-Statistics_UCM_319064_SubHomePage.jsp#

Australian Institute of Health and Welfare. (2011). *Cardiovascular disease Australia facts 2011.* Cardiovascular Disease Series. Cat. no. CVD 53. Canberra, ACT: AIHW. Retrieved July 24, 2014 from http://www.aihw.gov.au/WorkArea/DownloadAsset.aspx?id=10737418530

Bantle, J. P., et al. (January 2008). Nutrition recommendations and interventions for diabetes: A position statement of the American Diabetes Association. *Diabetes Care.* 31(Suppl1), S61–S78.

Canadian Diabetes Association. (2012). *Diabetes facts.* Retrieved February 11, 2013 from http://www.diabetes.ca/diabetes-and-you/what/facts/

Diabetes Canada. (2016). Diabetes Statistics in Canada. Retrieved May 1, 2018 from http://www.diabetes.ca/how-you-can-help/advocate/why-federal-leadership-is-essential/diabetes-statistics-in-canada

Evert, A. B., Boucher, J. L., Cypress, M., Dunbar, S. A., Franz, M. J., Mayer-Davis, E. J., Neumiller, J. J., Nwankwo, R., Verdi, C. L., Urbanski, P., Yancy, W. S. Jr. (October 9, 2013). Nutrition therapy recommendations for the management of adults with diabetes. *Diabetes Care.* Retrieved April 15, 2014 from http://care.diabetesjournals.org/content/early/2013/10/07/dc13-2042.full.pdf+html

Heart and Stroke Foundation. (Feb 4, 2008). *The heart truth official launch.* Retrieved June 4, 2008 from http://www.thehearttruth.ca/News/2008/02/launch/

Heart and Stroke Foundation. (January 25, 2010). *A perfect storm of heart disease looming on our horizon: 2010 Heart and Stroke Foundation annual report on the health of Canadians.* Retrieved July 24, 2014 from http://www.heartandstroke.com/atf/cf/%7B99452D8B-E7F1-4BD6-A57D-B136CE6C95BF%7D/Jan23_EN_ReportCard.pdf

Heart and Stroke Foundation. (2013). *Statistics.* Retrieved January 30, 2013 from http://www.heartandstroke.bc.ca/site/c.kpIPKXOyFmG/b.3644453/k.3454/Statistics.htm

Hypertension Canada and the HSFC/CIHR Chair in Hypertension Prevention and Control. (2016). *Hypertension in Canada.* Retrieved May 1, 2018 from http://www.hypertensiontalk.com/wp-content/uploads/2016/05/HTN-Fact-Sheet-2016_FINAL.pdf

Lavie, C. J., Milani, R. V., Ventura, H. O. (May, 2009). Obesity and cardiovascular disease: risk factor, paradox, and impact of weight loss. *Journal of the American College of Cardiology.* 53(21), 1925–1932.

Lee, D. S., Chiu, M., Manuel, D. G., Tu, K., Wang, X., Austin, P. C., Mattern, M. Y., Mitiku, T. F., Svenson, L. W., Putnam, W., Flanagan, W. M., Tu, J., (August 4, 2009; Epub 2009 Jul 20). Trends in risk factors for cardiovascular disease in Canada: Temporal, socio-demographic and geographic factors. *Canadian Medical Association Journal.* 181(3–4), E55–66.

Mayo Clinic. (August 10, 2012). *High cholesterol: Causes.* Retrieved January 30, 2013 from http://www.mayoclinic.com/health/high-blood-cholesterol/DS00178/DSECTION=causes

Miller, R., Wood, S. (August 24, 2011). Dr. William Kannel, long-time Framingham study director, dies. *Medscape*. Retrieved April 15, 2014 from http://www.medscape.com/viewarticle/748510

PHAC. (2009). *Tracking heart disease and stroke in Canada, 2009*. Ottawa, ON: Public Health Agency of Canada. Retrieved July 24, 2014 from http://www.phac-aspc.gc.ca/publicat/2009/cvd-avc/index-eng.php

PHAC. (May 28, 2010). *Report from the Canadian Chronic Disease Surveillance System: Hypertension in Canada, 2010*. Ottawa, ON: Public Health Agency of Canada. Retrieved February 14, 2013 from http://www.phac-aspc.gc.ca/cd-mc/cvd-mcv/ccdss-snsmc-2010/2-1-eng.php

PHAC. (2011a; June 28, 2011). *Minimizing the risks of cardiovascular disease*. Ottawa, ON: Public Health Agency of Canada. Retrieved July 24, 2014 from http://www.phac-aspc.gc.ca/cd-mc/cvd-mcv/risk-risques-eng.php

PHAC. (2011b). *Diabetes in Canada: Facts and figures from a public health perspective*. Ottawa, ON: Public Health Agency of Canada. Retrieved July 24, 2014 from http://www.phac-aspc.gc.ca/cd-mc/publications/diabetes-diabete/facts-figures-faits-chiffres-2011/index-eng.php

PHAC. (2011c). *Tracking Heart Disease and Stroke in Canada – Stroke Highlights 2011*. Retrieved May 1, 2018 from https://www.canada.ca/en/public-health/services/chronic-diseases/cardiovascular-disease/tracking-heart-disease-stroke-canada-stroke-highlights-2011.html

PHAC. (2016a). *Health Status of Canadians 2016: Report of the Chief Public Health Officer – How are we unhealthy? – Cardiovascular disease*. Retrieved May 1, 2018 from https://www.canada.ca/en/public-health/corporate/publications/chief-public-health-officer-reports-state-public-health-canada/2016-health-status-canadians/page-17-how-are-we-unhealthy-cardiovascular-disease.html

PHAC. (2016b). *Heart Disease in Canada*. Retrieved May 1, 2018 from https://www.canada.ca/content/dam/phac-aspc/documents/services/publications/diseases-conditions/heart-disease-maladies-coeur-eng.pdf

PHAC. (2017). *For professionals: Heart disease and conditions*. Retrieved May 1, 2018 from https://www.canada.ca/en/public-health/services/diseases/heart-health/heart-diseases-conditions/for-professionals-heart-diseases-conditions.html#a2

Statistics Canada. (January 14, 2010). *Diabetes*. Retrieved February 14, 2013 from http://www.statcan.gc.ca/pub/82-229-x/2009001/status/dia-eng.htm

Statistics Canada. (2011, October). *Mortality, summary list of causes 2008*. Retrieved July 24, 2014 from http://www.statcan.gc.ca/pub/84f0209x/84f0209x2008000-eng.pdf

Statistics Canada. (2017). *The 10 leading causes of death, 2013*. Retrieved May 1, 2018 from https://www.statcan.gc.ca/pub/82-625-x/2017001/article/14776-eng.htm

Tulchinsky, T. H., Varavikova, E. A. (2010). What is the "New Public Health"? *Public Health Reviews, 32*, 25–53. Retrieved April 15, 2014 from http://www.publichealthreviews.eu/show/f/23

5 Cancer

Learning Objectives

By the time you have finished this chapter you should be able to

- Explain what cancer is and what causes it
- Describe trends in incidence and mortality for the major cancers in Canada and suggest explanations for these trends
- Outline the major risk factors and tests for major types of cancer
- State the rationale for early detection of cancer
- Discuss how to efficiently and effectively screen for disease in a population
- Summarize actions an individual can take to decrease risk of contracting or dying from cancer

1 Overview

Cancer is the leading cause of death in Canada. Collectively, cancers accounted for 30% of all mortality in 2013. Heart disease and stroke accounted for 20% and 5%, respectively (Statistics Canada, 2017). Four major cancers (lung, breast, colorectal, and prostate) account for half of newly diagnosed cancers in Canadians. **Mortality** (death) rates are declining in Canada for all four of these major cancers (Canadian Cancer Society, 2017). We can attribute this trend to both improvements in *screening* and **early detection**, and the discovery and use of more effective and less toxic cancer **treatments** (Canadian Cancer Society, 2013a).

The *number* of new cases of cancer in Canada has risen steadily over the last three decades. This is partly because the Canadian population is increasing in number. Also, cancer is more common among older people, and the

Canadian population is aging. The **age-standardized incidence rate (ASIR)** takes account of these two factors. The Canadian cancer ASIR is about 550 per 100,000—that is, in a city of 100,000 people, about 550 people will get a new diagnosis of cancer this year. Lifetime prevalence of cancer in Canada is 47%, meaning that almost half of all Canadians will be diagnosed with cancer sometime during their life (Canadian Cancer Society, 2017). Non-melanoma skin cancer (discussed in more detail later in this chapter) is not included in this figure, or in most other cancer statistics. Non-melanoma skin cancer is the most common cancer diagnosed in Canadians, but it accounts for very few deaths (Canadian Cancer Society, 2012, p. 7).

> Do you remember from Chapter 3: Infectious Disease what "incidence" is?

Cancer is primarily a disease of older people. Eighty-nine percent of new cases occur in people age 50 and older, with about half of this incidence in people age 70-plus (Canadian Cancer Society, 2017). In Canada, more males die of cancer than females: about 39,000 deaths versus 36,000 deaths, respectively, in 2013 (Statistics Canada, 2017). Canadian age-standardized mortality rates for all cancers combined have decreased over the last several decades, with the rate decreasing more rapidly in males than in females (Canadian Cancer Society, 2017). This seems partly because male rates are higher, so there is more room for improvement. The lesser decline in female rates is also because male lung cancer rates leveled off in the 1980s and have declined since, while female lung cancer rates have only recently plateaued.

Cancer was the leading cause of *potential years of life lost (PYLL)* in 2009 (Canadian Cancer Society, 2013b). Diseases of the heart were the second leading cause of PYLL (Figure 5.1). The PYLL for an individual is calculated by subtracting age of death from life expectancy. For example, a person with a life expectancy of 70 years (determined from gender and year of birth) who dies at age 65 has a PYLL equal to 5. If the same person died at age 25, he would have 45 PYLL. Lung cancer accounted for 26% of all premature mortality caused by cancer, with the use of tobacco the most important cause. PYLL from cancer is higher for women than for men, because the PYLL for breast cancer is several times higher than that of prostate cancer, because of the relatively young age at which women die from breast cancer (Canadian Cancer Society, 2013b).

2 Mechanisms of Cancer

Cancer involves uncontrolled multiplication of cells. The different tissues of the body (skin, bone, lung, etc.) are made up of many small, specialized cells. Most cells have genetic material called DNA (although red blood cells don't). DNA

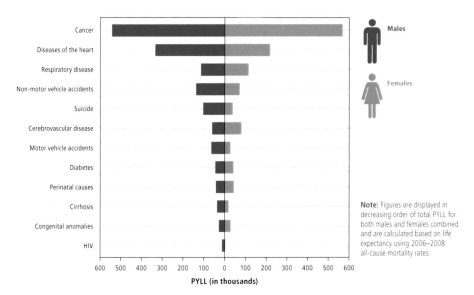

Cancer
Diseases of the heart
Respiratory disease
Non-motor vehicle accidents
Suicide
Cerebrovascular disease
Motor vehicle accidents
Diabetes
Perinatal causes
Cirrhosis
Congenital anomalies
HIV

Males

Females

Note: Figures are displayed in decreasing order of total PYLL for both males and females combined and are calculated based on life expectancy using 2006–2008 all-cause mortality rates.

600 500 400 300 200 100 0 100 200 300 400 500 600

PYLL (in thousands)

Analysis by: Chronic Disease Surveillance and Monitoring Division, CCDP, Public Health Agency of Canada
Data source: Canadian Vital Statistics Death database at Statistics Canada

Figure 5.1. Potential years of life lost (PYLL) for selected causes of death in Canada (2009).
Source: Canadian Vital Statistics database at Statistics Canada.

molecules contain "instructions" for making things the body needs, including copies of cells. Life starts with a single cell—the female egg (ova)—which is fertilized by the addition of genetic material from one sperm cell. This cell grows and divides many times, with cells becoming more specialized as the embryo develops. Throughout life, cell multiplication and division create extra cells needed for growth and repair. Multiplication is normally controlled; that is, it's "turned on" and "turned off" at the right times. Normal cells have a "biological clock," in that they are programmed to reproduce a certain number of times or for a certain time period and then to die.

Why do we have cancer?

Cancer occurs when ***mutations*** happen to DNA. The mutations cause the mechanism of normal cell growth to malfunction, which allows uncontrolled cell division.

In a normal cell, when DNA gets damaged the cell either repairs the damage or the cell dies. In cancer cells, the damaged DNA is not repaired, and the cell doesn't die like it should. Instead, the cell goes on making new cells that the body doesn't need. These new cells all have the same abnormal DNA as the first cell does. Growing out of control and invading other tissues are what makes a cell a cancer cell. (American Cancer Society, 2012)

Many cancer cells are killed by white blood cells, which are part of the immune system. Cancer cells that are not killed can progress and accumulate in clumps called *tumours.*

Cancer cells often travel to other parts of the body where they begin to grow and form new tumours. This happens when the cancer cells get into the body's bloodstream or lymph vessels.[1] Over time, the tumours replace normal tissue. The process of cancer spreading is called *metastasis.* No matter where a cancer may spread, it's always named for the place where it started. For example, breast cancer that has spread to the liver is called metastatic breast cancer, not liver cancer. Likewise, prostate cancer that has spread to the bone is called metastatic prostate cancer, not bone cancer. (American Cancer Society, 2012)

Tumours that *metastasize* are called *malignant* tumours.

Cancer-causing agents are called *carcinogens* (Figure 5.2). In addition, other agents can promote cancer growth. For example, the female hormone estrogen promotes breast cancer. Estrogen is not a carcinogen; it does not cause cancer, but it stimulates cancer growth. Many things act as carcinogens:

- **Chemicals** such as benzene or vinyl chloride, which can be ingested through food or water, can be inhaled, or can pass through the skin.
- **Radiation**, which includes ultraviolet radiation from the sun or tanning studios and X-rays from medical or dental work, uranium mining, nuclear power plants, or nuclear weapons. After the atomic bombing of the Japanese cities of Nagasaki and Hiroshima at the end of the Second World War, thousands died from radiation-induced cancers, including leukemia (cancers of the blood-forming organs) and breast cancer.
- **Pathogens**, such as hepatitis B, which can cause liver cancer. Some varieties of human papillomavirus (HPV) cause most cervical cancer.

---

1   The lymphatic system is a network of tubes that collects extra fluid from the extremities and returns this fluid to the heart.

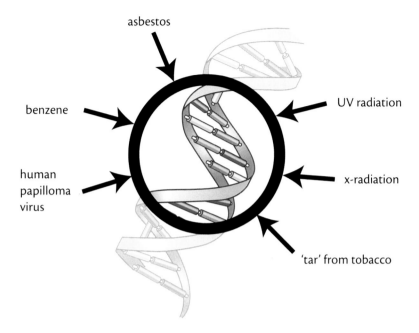

asbestos

benzene

UV radiation

human
papilloma
virus

x-radiation

'tar' from tobacco

Figure 5.2. Various environmental agents "attack" DNA. This causes damage (mutations) to this important biomolecule.

The different types of cancer vary in their location, extent, and responsiveness to treatment. Cancer can cause problems in several different ways:

- **Cancer cells often form a tumour, or mass of cells**. A few cancers (e.g., leukemia) do not form tumours.

   Not all tumours are cancer. Tumours that aren't cancer are called ***benign***. Benign tumours can cause problems—they can grow very large and press on healthy organs and tissues. But they cannot grow into (invade) other tissues. Because they can't invade, they also can't spread to other parts of the body (metastasize). These tumours are almost never life threatening. (American Cancer Society, 2012)

- **Cancers of the immune system make the body more vulnerable** to potentially fatal infections such as pneumonia.

- **Cancerous cells can also compromise normal physiological function** by using body supplies of energy and other nutrients intended for healthy cells.

- **Cells from malignant cancers can enter the lymph or blood vessels** and metastasize to other sites. Although we most commonly think of metastasis in terms of cancer, other diseases can metastasize, too, such as when the virus that causes influenza enters the body through the nose and mouth and then migrates down into the throat and chest.

By convention, we consider cancer to be cured if the patient is still living five years after the original diagnosis. Because people die of other causes than cancer, the **five-year survival rate** for cancer is usually expressed relative to the survival of that part of the general population that is similar to the patient in age, race, and gender. A survival rate of 80% for a certain type of cancer means that if we compared 100 patients with 100 non-patients, after five years the number of patients living would be 80% of the number of non-patients still living. Five years is a completely arbitrary figure, of course, but it is the standard definition. Overall, the five-year survival rate in Canada for all types of cancer combined is 60%. However, survival rates vary greatly; some types of cancer have survival rates of almost 100%, while survival rates are less than 20% for other types (Canadian Cancer Society, 2017).

> ### Will we ever find a cure for cancer or be able to prevent it?

Scientists are learning more and more about how cancer works at the cellular and molecular level. It seems likely that we will discover drugs that can cure at least some types of cancer.

For example, in order to metastasize, malignant cells break away from the primary tumour, attaching to and degrading proteins that make up the surrounding extracellular matrix (ECM), which separates the tumour from adjoining tissue. By degrading these proteins, cancer cells are able to breach the ECM and escape. The body resists metastasis by a variety of mechanisms, through the actions of a class of proteins known as metastasis suppressors. Scientists have identified about a dozen of these.

A critical event in metastasis is the growth of a new network of blood vessels, which is called tumour angiogenesis. Angiogenesis inhibitors, or drugs that would stop angiogenesis from happening, would therefore reduce metastases.

Cancer can be prevented. We can't guarantee any particular individual will not get cancer, but we can reduce the risk of particular cancers in a population. This is more effective for some types of cancer than for others. For example, lung cancer is strongly associated with tobacco smoking. The risk of lung cancer for non-smokers is only 5% to 10% of the risk for smokers. On the other hand, leukemia (cancer of the blood-forming organs) is not as well associated with changeable risk factors, so it is harder to prevent.

> Do you remember from Chapter 4: Cardiovascular Disease & Diabetes how *primary prevention* differs from *secondary prevention?*

Primary prevention of cancer involves reducing exposure to carcinogens. A key element in secondary prevention of cancer is **early detection.** The five-year survival rates for some types of cancer are much higher if the cancer is still localized when it is first detected, since these cancers can often be treated quite effectively.

The five-year survival rate for breast cancer is 87% if it is localized but drops to 47% if it has already spread when first diagnosed. Small tumours localized to the breast can be removed by lumpectomy, in which only the area of cancerous tissue is surgically cut away. This is the least invasive procedure, and leaves the breast looking normal. In advanced cases, the whole breast is removed, as well as the lymph nodes under the armpit. This is much more physically and psychologically traumatic, more expensive, more prone to medical complication, and has a poorer outcome because the cancer may have metastasized already.

Cancer research has been complicated by the fact that cancer typically has a long *latent period.*

> Do you remember from Chapter 3: Infectious Disease what a *latent period* is?

Some types of cancer, such as lung cancer, may have a latent period of 40 years. That is, a person can be exposed to a carcinogen, such as asbestos fibres, as a teenager and not show any indication of lung cancer until they are 55 years old. This long latent period makes it very difficult to establish a cause-effect relationship. How can you determine which of the thousands of compounds to which you have been exposed is responsible for your cancer? Furthermore, there are large individual differences in susceptibility to cancer. For example, some people will develop lung cancer following a single exposure to asbestos, while others work with asbestos every day for decades and never develop the disease.

3 Major Types of Cancer

3.1 Lung cancer

Lung cancer is the leading fatal cancer for both males and females. As mentioned earlier, male lung cancer rates leveled off in the 1980s and have declined since, while female lung cancer rates have only recently plateaued. Until 1993, breast cancer was the leading form of fatal cancer in females. Since then, age-standardized female mortality rates for breast cancer have declined steadily. Meanwhile, age-standardized female mortality rates for lung cancer continued to rise, then remained steady since about 2007 (Canadian Cancer Society, 2017).

Tobacco smoking is a major risk factor for lung cancer. Smoking accounts for about 27% of all cancer deaths (Canadian Cancer Society, 2013a). Of all lung cancer deaths that occur in people less than 70 years old, an estimated 63% are directly attributable to cigarette smoking. Cigarette smoking in North America increased in the years following World War I, held steady for a few years during World War II, then increased again to a peak in 1965. At that time, 62% and 37% of adult Canadian males and females, respectively, smoked. Cigarette smoking by Canadian adults, especially males, has decreased steadily since. In 2012, only 16% of Canadians identified as smokers (Health Canada, 2012).

The long latent period for lung cancer means that current lung cancer mortality doesn't compare well with current smoking prevalence. For example, lung cancer mortality for Canadian males continued to climb through the 1970s to a peak in 1988, at a time when smoking was on the decline. But when lung cancer is compared with tobacco consumption 20 years earlier, there is a good fit.

> Do you understand the preceding point?
> Could you illustrate it with a graph?

The most carcinogenic substances in tobacco are in the **tar**. Smoking low-tar cigarettes should reduce the risk for lung cancer, unless the smoker smokes more often or inhales more deeply.

Other products can cause lung cancer, too, including asbestos, fumes from metal smelting, and dusts from some types of wood and leather. Until recently, asbestos was widely used to insulate schools, hospitals, and office buildings. However, the health risk of inhaling asbestos fibres is now well recognized, and much of this insulating material is being removed. Asbestos and tobacco smoking have a multiplicative effect on lung cancer risk; that is, cigarette smokers and asbestos workers each have a several-fold increase in risk of lung cancer, but an asbestos worker who also smokes has a 60-fold increase in lung cancer risk relative to a non-smoker who is not exposed to asbestos.

The early signs and symptoms of lung cancer are not very specific, and so far screening has not been very successful with lung cancer. Chest X-rays don't detect tumours early enough, when they are small enough to make a difference to mortality. Compared to standard chests X-rays, a new X-ray procedure called low-dose computerized tomography (LDCT) is better at finding small abnormal areas in the lungs, and exposes the patient to lower doses of radiation. The National Lung Screening Trial gave over 55,000 smokers age 50 to 74 either a standard chest X-ray (the control group) or a LDCT (the experimental group) every year for three years. The subjects who got the LDCT were 20% less likely to die from lung cancer than the control group (American Cancer Society, 2016).

3.2 *Breast cancer*
Breast cancer is the most common non-skin cancer in females and the second leading cause of female cancer mortality in Canada (Canadian Cancer Society, 2012, p. 11).

The main risk factors for breast cancer are female sex, older age, and family history. If a woman's mother or sister had breast cancer, her own risk of cancer is increased by 50% to 300%.

> If you are female, think about your mother, her sisters (your aunts), your grandmothers, and your sisters.
>   a) How many of them have breast cancer?
>   b) Did they have it early or later in life?
>   c) Did they have it in one breast or both?
>   The more breast cancer there is in your family, especially early in life and/or in both breasts, the higher your own risk of breast cancer.

Female hormones, such as estrogen, promote breast tumour growth. **Estrogen** does not appear to *cause* the DNA mutations that trigger the development of human cancer. However, as one of its normal roles, estrogen promotes the proliferation of cells in the breast and uterus. If breast cells already possess a DNA mutation that increases the risk of developing cancer, both the normal and the mutated cells will proliferate.

- Women who start **menstruating** early or have a **late menopause** are at higher risk of breast cancer because their lifetime hormone exposure is greater. Women who have never had children are at greater risk compared with women who have given birth. Women whose first full-term pregnancy occurred past age 30 are at higher risk than women who gave birth before age 18 or 19. "A number of studies suggest that current use of **oral contraceptives** (birth control pills) appears to slightly increase the risk of breast cancer, especially among younger women. However, the risk level goes back to normal 10 years or more after discontinuing oral contraceptive use" (National Cancer Institute, 2012).

- **Hormone replacement therapy** appears more controversial. The issue seems to centre on the relative benefits and risks. The US Preventive Services Task Force "recommends against the use of combined estrogen and progestin for the prevention of chronic conditions in postmenopausal women" (Moyer, 2013). The prevention alluded to above speaks to estrogen's beneficial effects on bone density and serum cholesterol levels. The recommendation against using combined estrogen and progestin does not apply to women younger than 50 years who have had surgical menopause (i.e., had their ovaries removed) or to women who are considering hormone therapy for the management of menopausal symptoms, such as hot flashes or vaginal dryness.
- The drug **tamoxifen** blocks the action of estrogen in breast tissue, which reduces risk of both occurrence and recurrence of breast cancer. Unfortunately, tamoxifen mimics the effect of estrogen on uterine cells, thus increasing risk of uterine cancer. Scientists are looking for better cancer-blocking drugs (National Cancer Institute, 2010).
- **Breast implants** do not increase breast cancer incidence, but they do increase mortality because the implants impair early tumour detection.

Diet may play a role in breast cancer. Japanese immigrants to the United States and first-generation children of these immigrants have breast cancer rates similar to Caucasian Americans and much higher than native Japanese. Dietary fat may explain this. However, the largest prospective study done, involving over 89,000 nurses, showed no link between fat and breast cancer. Alcohol consumption is correlated with breast cancer; two drinks per day increases risk by 40% compared with drinking no alcohol. Alcohol apparently has its greatest effect on breast cancer before age 30.

Epidemiological evidence suggests that **regular physical activity** reduces risk of breast cancer in women. In a paper presented at the European Breast Cancer Conference in Glasgow, biostatistician Mathieu Boniol reported that an analysis of 37 studies involving more than four million women showed an hour of physical activity per day reduces risk of breast cancer by up to 12%. Researchers don't yet know the mechanism for this, but it doesn't seem to be related to the role of exercise in preventing overweightness (Press Association, 2014).

No interventions have proven to decrease the risk of developing breast cancer. Therefore, prevention centres on secondary prevention through monthly breast self-examination, regular physical examinations by a health professional, and *screening mammography* (a low-dose X-ray of the breast).

3.2.1 Multi-stage screening

Breast cancer offers a good opportunity to introduce the *11* approach (Figure 5.3). *Screening* for a disease is different from testing for a disease. We apply screening to apparently healthy populations, as compared with **testing** for diseases that we know or suspect they have.

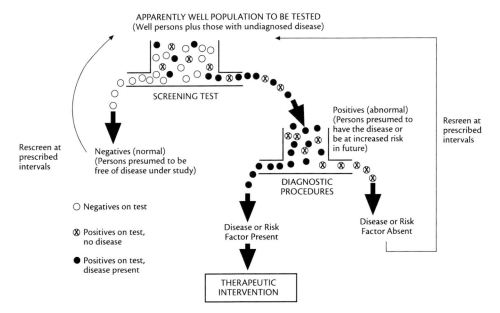

Figure 5.3. Multi-stage screening for suspected disease.

First-line screening tests should be low-cost, non-invasive, and low-risk. There are always some **false-positive** results—that is, people who are disease-free but who test positive, as if they have the disease. The Screening Mammography Program of British Columbia reports that for every 1,000 women screened, approximately 100 will have a positive mammogram, and 96 of these will be false positives. Only four will prove to have cancer.

This means we must use a second screening test to separate these false positives from the truly diseased people. This process can be repeated with a third or fourth test, each one more specific, and also usually more expensive, invasive, or risky. For example, if a woman has a positive screening mammogram, she is called back for a **diagnostic mammogram**, which uses a higher dose of radiation. If this is also positive, her physician may order a **biopsy** (a procedure in which a sample of cells from around the breast lump is taken) or an **ultrasound** scan. Overall, this multi-stage system is an effective and efficient way to use test populations and is used for other diseases besides breast cancer.

3.2.2 Mammogram controversy

In 2011, the Canadian Task Force on Preventive Care (CTFPC) made the following changes to its breast cancer screening recommendations (Breastcancer. org, 2011):

- Routine breast cancer mammogram screening for women with an average risk of breast cancer should start at *age 50* instead of 40.
- Women age 50 to 74 should be screened every *2 to 3 years* instead of every 1 to 2 years.
- MRI should *not* be used for breast cancer screening in women with average risk.
- Breast self-exam *isn't* recommended and doctors shouldn't routinely recommend it to women.

These recommendations apply to women at average risk for breast cancer. More aggressive screening may be appropriate for those at higher risk.

The recommendations to start screening at a later age and to screen less frequently were based on two things. First, the small extra benefit wasn't considered worth the cost and time to perform the extra mammograms. An estimated 2,100 women aged 40 to 49 would need to be screened every two to three years for 10 years to prevent one extra death from breast cancer. Second, when prevalence of a disorder in a population is low, the number of false positive results is high relative to the number of true positives. That is, a lot of the younger women would get an initial positive result, followed by extra testing, worry, and possibly unnecessary treatment.

The recommendation to drop breast self-examination (BSE) was based on absence of data showing that BSE lowered mortality from breast cancer and concern that many women would find lumps during BSE and get biopsies or other tests, only to find out the lumps were benign.

In 2009, the US Preventive Services Task Force (USPSTF) made recommendations similar to the CTFPC 2011 recommendations. In 2013, the Centers for Disease Control came out in support of this position. However, the American Cancer Society recommends annual screening mammograms for all healthy women starting at age 45 (American Cancer Society, 2017). In 2011, the American College of Obstetrics and Gynecology changed guidelines to recommend annual screening mammography beginning at age 40. (Previous ACOG guidelines recommended mammograms every one to two years starting at age 40 and annually beginning at age 50.)

Currently, the Canadian Cancer Society (2018) recommends that

- Women who are 40 to 49 years old should talk to their doctors about their risk of breast cancer and the benefits and risks of mammography.
- Women who are 50 to 69 should have a mammogram every two year.
- Women who are 70 or older should talk to their doctors about how often to have a mammogram.

The BC Cancer Agency recommends that women aged 50 to 74 without a family history of breast cancer should be screened every two years, while those with a "first-degree relative" (mother, daughter, or sister) with breast cancer should get annual screening from age 40 to 74 (BC Cancer Agency, 2018). A 25-year randomized clinical trial of almost 90,000 Canadian women concluded that screening mammography has no benefit in reducing death from breast cancer in women aged 40 to 49 (Miller, 2014).

Women will understandably feel confused by the discrepant expert recommendations. It seems likely to me that the various expert groups share the goal of best health outcomes for patients but are interpreting the relative risks and benefits differently. Women age 40 and older may wish to discuss the most appropriate approach with their personal health care provider.

3.3 Prostate cancer

The **prostate gland** is about the size of a walnut, situated near the bladder. Only males have a prostate gland. The prostate produces and secretes fluids that form part of the semen ejaculated during orgasm. Male hormones such as **testosterone** stimulate prostate growth. In Canada, prostate cancer is the most common non-skin cancer in men, and the third leading cause of male cancer mortality (Canadian Cancer Society, 2012, p. 10).

Prostate cancer incidence had been increasing steadily from 1970 to 1990. Then it increased dramatically because of the development and widespread adoption of a new test (the PSA test, which is explained below). The PSA detected cancers that had previously been undetected. Incidence declined in the latter part of the 1990s, presumably because the pool of previously undetected cancers was becoming depleted.

The main risk factors are **family history** and **older age**. Prostate cancer mainly occurs in older men. About 14% of American men are diagnosed with prostate cancer during their lifetime, but only about 3% of American men die from prostate cancer (American Cancer Society, 2013b).

Race is another risk factor for prostate cancer; it's more common in African-Americans than Caucasians, and less common in Asians.

Obesity is also a risk factor. "Obese men diagnosed with prostate cancer may be more likely to have advanced disease that's more difficult to treat" (Mayo Clinic, 2013).

> If you are male, think about your father, his brothers (your uncles), your grandfathers, your brothers.
> a) How many of them were treated for prostate cancer?
> b) How many of them died from prostate cancer?

People with prostate cancer may have no symptoms, or they may notice less rigid erections, a decrease in amount of fluid ejaculated, blood in the urine or semen, or severe pain in the back, pelvis, hips, or thighs. Prostate cancer can be detected with a digital rectal exam (Figure 5.4). The test I mentioned above measures blood levels of a protein called **prostate-specific antigen** (PSA). Elevated PSA levels may indicate prostate cancer, but other conditions, such as infection, can also raise PSA levels. As with breast cancer, false positives lead to many unnecessary procedures, such as biopsies and prostate surgeries. It may be more useful to watch how PSA levels change over time rather than act on an isolated score.

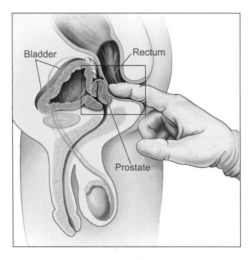

Figure 5.4. In a digital rectal exam, the clinician inserts a gloved, lubricated finger into the rectum and feels for lumps in the prostate.

Until recently, many doctors and professional organizations encouraged yearly PSA screening for men beginning at age 50. Some

organizations recommended that men who are at higher risk of prostate cancer, including African American men and men whose father
or brother had prostate cancer, begin screening at age 40 or 45. However, as more has been learned about both the benefits and harms of
prostate cancer screening ... a number of organizations have begun to
caution against routine population screening. Although some organizations continue to recommend PSA screening, there is widespread
agreement that any man who is considering getting tested should
first be informed in detail about the potential harms and benefits.
(National Cancer Institute, 2012d)

There are several options for treatment of prostate cancer. The gland may
be surgically removed. Or small radioactive **seeds** about the size of grains of
rice can be implanted into the prostate to kill the cancerous cells. **Cryotherapy**
(freezing the prostate) is an alternative. Patients can also use drugs to decrease
male hormone levels, which shrink the prostate and also the cancer.

3.4 Colorectal cancer

The **colon** is the major part of the large intestine. The **rectum** is the final part
of the colon, just before it exits the body through the anus.

A change in bowel movements (such as constipation or diarrhea) lasting
10 days or more may be one of the first symptoms of colorectal cancer. There may
be pain and tenderness in the abdomen. Blood in the stool is another important
warning sign (although this can also be caused by hemorrhoids). Blood is not
always visible but can be detected by chemically testing a stool sample. Fecal
blood screening for colorectal cancer is recommended in the United States
(Centers for Disease Control and Prevention, 2014b) and in Canada (Canadian
Cancer Society, 2014b).

Colorectal cancer proceeds in stages, the first being the appearance of non-
cancerous growths called **polyps** (growths that resemble small mushrooms)
inside the intestine. These growths are not malignant, but the longer they grow
and the larger they get, the more likely they are to develop into a cancer. In the
early stages, the abnormal cancerous cells are contained within the polyp and
can be removed. If the polyp is not removed, the cancer cells can eventually
invade the nearby colon tissue, growing into and beyond the walls of the colon
and rectum. At a still more advanced stage, the tumour sheds cells into the
circulatory system, which can spread cancer to other organs (John Hopkins
Medicine, 2014).

Known risk factors for colorectal cancer include **older age**, **male** sex, **inflam-matory bowel disease**, certain hereditary factors, and a **family history** of colorectal cancer or growths.

Lack of physical activity is another risk factor for colorectal cancer. One report notes, "… men who engage in exercise or sports at least five times a week are less likely to develop colon or rectal cancer than men who rarely or never exercise. The findings for women were similar. In addition, they found that the more time spent in sedentary activities, the more likely a person was to develop colon cancer." The mechanism for this effect is unclear (John Hopkins Health Alerts, 2012).

Age-standardized mortality rates have declined somewhat over the last three decades, but colorectal cancer remains the second leading cause of cancer mortality in Canadians overall—second-highest for men and third-highest for women (Canadian Cancer Society, 2012, pp. 9–11). The incidence of colorectal cancer is also higher in populations that eat a high-meat, high-fat, high-protein, low-fibre, low-calcium **diet**.

3.5 Cervical cancer

The *cervix* is the outer portion of the uterus, where it meets the vagina. Almost all cervical cancers are caused by infection with high-risk types of **human papilloma viruses** (HPV). Most infections with high-risk HPVs do not cause cancer and go away within one to two years. However, longer-lasting infections increase risk of cancer (National Cancer Institute, 2012b). We will consider HPV infection in more detail in Chapter 11: Sexually Transmitted Infections. Other, less important risk factors for cervical cancer include smoking, family history of cervical cancer, weakened immune system, chlamydia infection (a sexually transmitted infection; more in Chapter 11), long-term use of birth control pills, first full-term pregnancy younger than age 17, and more than three full-term pregnancies (American Cancer Society, 2013a).

Cervical cancer proceeds in well-defined stages. Before any cancer appears, a test can detect abnormal changes in cells on the surface of the cervix. Some of the cells are collected and examined under the microscope. The cervical smear test is also known as the *Pap test,* after George Papanicolaou, the pathologist who devised it in the 1930s. Mild abnormalities may revert back to normal or may proceed to more advanced stages of cervical cancer.

The BC Cancer Agency recommends women get a Pap test at age 21 or three years "after first sexual contact." This includes touching as well as intercourse, because the human papilloma virus (HPV) is transmitted through sexual *contact*, not just sexual *intercourse* (BC Cancer Agency, 2013). Almost 80% of British

Columbia women aged 20 to 69 had a Pap test in a recent three-year period (BC Cancer Agency, 2013). Some groups—for example, Indigenous women, immigrants, and women with very low socioeconomic status—are less likely to have Pap tests (CBC, 2013). In Australia, the number of Indigenous women who have Pap tests is about half the national average (Binns & Condon, 2006). In the USA, poor women have higher rates of cervical cancer, perhaps because they have less access to quality health care that includes regular Pap tests (American Cancer Society, 2013a).

The Canadian Task Force on Preventive Health Care (2013) reports that Pap tests

> reduced mortality and morbidity among women aged 30–69 years; the task force strongly recommends screening for women in this age group at 3-year intervals ... Pap tests may have a small effect in reducing mortality and morbidity associated with cervical cancer among women aged 25–29 years; however, among women less than 25 years of age, we found no benefit to outweigh the potential harms. Screening may stop in women aged 70 years and older after 3 successive negative Pap test results.

3.6 Skin cancer

Skin cancer is common. The most common form of skin cancer (basal cell carcinoma) is highly treatable. About one of every 1,000 people with this type of cancer die from it, which is a mortality rate of 0.1% (IQWiG, 2011). Basal cell carcinomas almost never spread. These skin cancer lesions grow slowly, are usually painless, and may not look that different from your normal skin. There may be a bump that is pearly or waxy, white, light pink, flesh-coloured, or brown (Berman, 2011).

The most dangerous form of skin cancer is **malignant melanoma**, with a five-year mortality rate of 15% in men and 10% in women. Both incidence rate and mortality rate are rising in Canada (Grant, 2014). Experts generally attribute this to increased exposure to solar radiation but are uncertain whether the root cause is behavioural (people being less careful to protect themselves, e.g., with sunscreen) or environmental (because the protective ozone layer of the atmosphere is deteriorating).

Be on the lookout for changes in moles or freckles. Watch for any change in shape, darkening, tenderness, pain, itching, or bleeding. See your physician if you notice anything unusual. Use the A-B-C-D-E approach to help detect melanomas early (IQWiG, 2011):

Asymmetry	asymmetrical shape, rather than round or oval
Border	irregular border
Colour	colour change, maybe to white, blue, or red
Diameter	larger than 6 mm (the diameter of a pencil)
Evolving	changes shape, size, or colour, becomes raised, bleeds, grows wet, itches, and/or forms a scab or crust

Considerable attention has centred on the role of suntan studios in skin cancer. The lamps used in suntan booths expose the subject to UV light, and UV light increases risk of skin cancer. UV radiation also accelerates the aging of the skin by breaking down connective tissue fibres that give the skin its normal elasticity. In a 2014 Canadian survey, 4.5% of respondents over age 12 reported using tanning beds, the equivalent of 1.35 million Canadians. Seventy percent of the users were female, with half of these younger than age 35 (Qutob et al., 2017). By 2016, all 10 of Canada's provinces had passed laws that banned tanning beds for minors (Chai, 2017).

> What is *your* relationship to the sun?
> a) Do you like lying in the sun? Playing outdoors on sunny days?
> b) Do you use sun protection (hat, shirt, sunglasses, sunscreen)?
> c) Do you prefer shade to sun when you are outside?
> d) Do you want your skin to be dark or light
> e) Do you go to tanning salons?

4 Treating Cancer

Cancer treatment depends largely on when the cancer is discovered—early in its development or later. Current treatments include the following:

- **Surgical removal:** Localized cancers can be removed surgically. The surgeon tries to cut out the entire tumour and sometimes the adjacent lymph nodes as well, to reduce the possibility of metastatic transfer of the cancer to other body sites. For example, small breast lumps can be removed while preserving the rest of the breast tissue. Surgery for larger, more advanced tumours may remove an entire breast, or the breast plus the lymph nodes under that armpit.
- **Radiation therapy:** This is another approach to localized cancer. Radiation beams are focused on the tumour from several directions, causing a much higher dose of ionizing radiation at the tumour that at the various layers of healthy tissue through which the beams pass. The radiation kills the cancer cells by damaging their DNA.

- **Chemotherapy:** This is an option when the cancer may have spread. Traditional chemotherapy works by killing cells that divide rapidly. This affects not just cancer cells but also normal cells that divide rapidly, such as those in the skin and the lining of the gastrointestinal tract (stomach, intestines, etc.). For this reason, chemotherapy often causes hair loss, nausea, and fatigue in those undergoing treatment. Molecular targeted therapy is a different chemotherapy approach, based on interfering with specific molecules on cancer cells that are different than normal cells, rather than interfering with all rapidly dividing cells.
- **Hormone therapy:** This works for cancers in which hormones help the cancer grow, such as breast cancer and prostate cancer. For example, therapeutic drugs aim to either block the estrogen receptor or lower the woman's estrogen level (American Cancer Society, 2014).
- **Photodynamic therapy:** This starts with injection of a drug that makes cells sensitive to light. Cancer cells absorb the drug over a couple of days. Then the practitioner shines a laser beam at the tumour, killing the sensitized cells.
- **Immunotherapy:** This helps the body's immune system fight cancer. The microenvironment around tumours contains many suppressor cells that interfere with the activation and proliferation of another type of immune-system cell (T-cells) that attacks tumours. Scientists have recently identified a molecule that exists on the surface of the suppressor cells but not on other immune-system cell types. This discovery should allow scientists to make an antibody that will bind to and get rid of the suppressor cells (Sciencedaily.com, 2014).
- **Gene therapy:** This is an experimental treatment that may replace chemotherapy. Gene therapy uses genetic material to modify cells. For example, introducing tumour suppressor genes into rapidly dividing cells may slow or stop tumour growth. In future human clinical application, a simple blood or tissue sample might identify which cancer-causing genetic mutation(s) a patient has. Then the oncologist (cancer doctor) would prescribe specific pills to target those mutations. This targeted treatment would be less toxic than traditional chemotherapy, causing less damage to the body's healthy cells and fewer side effects (Diaz, 2014). Targeted gene therapy may also change the language of cancer. Instead of categorizing cancers by site (lung, breast, liver, etc.), they would be grouped by the specific mutation involved, as often the same mutation produces cancers at diverse body sites (Diaz, 2014).

5 Preventing Cancer

According to the Canadian Cancer Society (2013a), about half of cancers can be prevented. *Primary prevention* attempts to prevent cancer from starting by modifying an individual's lifestyle. Although the exact cause and mechanisms of cancer are not known, a risk factor approach is useful. It is estimated that 80% of all cancers are *environmentally* caused, if one includes diet, smoking, voluntary exposure to radiation, and so on together with other environmental factors, such as unintentional exposure to carcinogens in air and water. Following are some examples of primary prevention:

- **Don't use tobacco products.** This includes cigarettes, cigars, pipes, and chewing tobacco.
- **Decrease exposure to ultraviolet light.** Avoid indoor tanning. Minimize time spent in the sun, especially from 10:00 a.m. to 3:00 p.m., when the sun's rays are most intense. Wear a shirt, a broad-brimmed hat, and sunglasses. Use sunscreens with a sun protection factor (SPF) of at least 15 (Centers for Disease Control and Prevention, 2014a). Apply sunscreen 20 minutes before going out into the sun. Be sure to use a sufficient quantity; an average-sized adult in a bathing suit should use one ounce per application, repeated every two hours, or more frequently if you are swimming or perspiring heavily (United States Environmental Protection Agency, 2006). Some facial cosmetics contain sunscreens. Sun protection is especially important in children and young adults, as a significant percent of lifetime exposure occurs before age 18. Be aware that certain medications (including some antibiotics, birth control pills, diuretics, antihistamines, and antidepressants) increase the skin's sensitivity to the sun's rays.
- **Minimize exposure to X-rays.** This is not really a concern to the general public, as the dosages used in medical and dental X-rays are very low. This recommendation is aimed more at medical or dental professionals, uranium miners, and nuclear power plant workers, who receive occupational exposure to X-radiation.
- **Minimize exposure to environmental carcinogens.** At work, ask your health and safety representative for information. Read the material safety data sheets (MSDS) that the law requires to be provided for any chemical used in the workplace. Get involved with an environmental group to learn more about carcinogens in your local air and water.
- **Reduce the amount of fat you eat.** High-fat diets have been associated with cancers of the colon, rectum, breast, prostate, and uterus.

- **Eat more fibre.** This appears to lower risk of colorectal and perhaps stomach cancer. Fruits, vegetables, and whole grains are good sources of fibre.
- **Get sufficient beta-carotene (a precursor of vitamin A) and vitamin C.** This may lower risk of certain types of cancer, including those of the mouth, esophagus, and stomach. Beta-carotene is found in yellow and dark green vegetables, including cantaloupes, carrots, broccoli, mangoes, spinach, sweet potatoes, and squash. Rich sources of vitamin C include citrus fruits and juices (and other juices which have vitamin C added; read the label), strawberries, and green or red peppers. In addition, there appears to be a substance in vegetables of the cabbage family that reduces risk of colon cancer. This includes cabbage, broccoli, cauliflower, Brussels sprouts, rutabagas, and turnips.
- **Avoid smoked, barbecued, and salted foods.** These types of foods increase risk of stomach cancer. A potent carcinogen forms when fat drips onto hot coals or rocks. Smoke or flare-ups can carry this carcinogen back up and deposit it on the meat. Smoked meats such as ham, bacon, sausage, hot dogs, and luncheon meat contain carcinogenic **nitrites** and **nitrates**. Salt can initiate the cancer process by irritating cells lining the digestive tract. It is safer to bake, roast, broil, stew, poach, or microwave foods.
- **Don't eat mouldy peanuts.** This includes peanut butter, seeds, and corn. The mould on these foods contains powerful carcinogens.
- **If you drink alcohol, limit it to two or fewer drinks per day.** This is especially true if you also use tobacco products. Alcohol increases risk of liver cancer, and in combination with carcinogens in tobacco, it increases susceptibility to cancers of the mouth, larynx, esophagus, and upper respiratory tract.
- **Watch your weight.** Keep it close to ideal.
- *Secondary prevention* is also useful. **Get recommended checkups and do self-examinations.** This is not as simple as a complete yearly physical examination. Rather, specific risk groups should be screened at appropriate intervals with tests for specific types of cancer. The Additional Resources section near the end of this chapter gives contact information for the BC Cancer Control Agency and the Canadian Cancer Society, where you can obtain recommendation for what checkups to get when, and other information about cancer.

> Look over the preceding list of 12 prevention points.
> How many of these are things that you already do?

6 Conclusion

Many people fear cancer. A measure of healthy respect for cancer is certainly reasonable, but fear of cancer causes some people to deny early symptoms of the disease and delay seeking medical attention. Sometimes days can make the difference between life and death. Some types of cancer can now be treated quite successfully, especially if detected early. Very active research is beginning to unravel the mechanisms of cancer, and it may be possible in the future to cure or prevent cancer. In the meantime, a number of risk factors for cancer have been identified, and many of these can be reduced by practising good health habits, and through concerted political and economic action to reduce our exposure to carcinogens in our air, water, and food.

Study Questions

1.   What is cancer?
2.   In general terms, what causes cancer?
3.   For what type of cancer is mortality highest in Canada?
4.   What lifestyle factor contributes the most to premature mortality from cancer?
5.   What is the difference between a benign tumour and a malignant one?
6.   Discuss each of the following types of cancer. For each, outline risk factors and methods of early detection.
     - Lung
     - Breast
     - Prostate
     - Colon/rectal
     - Cervical
     - Skin
7.   What is the difference between primary and secondary prevention?
8.   Explain the multi-stage screening approach to cancer detection. Why is this approach better than, say, giving women breast biopsies every year?
9a. What does the Canadian Cancer Society say about screening mammography for normal-risk women aged 40 to 49?
9b. Explain why experts do *not* recommend screening mammography for young females (e.g., under age 40).
10. Compare screening for breast cancer with that for prostate cancer.
11. Briefly describe the main treatments for cancer.
12. Describe the things a person can do to decrease the risk of dying from cancer. Refer to specific cancers in your answer.

Glossary

benign tumours—tumours that are composed of cells similar to the surrounding cells and that are enclosed in a capsule that prevents them from spreading to other parts of the body

cancer—the uncontrolled division and growth of cells that spreads to other parts of the body

carcinogens—cancer-causing agents

cervix—the outer portion of the uterus, where it meets the vagina

latent period—the incubation period for a disease, or the period between initial exposure to the disease-causing agent and the development of signs or symptoms of the disease

malignant tumours—tumours that metastasize, or spread from the site where they originate to another place in the body

mammography—an imaging technique for the breast that uses low-dose X-rays

metastasis—the spread of a disease (such as cancer) from the place where it originates to another place in the body

metastasize—the verb form of *metastasis*

multi-stage screening—a technique that is applied to apparently healthy populations. (Note: screening ≠ testing.) It starts with simple, inexpensive, less invasive tests. People with positive findings on these screens are given further screening, with more expensive, sophisticated, and invasive tests.

mutation—the act or process of being altered or changed

Pap test—a test that involves inspection of a sample of cells from the cervix to look for evidence of cancer

potential years of life lost—a number that is equal to life expectance minus age at death

primary prevention—preventing a disease from occurring, for example, by vaccination for infectious diseases or by modification of risk factors for diseases such as cancer

screening—examining an apparently healthy population for disease or risk factors for disease

secondary prevention—early detection and treatment of a disease

testing—examining a population with known or suspected disease

tumour—a mass of cells

Additional Resources

BC Cancer Control Agency

www.bccancer.bc.ca

Click on the tab "Patient/Public Info" to view links to *prevention* and *screening programs.*

Canadian Cancer Society
  http://www.cancer.ca/
John Hopkins Medicine Health Library
  Illustrated instructions for breast self-examination are available at http://
  www.hopkinsmedicine.org/healthlibrary/conditions/breast_health/how_
  to_perform_a_breast_self-examination_bse_85,P00135/
Screening Mammography Program of British Columbia
  Offers free mammograms for all women aged 40 to 79. Contact (604) 877-
  6187 in the Lower Mainland or 1 (800) 663-9203 for information or an appointment. More information (and an email link) is available at http://www.
  smpbc.ca/default.htm

References

American Cancer Society. (March 21, 2012). *What is cancer?* Retrieved April 14, 2014
  from http://www.cancer.org/cancer/cancerbasics/what-is-cancer

American Cancer Society. (2013a; April 24, 2013). *Cervical cancer overview.* Retrieved
  April 27, 2013 from http://www.cancer.org/cancer/cervicalcancer/overviewguide/
  cervical-cancer-overview-what-causes

American Cancer Society. (2013b; August 26, 2013). *What are the key statistics about
  prostate cancer?* Retrieved April 14, 2014 from http://www.cancer.org/cancer/pros-
  tatecancer/detailedguide/prostate-cancer-key-statistics

American Cancer Society. (January 31, 2014). *Hormone therapy for breast cancer.* Retrieved May 31, 2014 http://www.cancer.org/cancer/breastcancer/detailedguide/
  breast-cancer-treating-hormone-therapy

American Cancer Society. (2016). Can lung cancer be found early? Retrieved May 1, 2018
  from https://www.cancer.org/cancer/lung-cancer/prevention-and-early-detection/
  early-detection.html

American Cancer Society. (2017). American Cancer Society Guidelines for the Early
  Detection of Cancer. Retrieved May 1, 2018 from https://www.cancer.org/healthy/
  find-cancer-early/cancer-screening-guidelines/american-cancer-society-guidelines-
  for-the-early-detection-of-cancer.html

American College of Obstetrics and Gynecology. (July 20, 2011). *Annual mammograms
  now recommended for women beginning at age 40.* Retrieved June 8, 2014http://
  www.acog.org/About_ACOG/News_Room/News_Releases/2011/Annual_Mam-
  mograms_Now_Recommended_for_Women_Beginning_at_Age_40

BC Cancer Agency. (2013). *Cervical cancer screening program.* Retrieved April 14, 2014.
  http://www.bccancer.bc.ca/PPI/Screening/Cervical/default.htm

BC Cancer Agency. (2018). Who should get a mammogram? Retrieved May 1, 2018 from
  http://www.bccancer.bc.ca/screening/breast/get-a-mammogram/who-should-get-
  a-mammogram

Berman, K. (July 26, 2011). Basal cell carcinoma. *MedLine Plus.* Retrieved April 14, 2014
  from https://www.nlm.nih.gov/medlineplus/ency/article/000824.htm

Binns, P. L., Condon, J. R. (2006). Participation in cervical screening by Indigenous
  women in the Northern Territory: A longitudinal study. *Medical Journal of Australia.* 185(9), 490–494.

Breastcancer.org. (November 21, 2011). *Canadian task force changes breast cancer screening recommendations.* Retrieved June 8, 2014 from http://www.breastcancer.org/research-news/20111121

Canadian Cancer Society. (2013a). *Canadian cancer death rate down.* Retrieved January 15, 2013 from http://www.cancer.ca/Canada-wide/About%20us/Media%20centre/CW-Media%20releases/CW-2012/Canadian%20Cancer%20Statistics%202012.aspx

Canadian Cancer Society. (2014b). *Screening for colorectal cancer.* Retrieved April 14, 2014 from http://www.cancer.ca/en/prevention-and-screening/early-detection-and-screening/screening/screening-for-colorectal-cancer/?region=sk

Canadian Cancer Society. (2017). *Canadian Cancer Statistics 2017.* Toronto, Ontario: Canadian Cancer Society. ISBN 0835-2976.

Canadian Cancer Society. (2018). Screening for breast cancer. Retrieved May 1, 2018 from http://www.cancer.ca/en/cancer-information/cancer-type/breast/screening/?region=on

Canadian Cancer Society Steering Committee on Cancer Statistics. (2012). *Canadian Cancer Statistics 2012.* Toronto, ON: Canadian Cancer Society.

Canadian Task Force on Preventive Health Care. (January 7, 2013). Recommendations on screening for cervical cancer. *Canadian Medical Association Journal.* 185(1).

CBC News Staff. (January 7, 2013). Stop Pap tests in women under 25, Canadian panel advises. *CBC News.* Retrieved April 14, 2014 from http://www.cbc.ca/news/health/stop-pap-tests-in-women-under-25-canadian-panel-advises-1.1306763

Centers for Disease Control. (October 31, 2013). *What screening tests are there [for breast cancer]?* Retrieved June 8, 2014 from http://www.cdc.gov/cancer/breast/basic_info/screening.htm

Centers for Disease Control and Prevention. (2014a; January 22, 2014). *Skin cancer.* Retrieved April 14, 2014 http://www.cdc.gov/cancer/skin/basic_info/prevention.htm

Centers for Disease Control and Prevention. (2014b; February 26, 2014). *Colorectal (colon) cancer.* Retrieved April 14, 2014 from http://www.cdc.gov/cancer/colorectal/basic_info/screening/

Chai C. (January 19, 2017). Here's the No. 1 reason why 1.35M Canadians are still using tanning beds. *Global News.* Retrieved May 10, 2018 from https://globalnews.ca/news/3192162/heres-the-no-1-reason-why-1-35m-canadians-are-still-using-tanning-beds/

Diaz, M. (March 4, 2014). Gene therapy: Cancer treatment revolution. *Newsmax Health.* Retrieved June 15, 2014 from http://www.newsmaxhealth.com/Headline/cancer-treatment-IV-chemotherapy/2014/03/04/id/555871/

Grant, K. (May 28, 2014). Skin cancer is on the rise. *The Globe and Mail.* pp. A6 & A7.

Health Canada. (2012). Canadian Tobacco Use Monitoring Survey 2012. Retrieved May 1, 2018 from https://www.canada.ca/en/health-canada/services/publications/healthy-living/canadian-tobacco-use-monitoring-survey-ctums-2012.html

IQWiG (Institute for Quality and Efficiency in Health Care). (August 4, 2011). *Fact sheet: Preventing and detecting skin cancer.* Retrieved April 14, 2014 from ttps://www.ncbi.nlm.nih.gov/pubmedhealth/PMH0014907/

John Hopkins Health Alerts. (April 11, 2012). Does regular exercise reduce the risk of colon cancer? Retrieved April 14, 2014 from http://www.johnshopkinshealthalerts.com/alerts/colon_cancer/exercise-colon-cancer_6153-1.html

John Hopkins Medicine. (2014). *Colorectal cancer: From polyp to cancer.* Retrieved April 14, 2014 from http://www.hopkinscoloncancercenter.org/CMS/CMS_Page.aspx?CurrentUDV=59&CMS_Page_ID=0B34E9BE-5DE6-4CB4-B387-4158CC924084

Mayo Clinic Staff. (August 13, 2013). *Prostate cancer risk factors.* Retrieved April 14, 2014 from http://www.mayoclinic.org/diseases-conditions/prostate-cancer/basics/risk-factors/con-20029597

Miller, A. B., Wall, C., Baines, C. J., Sun, P., To, T., Narod, S. A. (2014). Twenty five year follow-up for breast cancer incidence and mortality of the Canadian National Breast Screening Study: randomised screening trial. *British Medical Journal*, 348, 366–375.

Moyer, V. A. (2013). Menopausal hormone therapy for the primary prevention of chronic conditions: US Preventive Services Task Force Recommendation Statement. *Annals of Internal Medicine.* 158(1), 47–54.

National Cancer Institute. (October 15, 2010). *Estrogen receptors/SERMs.* Retrieved April 14, 2014 from http://www.cancer.gov/cancertopics/understandingcancer/estrogenreceptors

National Cancer Institute. (2012a). *Lung cancer screening.* Retrieved January 30, 2013 from http://www.cancer.gov/cancertopics/pdq/screening/lung/Patient/page3

National Cancer Institute. (2012b). *HPV and cancer.* Retrieved February 11, 2013 from http://www.cancer.gov/cancertopics/factsheet/Risk/HPV

National Cancer Institute. (2012c; March 21, 2012). *Oral contraceptives and cancer risk.* Retrieved April 14, 2014 from http://www.cancer.gov/cancertopics/factsheet/Risk/oral-contraceptives

National Cancer Institute. (2012d; July 24, 2012). Prostate-specific antigen (PSA) test. Retrieved April 14, 2014 from http://www.cancer.gov/cancertopics/factsheet/detection/PSA

Press Association. (March 20, 2014). Active women can reduce risk of breast cancer by 12%, say researchers. *The Guardian.* Retrieved April 14, 2014 from http://www.theguardian.com/society/2014/mar/20/active-women-reduce-risk-breast-cancer-12-per-cent-research

Qutob, S. S., O'Brien, M., Feder, K., McNamee, J., Guay, M., Than, J. (2017). Tanning equipment use: 2014 Canadian Community Health Survey. Statistics Canada. Retrieved May 10, 2018 from http://www.statcan.gc.ca/pub/82-003-x/2017001/article/14696-eng.pdf

Sciencedaily.com. (May 25, 2014). Cancer immunotherapy: Potential new target found. Retrieved May 31, 2014 from http://www.sciencedaily.com/releases/2014/05/140525154726.htm

Statistics Canada. (2012). *Leading causes of death in Canada, 2009.* Retrieved January 15, 2013 from http://www.statcan.gc.ca/pub/84-215-x/2012001/int-eng.htm

Statistics Canada. (2017). *The 10 leading causes of death, 2013.* Retrieved May 1, 2018 from https://www.statcan.gc.ca/pub/82-625-x/2017001/article/14776-eng.htm

United States Environmental Protection Agency. (September 2006). *Sunscreen: The burning facts.* EPA 430-F-06-13. Retrieved April 15, 2014 from http://www2.epa.gov/sites/production/files/documents/sunscreen.pdf

6 Physical Activity

Learning Objectives

By the time you have finished this chapter you should be able to

- Differentiate between "fitness," "exercise," and "activity"
- List the components of health-related and performance-related fitness
- Describe the health benefits and risks of physical activity
- Discuss the type of evidence for these benefits and risks
- Explain how to develop aerobic fitness, muscle strength and endurance, and flexibility

1 Overview

Contemporary Canadian society is quite sedentary. Motor vehicles predominate as modes of transportation. The average household has many labour-saving appliances, such as electric vacuum cleaners, automatic washing machines, and coffee grinders. We spend a lot of "screen time," that is, time on computers, smart phones, and similar devices.

- One source estimates that Canadian children spend an average of *7.5 hours a day* in front of screens (Jones, 2015). The picture in the USA seems similar: 7.2 hours of screen time daily for 8- to 18-year-olds (Campaign for a Commercial-Free Childhood). By contrast, the Canadian Society for Exercise Physiology recommends for those age 5 to 17 no more than 2 hours per day of recreational screen time (CSEP, 2018).

- Several separate surveys give estimates of North American adults' average screen time that range from *31 to 40 hours per week* (Marlow, 2010; *CBC News,* 2012; Thompson, 2012).

> How much screen time do *you* get in a week?
> It may be easier to think about per day, and then multiply by seven.

2 Physical Activity of North Americans

The Canadian Society for Exercise Physiology recommends for those 18 years and older at least 150 minutes of moderate- to vigorous-intensity aerobic physical activity per week, in bouts of 10 minutes or more. The Society also recommends at least two days per week of muscle- and bone-strengthening activities using major muscle groups (CSEP, 2018).

Many North Americans are not meeting these recommended minimum levels of activity. Statistics Canada (2016) reports that 54% of Canadians age 12 and above get *some* leisure time physical activity. These self-reports of activity are highest among those age 12 to 19 (70%) and decline progressively with increasing age. In the USA, only 30% of high school students get at least 60 minutes of physical activity daily. Only 21% of American adults get the recommended weekly 150 minutes of moderate-intensity aerobic activity and two muscle-strengthening sessions (CDC, 2014).

Furthermore, self-reports of activity may be inaccurate. As part of the 2007 to 2009 Canadian Health Measures Survey, a sample of Canadians aged 20 to 79 were asked to wear an **accelerometer,**[1] a device that measures body movements. The information from those subjects who produced "valid data" (by wearing the accelerometer for at least 10 hours a day for at least four of the seven days) showed that only *15%* (17% of men and 14% of women) met the exercise recommendation (that is, accumulated 150 minutes per week of moderate to vigorous physical activity in 10-minute bouts). *Only 5%* accumulated 150 minutes on a regular basis—at least 30 minutes on at least five days a week. The researchers concluded that, "The CHMS accelerometry data indicate that Canadians are less active than self-reported estimates suggest" (Colley et al., 2011, p. 6).

Inactivity habits start early in life. Two Statistics Canada reports based on accelerometer measures of activity indicate that only 24% of 3- and 4-year-olds and only 30% of 5-year-olds get an hour or more of daily moderate to vigorous physical activity. Boys are, on average, more active than girls. In addition, "children of lower-income families were significantly less likely to meet the activity targets for their age group" (Canadian Press, 2016).

---

1   An accelerometer is a small device that responds to movement. The commercially available Fitbit and similar products use accelerometers to track movement.

Do *you* get 30 minutes of moderate to vigorous activity at least five days a week?

    If not, what are the main barriers for you?

    Time is a barrier a lot of people mention. Reflect back on your thoughts from the previous page. You spend how much screen time, but you don't have enough time for a little physical activity? What do you think this says?

It is becoming clear that **prolonged sitting** is an independent health risk factor. That is, even if you get more than the minimum recommended amount of physical activity in a day, if you sit for much of the rest of the day, your risk of disease and death increase (Whiteman, 2016). So, activity guidelines now include the recommendation of "limited sitting for extended periods" (CSEP, 2018). A recent epidemiological study showed lowest mortality rates among those whose sitting periods lasted 30 minutes or less (Diaz et al., 2017). This suggests that rising from the seated position every 30 minutes and moving around a bit could help reduce the health risks associated with prolonged sitting.

3 Activity, Exercise, and Fitness

The terms "activity," "exercise," and "fitness" are often used interchangeably. However, they have different meanings.

- Physical *fitness* is a *capacity*. It is the extent to which the body can respond to the demands of physical effort. Fitness can be measured; for example, you can note how far you can run in a given time or how many times you can lift a certain weight.
- *Exercise* is the *process* of planned, structured, and repetitive physical activity done to maintain or improve one or more component of physical fitness. Many activities can be considered exercise if they are part of a plan and are appropriate for the intended goal.
- *Activity* is any voluntary movement that expends calories. Running on the treadmill and lifting weights are activity. Walking to work or school is also activity. So is raking leaves, washing the car, playing Frisbee, walking the dog, dancing in a club, shooting baskets, or rollerblading.

If you think about activity as something broader than exercise, does the amount of moderate to vigorous activity you get in a week increase?

    If so, what do you think this says about messaging around the promotion of physical activity to the general Canadian public?

- **Health** is something else, something that probably includes physical fitness, activity, and exercise, but also much more.

> What do you remember about health from Chapter 1: The Concept of Health?

4 Components of Physical Fitness

Health-related fitness is usually viewed as having four components (Figure 6.1):

- Cardiorespiratory fitness (also known as aerobic fitness or sometimes just endurance)
- Muscular strength and endurance
- Flexibility
- Body weight and composition

We will discuss the first three components in this chapter. The fourth is covered in a separate chapter.

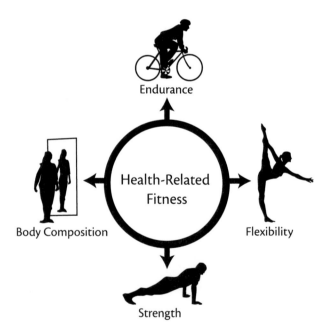

Figure 6.1. The four components of health-related fitness. Some writers show "muscular strength" and "muscular endurance" as separate components.

Performance-related fitness has additional elements, including speed and power, agility, and anaerobic power and capacity. These elements are important for high performance in sports, and in some very physically demanding jobs, but are not related to conventional health measures such as longevity or vitality.

5 Benefits of Exercise

Aerobic fitness is arguably the most important health-related component. Aerobic fitness comes from rhythmic, sustained movements of large muscle groups. Such activity elevates heart rate, breathing rate, metabolic rate, and body temperature. Cycling, running, hiking, swimming, skating, swimming, basketball, tennis, soccer, calisthenics, and some types of dancing are all examples of aerobic activities (Figure 6.2).

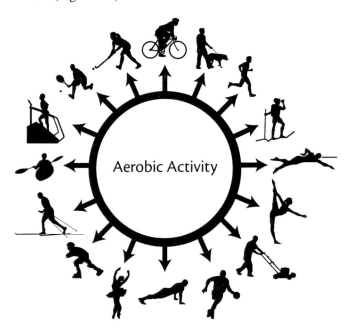

Figure 6.2. Some of the many forms of aerobic activity.

Can you improve your vital organs with exercise?

Yes, definitely. One of the basic truths of biological science is that organisms adapt (within limits) to the demands placed on them.

Regular physical activity and exercise are associated with decreased risk of developing coronary heart disease, stroke, Type II diabetes, and some forms of cancer (e.g., colon, breast). Activity and exercise are also associated with delayed all-cause mortality and increased cognitive function, energy, and feelings of well-being (Garber et al., 2011, pp. 1335 and 1337).

> What kind of evidence is this? (See Chapter 2: Evaluating Health Claims.)

Exercise and physical activity can

- Reduce blood pressure
- Improve lipoprotein profile (see Chapter 4: Cardiovascular Disease and Diabetes)
- Increase cellular sensitivity to insulin (see Chapter 4)
- Prevent and improve mild to moderate depressive disorders and anxiety
- Improve bone mass, muscle strength, and body composition, and reduce risk of falling (Garber et al., 2011, pp. 1335, 1337, and 1342).

How long will you live if you never exercise?

It is not possible to predict the lifespan of any *individual*. However, *population* data show that, in general, people who are less physically active die younger. A National Institutes of Health study (NIH, 2012) analyzed self-reports of health, weight, and physical activity levels for over 650,000 people (most of them over age 40). The report concluded that those who reported 2.5 hours of moderate-intensity activity per week lived, on average, 4.5 years longer than those who reported no physical activity—regardless of their body weight.

The combination of 2.5 hours of moderate-intensity weekly activity and normal body weight was associated with a 7.2-year increase in life expectancy (NIH, 2012).

Resistance training increases the thickness, density, and strength of muscle, bone, tendon, and ligament tissue. This allows muscles to generate more tension, and makes all of these tissues more resistant to injury. Musculoskeletal fitness improves the ability to perform activities of daily living with ease, grace, and safety. Improved musculoskeletal fitness increases **mobility** and **functional independence**, especially in older adults. Increased muscular endurance may reduce incidence of falls and the associated injuries and illness.

Weight-bearing or resistance training exercises increase the density and strength of bones. As such, they are important in the prevention and treatment of *osteoporosis*, a condition in which bones lose mineral content and become more vulnerable to fracture. Osteoporosis is especially common in post-menopausal women. A relatively minor accident, such as tripping on an electrical cord or carpet and falling to the floor, can fracture the thigh bone at the hip.

Increased muscle size and tone are, for many people, related to improved **self-image**. This is a tricky issue. Improved self-image, self-confidence, and self-efficacy (the belief you can take charge of your life and effect change) are important determinants to effecting positive health behaviours. However, the strong emphasis contemporary society places on appearance (young, slim, muscular, fit, beautiful) causes other problems. One such problem is misuse of **anabolic steroids**, hormones that enhance the body's ability to build muscle. Steroid use by athletes seeking a competitive advantage is a well-recognized issue. It is even more distressing to see the increase in steroid use by youths whose motivations are "to get big," "to look better," or "to be more popular."

What about *you*?
What are the reasons you spend time being physically active?

---

6 Nature of the Evidence

Many **epidemiological studies** have shown that exercise, occupational activity, or recreational activity is associated with lower cardiovascular disease incidence and mortality. The Framingham Heart Study was one such study (see Chapter 2: Evaluating Health Claims and Chapter 4: Cardiovascular Disease and Diabetes). A classical epidemiological study found that drivers of double-decker buses in London, England, had higher heart disease rates than the conductors on the same buses (Morris et al., 1953), purportedly because the drivers sat all day, while the conductors walked around both levels of the bus checking riders' tickets. One problem with epidemiological studies is that the *association* between activity and disease does not prove the activity protects against disease. For example, maybe the London bus drivers had more heart disease than the conductors because driving is stressful rather than because of the occupational walking done by the conductors.

Health effects of moderate activity have also been shown **experimentally;** that is, subjects who increased their activity showed decreases in blood pressure, improved blood lipids, and so on. In research studies, both activity and exercise are usually **self-reported,** often *retrospectively;* that is, subjects are asked to say how much exercise they did in the past week, month, or year. Retrospective data are relatively easy to collect and can be obtained with a single interview. But there are two problems with the accuracy of this kind of data. The first problem is **honesty**. Surprisingly, even in confidential or anonymous studies, inactive people exaggerate the amount of exercise they do. Maybe they feel guilty and this is a way of helping them feel better about themselves.

The second problem is **memory**. Participants in retrospective studies may not remember accurately, especially events that happened some time ago. The memory problem is largely solved with a *prospective* design—that is, by giving people a diary at the start of the study and asking them to record what exercise or activity they do each day. Researchers may have to wait years for the effects to unfold before they can analyze the results. Despite this barrier, some prospective studies of the effects of physical activity on mortality have been successfully completed and published.

Sluik et al. (2012) followed a cohort of almost 6,000 people with diabetes mellitus for a median period of 9.4 years. During this period, 755 of the participants died. Those who were moderately active had the lowest mortality risk (only 62% as likely to die as those who were physically inactive).

Ruiz et al. (2008) measured fitness in a cohort of almost 9,000 men enrolled in a famous fitness centre in Dallas, Texas. Over an average of 18.9 years follow-up, 503 men in the cohort died. The study suggested muscular strength and cardiorespiratory fitness had favourable and independent effects on mortality risk; the death rate in those with high levels of both muscular and cardiorespiratory fitness was 60% lower than in the group with the lowest levels of both fitness components.

7 Risks of Exercise/Physical Activity

With all the talk about the benefits of exercise, the risks of exercise are often overlooked. The most common health risk associated with exercise is injuries, usually to the musculoskeletal system. **Traumatic injuries**, such as a sprained ankle or a fractured arm, happen suddenly. **Overuse injuries**, such as shin splints, tennis elbow, and runner's knee, develop over weeks as a result of accumulated strain. Overuse injuries are rarely life threatening. They are usually caused by increasing the amount of exercise too drastically, for example, a person who starts playing tennis and immediately plays three hours a week with no pre-season conditioning. Most sports injuries heal on their own within a few days, or perhaps weeks, of rest.

Another common risk associated with exercise is **general overstress**, which can lead to injury or to illness, such as influenza. Although exercise helps many people manage stress, exercise itself is a stressor. I remember a middle-aged man who approached me for advice regarding training for a marathon race. He was a busy corporate executive, working toward his MBA degree at night school, coaching the soccer team of one of his teenage children, and considering adding five to 10 hours of running per week to his schedule. This person was clearly over-committed already, and an exercise program might have pushed him over the edge.

Another risk of exercise is **temperature injury**, either from being too hot or too cold. Prolonged exercise can cause dehydration as a result of sweat loss, which can result in heat exhaustion or heat stroke. On the other hand, exercise in cool, damp, or windy conditions can result in **hypothermia**, or excess loss of body heat. Overheating and overcooling are both potentially fatal.

There are a number of more serious, but fortunately rare, medical risks associated with exercise for some people. Unaccustomed vigorous exercise can trigger "cardiovascular events" such as heart attack and sudden death, especially in people with coronary heart disease or when exercising with extra environmental stressors such as high environmental temperatures (Garber et al., 2011, p. 1348). Warning signs and symptoms, such as chest pain or shortness of breath, may or may not precede such exercise-induced events. Sometimes individuals miss or ignore these warning symptoms. Risks can be reduced if health care practitioners evaluate their patients carefully and educate them about warning signs and symptoms (Garber et al., 2011, p. 1348).

> ### *Can vigorous training at a young age* **shorten** *life span?*

This *can* happen, but it is not typical. Daily physical activity is strongly associated with improved cardiovascular health and positive effects on lifespan. However, there is some evidence that "chronic excessive sustained endurance exercise" can cause adverse structural changes to the heart and the large arteries, or blood vessels (O'Keefe et al. 2012; Patil et al., 2012; note these two papers are published by the same group of authors). These authors are referring to marathons, ultra-marathons, Iron Man triathlons, and very long-distance bicycle racing.

The authors make several qualifying statements:

- The "concept is still hypothetical and there is some inconsistency in the reported findings" (O'Keefe et al., 2012).
- "Not all veteran extreme endurance athletes develop pathological remodeling, and indeed lifelong exercisers generally have low mortality rates and excellent functional capacity" (Patil et al., 2012).
- Their subjects were "veteran athletes," not teens.
- They do not know how many months or years of "excessive" exercise to consider "excessive," or to what extent early damage might be subsequently repaired.

My sense is still that, for most people, the benefits of exercise, including vigorous exercise by teens, greatly outweigh the risks. I will be interested to see what additional information comes out on this topic over the next decade.

Finally, for some people exercise can become a **compulsion**. I had a friend who developed this problem. He worked in an office in a junior management position. After work and on the weekends, he trained to compete in triathlons. He exercised for hours a day, some days swimming, others cycling or running, or a combination of these. Even when it was dark, wet, and cold outside, or when he was tired or didn't feel like exercising, he still kept to his program. If he missed a training session, he felt guilty. One weekend, he and his girlfriend went on vacation. After they unpacked, he went for a four-hour bicycle ride. When he returned, his girlfriend confronted him: "All you do when we're together is exercise, eat, and sleep. You're even too tired most of the time for sex. You've got to choose between me and your stupid triathlon training!" Well, he did choose—he broke up with his girlfriend! A couple of months later, he realized how unhealthy and unbalanced his life had become, and for six months he deliberately did no exercise as a way to cure himself of his "addiction."

8 How to Develop Aerobic Fitness

> *How many minutes a day of exercise do people need to live a healthy lifestyle? How many days a week? What type of exercise?*

The Canadian Society for Exercise Physiology (CSEP; 2018) recommends that adults age 18 and older "should accumulate at least 150 minutes of moderate- to vigorous-intensity aerobic physical activity per week, in bouts of 10 minutes or more."

Aerobic means "with air." This kind of exercise involves large muscle groups, used in a rhythmic and sustained fashion. The energy for such activity derives mainly from stored fats and carbohydrates in combination with oxygen. The lungs draw in air. In the lung, oxygen moves into the blood. The heart pumps the oxygenated blood out to all tissues, including muscles. Muscles take up and use the oxygen (Figure 6.3). Walking, hiking, jogging, and running are all aerobic.

- Sprinting (running very fast) is not aerobic, as it is too high-intensity.

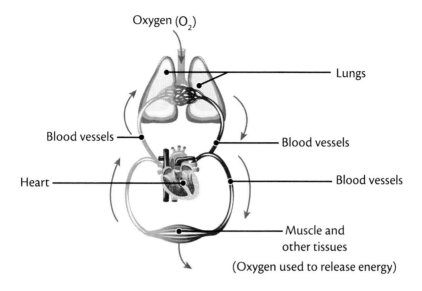

Figure 6.3. A diagrammatic representation of the main elements of the aerobic system.

- Playing cards or billiards uses aerobic energy, but the intensity level of these activities is too low to provide training stimulus.
- Normally, strength training is not aerobic. The intensity is high enough, but the sustained duration is not long enough.
- Resistance training (using weights, pulleys, push-ups, etc.) *can* be done in an aerobic fashion if one moves quickly from one exercise to the next. This is called **circuit weight training** and typically consists of 30 seconds of exercise followed by 30 seconds of moving to the next station and getting ready for it, another 30 seconds of a different exercise, then moving to the next station, and so on. This must be sustained for a period of at least 10 minutes.

Other forms of aerobic exercise include bicycling, swimming, skating, dancing, and many sports, such as soccer, basketball, tennis, badminton, and volleyball. Other team sports, such as baseball, use little aerobic energy because most players (except the pitcher and catcher) are active for only brief periods, separated by long periods of waiting. Meaningful aerobic benefits also occur for most people (probably not those who are already very physically fit) from activities around the home, such as gardening, raking leaves, cutting the lawn (especially with a non-motorized push mower), washing the car, and sweeping or vacuuming floors.

> Can *you* think of other sports that fit this description?

The CSEP recommendations for this age group continue, "It is beneficial to add **muscle and bone strengthening activities** using major muscle groups, at least two days per week," and add, "more physical activity provides greater health benefits."

You should plan on exercising **three to five times per week**, with no more than two days between exercise sessions.

You are more likely to stick with a program if you choose a time of day that **fits your schedule** and **pick activities you enjoy**.

Pick **appropriate exercises**. For example, hockey or football may be appropriate for a young person but are probably inappropriate for older individuals because of the risk of injury. Basketball may be fine for a university student, but 10 years later this same individual may find basketball inappropriate because it is too difficult to organize nine friends for a game. Cycling on the road may be great for the summer, but in the dark, cold, wet days of winter it may be too uncomfortable and dangerous to be appropriate.

Short bouts of exercise can be effective in promoting aerobic fitness, weight loss, HDL cholesterol, and so on—benefits formerly believed to occur only when training sessions were at least 15 to 20 minutes long. The key seems to be to accumulate at least 30 minutes of activity daily.

9 How to Develop Muscular Fitness

> *How do muscles work?*

You have three types of muscle in your body: cardiac muscle (in the heart), smooth muscle (e.g., in the digestive system and airways of the lungs), and skeletal muscle (connecting bones to each other and producing movement). I will take this question as asking about skeletal muscle.

Think of muscles as having three components: signaling, contractile mechanism, and energy supply (Figure 6.4).

- **Signals** start either in the brain, when you "tell" your body to move, or in your spinal cord, for reflex movements. Nerves carry these signals to the appropriate muscles, where a combination of chemicals and electrical impulses "tell" the muscle to contract.

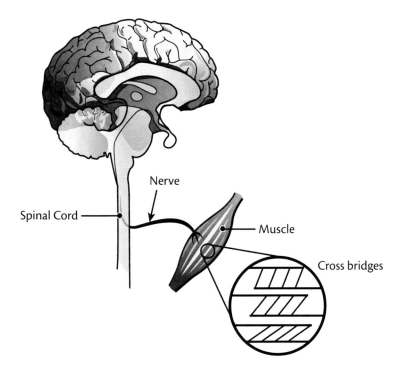

Figure 6.4. Nerve signals activate skeletal muscle, which then generates tension with the formation of cross-bridges between adjacent strands of protein.

- The **contractile** mechanism consists of strands or threads of two kinds of proteins that lie parallel to each other. When signalled to contract, little "bridges" form between the two types of proteins, and then the bridges rotate. This pulls one protein past the other, like an oar pulling a boat forward in the water, and the muscle shortens. The shortening of the muscle causes the bones to rotate at joints, and this produces movement. When the contract signal is over, the cross-bridges go away, and the proteins return to their original position.
- **Energy** is supplied from three sources.
  - *The immediate source* is small molecules stored right in the muscle. These molecules store energy in a chemical bond. When the bond is broken, the energy is released.
  - *The secondary source* is the metabolism (chemical breakdown) of glycogen (a storage form of sugar) and fatty acids (a storage form of fat) that are stored in the muscle. The energy thus provided is used to re-form the high-energy bond in the molecules used as the immediate energy source.

• *The third source* is from the blood. When muscle levels of glycogen and fatty acids drop, these compounds are resupplied via blood flowing through the muscle. Glycogen and fatty acids come from food that is consumed, broken down, absorbed, and metabolized. You will learn more about this in Chapter 7: Nutrition.

Resistance training comes in many forms, including **calisthenics** (e.g., push-ups and sit-ups), tubing, stacks of **weights** connected by cables and pulleys, and free weights (circular metal plates put on the ends of short one-handed dumbbells or longer two-handed bars). Experienced body builders and power lifters tend to prefer free weights. However, there is more risk of injury when handling free weights, so novices may be better advised to use other forms of resistance.

Strive for **balanced strength**, between the right and left sides of the body, between opposing pairs of muscles, and between the upper and lower body. Traditionally, resistance training has focused on the large muscles of the limbs, such as the biceps and triceps (the front and back, respectively, of the upper arm). More recently, the importance of building **core strength**, by working the abdominal, back, and other trunk muscles, has become recognized.

Do at least one exercise for each major muscle group. Sequence the exercises so you train the large muscles first. If you start with the small wrist and forearm muscles, your arms may be too tired to hold the weight for the later exercises. Perform each exercise through the full range of movement.

There is an almost unlimited combination of repetitions and sets of exercises. The basic recommendation is moderate-intensity resistance training, with one set of exercises for major muscle groups (chest, shoulders, back, hips, legs, trunk, and arms) done two to three days per week (Garber et al, 2011, p. 1343). This would take 20 to 30 minutes—longer if the weight room is busy and you have to wait your turn for a piece of equipment, and even longer if you spend a lot of time looking at yourself in the mirror!

Because the muscle rebuilding process takes about 48 hours, strenuous resistance training workouts are usually scheduled with at least one day of rest between them. Alternatively, the serious body builder might exercise her back and shoulders one day, legs and abdominals the next day, chest and arms the third day, and so on.

> What do *you* think about the preceding section?
>   In what ways is this consistent with, and in what ways is it different from, what you have learned about muscular fitness elsewhere?

10 How to Develop Flexibility

There isn't much scientific evidence regarding the benefits of flexibility or the optimal method to develop flexibility. This deficiency is partly due to imprecise use of terms; flexibility, stretching, mobilization, and warm-up are often incorrectly interchanged. ***Flexibility*** refers to the ***range of motion (ROM)*** at a joint. Improved range of motion at joints develops over time due to increased length of the connective tissue part of muscle and the capsules that surround joints. More-flexible joints require less energy to move through their range. In the athlete, good flexibility allows for better technique. For example, flexible shoulders give the golfer a higher back swing, the paddler a longer stroke, and the gymnast a stable hand stand. "No consistent link has been shown between regular flexibility exercise and a reduction of musculotendinous injuries, prevention of low back pain, or DOMS [delayed onset muscular soreness]" (Garber et al., 2011, p. 1344).

Stretching is exercise done to improve flexibility. There are several forms of stretching. The simplest and safest is ***static stretching***, in which the body moves slowly into the stretch and then holds it. Go to the limit of your range of motion, and perhaps a bit further. Try to relax into the stretch. Slow, relaxed breathing helps. Don't strain. You should feel tension, but not pain. Hold for 30 seconds. Repeat with the other side. If you contract the opposing muscle group while maintaining the stretch it helps the muscle being stretched to relax. In the seated toe touch, this would mean contracting your quadriceps muscles to help the hamstrings to relax. A stretching session for 10 or 12 major joints would take about 15 minutes. It should ideally be done daily, or at least every day you do vigorous aerobic or resistance exercise.

Stretching can also be done with bouncing or bobbing motions, but this is a riskier technique than the slow stretch. However, since many sports involve rapid stretching of muscles, it makes sense for athletes to include rapid stretching, too, probably near the end of the warm-up—that is, *after* the static stretching.

Also, it's a good idea to **cool down** gradually after resistance training or aerobic exercise, rather than dashing off to your car or the showers. This is a good time to stretch for the purpose of developing flexibility; muscles lengthen more effectively when they are warm, and holding them in a lengthened position as they cool down optimizes maintenance of this increased length.

Flexibility is the most neglected component of most people's exercise program. Unlike aerobic and resistance training, which produce exertion, perspiration, and fatigue, the effects of stretching are subtle and take a calmer, more patient mind to enjoy. For many people, stretching is like flossing your teeth—there is no inherent pleasure, it's just something to do because it's good for you. Maybe this is part of the "hurry up" syndrome that afflicts modern society. Maybe it's the culture of "no pain, no gain." Nevertheless, if you set aside the time to stretch and adjust your attitude, stretching can be fun.

11 Prevention of Activity-Related Injuries

If you are over 35 years old and have been sedentary for some time, or under 35 but have heart disease, lung disease, or metabolic disease (e.g., diabetes), or major risk factors for such diseases, you should **obtain a medical evaluation** before beginning regular fitness activities.

People with known or suspected disease should exercise under the supervision of an exercise specialist, at least initially, until they learn to pace themselves appropriately. Everyone, with or without disease, should increase activity level gradually over the first several months.

If you are resuming exercise after some time of inactivity because of illness, injury, travel, or another reason, you should not start right back at the same level you were when you stopped. **Fitness is lost at roughly the same rate as it is acquired.** That is, if you have stopped exercising for two weeks, you should start exercising at about the same level you were two weeks before you stopped. If you have been inactive for more than a few weeks, remember to start slowly to allow the muscles and joints time to readapt to the stresses of your activity.

It's a good idea to spend some time (up to 15 minutes for beginners, and as little as five minutes for those who are further along in their fitness program) warming up before running, resistance training, or other strenuous exercise. Start with mild whole body activity, such as brisk walking. Then do gentle movements, such as slow shoulder circles. Then gently stretch the muscles, for example, by clasping your hands together behind your back while standing, straightening your arms, and drawing your shoulders back and down. Work your way through the various joints (going from head to toe may help you remember to include all the major joints). The **warm-up** stimulates joints to secrete a lubricating fluid, improves coordination between the nervous system and musculoskeletal system, decreases stiffness in soft tissue, and readies the metabolism for harder work. The **mobilization** exercises, such as the shoulder circles, increase blood and nutrient supply to tissues around the joints.

Maintain **correct technique**. For example, when doing a biceps curl (holding the weight in your hands and flexing your elbows), avoid lifting such a heavy weight that your back arches and you sway back and forth. Lift with smooth, controlled movements.

Some soreness is common the day or two after a resistance training session. This is not due to lactic acid, as this all diffuses out of the muscle within an hour or so following exertion. Rather, the soreness is probably caused by microscopic damage to connective tissue in muscle. Usually it goes away on its own with time and is less likely to occur at a given level of resistance as one develops more strength. Light to moderate activity, stretching, massage, and heat packs or hot baths may all help to minimize post-exercise soreness.

Cross-training adds variety to a training program, which decreases the psychological and physical strain of repetitive movement. So instead of all your physical activity being just running, or just cycling, or just playing basketball, or just lifting weights, vary your type of activity over the week.

Rest is as important as exercise in developing and maintaining fitness. The body needs time to recover between exercise sessions. If you are feeling tired or unwell, it is probably better to rest for a couple of days and then resume exercising. Several signs and symptoms may indicate your body needs more recovery than you are allowing it. These include:

- Persistent pain, especially in or around a joint
- Increased difficulty performing a familiar amount of exercise
- Increased susceptibility to infections, such as influenza, staphylococcus, or acne
- General feeling of tiredness, lack of energy, or lack of enthusiasm

> Think back to an activity-related injury *you* might have had. What could you have done differently that might have prevented it?

12 Treatment of Activity-Related Injuries

Most activity-related injuries are simple strains to muscle or connective tissue. They get better on their own in a few days or weeks and require little or no medical intervention.

Canadian practitioners (e.g., doctors or physiotherapists) typically take a **conservative approach** to injury management. That is, rather than taking drastic action at first, unless it's clearly an emergency, they start with simple, basic measures, which usually work. If, over time, the patient does not show good progress, *then* they will investigate and treat more intensively.

The conservative model for activity-related injuries goes through the following steps, in this order:

1. **Rest:** This does not mean complete bed rest. This means staying active but protecting the injured part (e.g., with taping or a sling).
2. **Imaging:** Internal images, such as X-rays, CAT scans, or MRIs, may be taken to rule out anything like a broken bone. These images are usually negative (i.e., they don't show the presence of any such disorder).

3. **Medication:** Medication for pain and inflammation isn't usually necessary, but it's relatively safe, and it helps the individual get back to activity a bit faster. Medication typically consists of plain analgesics such as Tylenol (without codeine or other narcotics) or non-steroidal anti-inflammatories such as ibuprofen (Advil).

4. **Modalities:** This includes simple things such as cold or heat and more sophisticated things such as laser or ultrasound treatment. These modalities are not intended to "fix" the injury, but to help the natural healing process and help the individual do the movements and exercises needed for rehabilitation.

5. **Gentle mobilization:** Gentle back and forth movements within the pain-free range of motion help prevent loss of mobility (or regain lost mobility).

6. **Progressive strengthening:** This starts at low velocity and with low loads, and builds up over weeks (and months, if necessary).

7. **Aerobic conditioning:** This can be done while protecting the injured part, similar to cross-training. For example, a runner with a sore foot might be okay to ride a stationary bicycle.

8. **Address injury cause:** Before the individual returns to full activity, assess his technique, equipment, training methods, and so on to try to understand what caused the injury, and then modify accordingly.

9. **Sport-specific activities:** Once a foundation of range of motion, strength, and endurance is built, the individual moves on to movements and drills that simulate her specific sport or activity. If these go well, she is ready to return to activity—but gradually, to avoid an early recurrence of injury.

> Think back to an activity-related injury *you* might have had.
> How does this series of steps in management of activity-related injuries fit with the way your injury was managed?

13 Conclusion

There are a number of well-established health benefits of regular physical activity. The potential risks of exercise can be minimized by screening, instruction, and supervision. Although some Canadians have incorporated regular physical activity into their lifestyle, overall we are an increasingly sedentary society. Instead of preaching to the converted or wasting money on the hard-core couch potato, interventions should be focused where they will be most beneficial. At the societal level, the greatest good may come from getting those who are completely sedentary to start a little activity, and those who are only a little inactive to become a little more active.

Study Questions

1a. Approximately how many hours per week do Canadians spend on "screen time"—watching TV, using the Internet, and so on?

1b. What percentage of Canadians regularly get 150 minutes (2.5 hours) per week of moderate to vigorous physical activity?

2a. Explain the differences in the terms "physical fitness," "physical activity," and "exercise."

2b. A person regularly walks in the park for 30 minutes a day. Is this "exercise" or "activity"? Explain.

3. List the components of "health-related fitness."

4. Outline the physical and psychological benefits of regular exercise.

5. How do self-reported physical activity data compare with objective measures of physical activity made with accelerometers?

6a. What is the difference between a "retrospective" and a "prospective" study?

6b. Which is more likely to give accurate data? Why?

7. What problem with epidemiological studies of physical activity are avoided with an experimental study?

8. Outline the risks of exercise/activity.

9. What is the most neglected part of most people's exercise?

10. List at least six different activities that can produce aerobic fitness gains.

11. Summarize the recommendations regarding aerobic conditioning.

12. Outline the principles of safe, effective resistance training.

13. Describe how, when, and how often stretching exercises should be done.

14. Give recommendations to help minimize risk of injury during physical activity.

15. List at least three signs or symptoms of possible overtraining.

16. Outline the steps in treatment of activity-related injuries.

Glossary

activity—any voluntary movement that expends calories

aerobic fitness—also known as cardiorespiratory fitness, endurance, or stamina, this is the type of fitness needed to do sustained rhythmic contraction of large muscle groups at moderate to moderately high intensity

exercise—planned, structured, repetitive physical activity done to maintain or improve one or more component of physical fitness

flexibility—range of motion at a joint

health—more than the absence of disease or infirmity; a complete state of mental, physical, and social well-being

osteoporosis—a condition in which the bones lose mineral content and become more vulnerable to fracture

physical fitness—the extent to which the body can respond to the demands of physical effort

prospective—looking forward in time; prospective studies follow a person or persons from a starting point forward to some future time

range of motion (ROM)—the space through which a limb or joint can move, often expressed in terms of degrees of arc

retrospective—looking backwards in time; retrospective studies attempt to reconstruct the history of a group of subjects by questionnaires, review of medical and employment records, and so on

static stretching—moving slowly into a stretched position and then holding the stretch

References

Campaign for a Commercial-Free Childhood (no date). Selected research on screen time and children. Retrieved May 4, 2018 from www.commercialfreechildhood.org

Canadian Press. (September 21, 2016). Statistics Canada studies highlight importance of daily physical activity for kids. Retrieved April 12, 2018 from https://toronto.ctvnews.ca/statistics-Canada-studies-highlight-importance-of-daily-physical-activity-for-kids-1.3082298

CBC News. (September 4, 2012). Canadian online, TV and radio use rises in 2011. Retrieved February 28, 2013 from http://www.cbc.ca/news/business/story/2012/09/04/crtc-telecom-usage-report.html

CDC (Centers for Disease Control and Prevention). (2014). *Facts about Physical Activity.* Retrieved April 12, 2018 from https://www.cdc.gov/physicalactivity/data/facts.htm

CSEP (Canadian Society for Exercise Physiology). (2018). *Canadian 24-Hour Movement Guidelines.* Retrieved April 12, 2018 from http://csepguidelines.ca/

Diaz, K. M., Howard, V. J., Hutto, B., Colabianchi, N., Vena, J. E., Safford, M. M., Blair, S. N., Hooker, S. P. (2017). Patterns of sedentary behavior and mortality in US middle-aged and older adults: a national cohort study. *Annals of Internal Medicine.* 167(7):465–475.

Colley, R. C., Garriguet, D., Janssen, I., Craig, C. L., Clarke, J., Tremblay, M. S. (2011). Physical activity of Canadian adults: Accelerometer results from the 2007 to 2009 Canadian Health Measures Survey. *Statistics Canada.* Retrieved February 28, 2013 from http://www.statcan.gc.ca/pub/82-003-x/2011001/article/11396-eng.htm

Garber, C. E., Blissmer, B., Deschenes, M. R., Franklin, B. A., Lamonte, M. J., Lee, I-M., Nieman, D. C., Swain, D. P. (2011). Quantity and quality of exercise for developing and maintaining cardiorespiratory, musculoskeletal, and neuromotor fitness in apparently healthy adults: Guidance for prescribing exercise. *Medicine and Science in Sports and Exercise.* 43(7), 1334–1359.

Jones R. (2015). Alarming facts about kids and screen time. *ParticipACTION blog.* Retrieved May 4, 2018 from https://www.participaction.com/en-ca/blog/technology/alarming-facts-about-kids-and-screen-time

Marlow, I. (March 22, 2010). Canadians' Internet use exceeds TV time. *The Globe and Mail.* Retrieved February 28, 2013 from http://www.theglobeandmail.com/technology/canadians-internet-use-exceeds-tv-time/article4352565/

Morris, J. N., Heady, J. A., Raffle, P. A. B., Roberts, C. G., Parks, J. W. (1953). Coronary heart disease and physical activity of work. *Lancet.* 265(6795), 1053–1057.

NIH. (November 6, 2012). NIH study finds leisure-time physical activity extends life expectancy as much as 4.5 years. *NIH News.* US Department of Health and Human Services: National Institutes of Health. Retrieved January 22, 2013 from http://www.nih.gov/news/health/nov2012/nci-06.htm

O'Keefe, J. H., Patil, H. R., Lavie, C. J., Magalski, A., Vogel, R. A., McCullough, P. A. (2012). Potential adverse cardiovascular effects from excessive endurance exercise. *Mayo Clinic Proceedings.* June 2012. 87(6), 587–595.

Patil, H. R., O'Keefe, J. H., Lavie, C. J., Magalski, A., Vogel, R. A., McCullough, P. A. (2012). Cardiovascular damage resulting from chronic excessive endurance exercise. *Missouri Medicine.* Jul–Aug. 109(4), 312–321.

Ruiz, J. R., Suie, X., Lobelo, F., Morrow, J. R., Jr, Jackson, A. W., Sjostrom, M., Blair, S. N. (2008). Association between muscular strength and mortality in men: Prospective cohort study. *British Medical Journal.* 337(7661), 92–95.

Sluik, D., Buiksse, B., Muckelbauer, R., et al. (2012). Physical activity and mortality in individuals with diabetes mellitus. *Archives of Internal Medicine.* 172(17), 12851295.

Statistics Canada. (2016). Physical activity during leisure time, by age group and sex. Retrieved May 4, 2018 from http.//www.stsatcan.gc.ca/tables-tableaux/sum-som/l01/cst01/health77b-eng.htm

Thompson, H. (January 16, 2012). *Average American watches almost 33 hours of television each week.* Retrieved February 28, 2013 from http://www.digitalhome.ca/2012/01/average-american-watches-almost-33-hours-of-television-each-week/

Whiteman H. (2016). Prolonged sitting: 'Exercise does not offset health risks,' say AHA. *Medical News Today.* Retrieved May 4, 2018 from https://www.medicalnewstoday.com/articles/312356.php

7   Nutrition

Learning Objectives

By the time you have finished this chapter you should be able to

- State the functions and main dietary sources of protein, fats, carbohydrates, fibre, iron, and calcium
- Outline how public health agencies have tried to give basic nutritional advice to the general public
- Explain how we know if people are "eating right"
- Summarize the dietary recommendations for people living in developed countries
- Compare the current Canadian diet to these recommendations
- Describe the advantages and challenges of vegetarian diets
- Comment on the health benefits and risks of eating organic foods
- Describe the health concerns around genetically modified foods
- Identify nutritional priorities for the developing world

1 Overview

Nutrition is the area where we encounter some of our most strongly held and passionately defended beliefs. Nutrition plays an important role in health by providing raw materials that support tissue growth, repair, and normal function. Nutrition can also become a health problem when we consume too much of certain nutrients, or when pathogens, *toxins* (poisons), or *carcinogens* (cancer-causing agents) are consumed in our food.

Digestion, the process that breaks down the foods and beverages we ingest, starts in the mouth, with chewing and enzymes in saliva (Figure 7.1). It continues

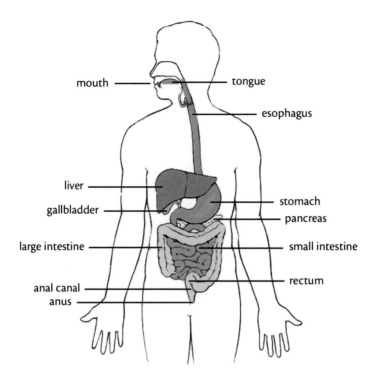

mouth

tongue

esophagus

liver

gallbladder

stomach

pancreas

large intestine

small intestine

anal canal

rectum

anus

Figure 7.1. The human digestive system.

with stomach acids, then in the small intestine with secretions from the pancreas, gall bladder, and intestinal wall. In the small intestine, most nutrients are absorbed into the blood, which carries them to the liver, the main site of ***metabolism.*** Metabolism is the complex set of chemical changes in living cells that provides energy and material for vital processes. ***Nutrition*** means the act or process of nourishing or being nourished. In this chapter, we will use the word ***diet*** to mean food and drink regularly provided and consumed.

2 The Main Categories of Nutrients
Nutrients have been grouped into six categories:

1. Fats
2. Carbohydrates
3. Proteins
4. Vitamins
5. Minerals
6. Water

Fats, carbohydrates, and proteins provide energy to support the body's vital functions and to do physical activity.

Water is the most vital nutrient. We can survive for weeks without food but will die in days without water. The human body is about 60% water by weight, and it is in this watery world that many metabolic reactions occur. Water is lost every day in urine, feces, and sweat. Water is used in digestion and forms the bulk of body fluids such as blood.

Carbohydrates are metabolized to glucose, which circulates in the blood as a ready energy source. Only a limited amount of carbohydrate is stored in the body, mostly in the liver and skeletal muscles, and it is largely depleted after a couple of hours of aerobic exercise.

Fats are essential components of cell membranes and some types of hormones. Body fat also provides insulation from heat loss and padding for internal organs. Fats have the highest **nutrient density**, with about 9 kcal/gram. Carbohydrates and proteins each yield about 4 kcal/gram.

Proteins are chains of *amino acids*. Proteins are not normally used for energy, but in extreme times (e.g., fasting, starvation, prolonged physical activity), they can be. The usual role of proteins is growth and repair of tissue.

The **vitamins** and **minerals** have been called **micronutrients** because we only need milligrams (thousandths of a gram) or micrograms (millionths of a gram) daily. The mineral **calcium** is essential for strong bones and teeth, while the mineral **iron** forms a central part of red blood cells. **Vitamins C, E, and beta-carotene** (the precursor to vitamin A) act as **antioxidants**, protecting against the effects of aging, lesions in the arteries, and cancer. Vitamins and minerals also play key roles at various points in metabolic chemical reactions.

> *What vitamins and minerals should I be taking? Which brands are best?*

The point of view expressed most often by health educators on this topic is that food is a better way to meet your nutrient needs than supplements. Regular meals of fresh, minimally processed foods will probably provide all, or most, of the necessary nutrients. There may be certain exceptions. See Section 6 for more about iron, calcium, and vitamins A and C.

3 What Is a Healthy Diet?

A simple answer might be "a diet that keeps people healthy." This can be defined in terms of **preventing deficiency diseases**. A diet with no vitamin C leads to the disease called scurvy. Add sufficient vitamin C (e.g., by eating oranges or other citrus fruits), and scurvy doesn't develop.

What about other diseases such as cardiovascular disease, diabetes, and cancer? These are not nutrient-deficiency diseases, but they are related to nutrition. That is, these multi-factorial diseases are not *caused* by nutrition, but nutrition affects *risk* of developing disease and can help in the primary or secondary prevention of these diseases.

Nutritional science uses lots of terms and acronyms that can be quite confusing to the student new to the field:

- Dietary reference intakes (DRI)
- Recommended daily allowances (RDA)
- Estimated average requirement (EAR)
- Acceptable macronutrient distribution range (AMDR)
- Adequate intake (AI)
- Tolerable upper intake level (UL)

The Additional Resources section at the back of the chapter contains Internet links to tables that contain values for these variables.

In this chapter, we'll largely sidestep the terminology and discuss nutritional recommendations and nutritional status in qualitative and comparative terms. That is, instead of saying, "experts say you should get at least 600 mg of calcium a day," we will point out that many Canadians and Americans are not getting enough calcium in their diet, and identify some of the main food sources of calcium.

Over the last 60-plus years, public health agencies in North America have tried to give basic nutritional advice to the general public. Health Canada (2006, p. 47) cautions that

> Food guides are educational tools intended to ... help individuals obtain adequate nutrient intakes ... Population surveys may report the proportions of the population with usual intakes that meet or do not meet the recommendations for each of the food groups ... However, the results cannot be used to assess adequacy of the nutrient intakes of the population.

The **Four Food Groups** was the concept behind an early food guide. A one-page chart indicated how many servings per day you should eat from each food group:

1. Milk and dairy products
2. Meats and alternatives
3. Fruits and vegetables
4. Grains and cereals

It was intended as a "foundation diet"; that is, the US Department of Agriculture expected people to consume more food than the plan recommended, which would provide more energy and other nutrients. The Four Food Groups concept is outdated because it focused on nutrient *deficiencies*, whereas most current nutritional concerns are *excesses*.

In 1992, Canada replaced the Four Food Groups with *Canada's Food Guide to Healthy Living*. The same four categories of food were used, but they were shown as a rainbow. The longer stripes on the outside of the rainbow (grains and vegetables/fruits) implied you should eat more servings of these than you should eat of the more **calorie-** and protein-dense inner categories. There was also a more explicit message to choose lower-fat foods.

In 2007, the *Canada Food Guide* was produced. It still uses the same four food groups, but it is much longer (six pages in printer-friendly form) and more comprehensive. It finally accounts for age and gender differences. It provides clear advice on portion sizes. It includes more culturally relevant foods. It advises consuming less processed foods (for example, have vegetables and fruit more often than juice, and prepare vegetables and fruit with little or no added fat, sugar, or salt). Finally, it emphasizes the importance of combining regular physical activity with healthy eating.

4 Nature of the Evidence

How do we know if people are eating right? This seems like a simple question, but it embodies multiple issues. Let's unpack this idea. First, what is "eating right"? It's not the same as eating enough, especially in developed countries where the main nutritional problems are eating too much (see Section 5 below). Next, we need a way to measure *what* people are eating. At the **individual level**, we could weigh and count everything a person eats, much as a high-performance athlete or astronaut would: one hard-boiled egg, one apple, one 200-ml glass of 2% milk, and so on. Then we could look up the nutrient content of each food item. Tables with these values are available (see the Additional Resources section near the end of this chapter). Computerized nutritional calculators are also available.

This same method can be used with **institutional populations** (e.g., people in hospitals, prisons, or the armed forces). The assumption is that the institutional setting provides a measure of control over and confidence about what people are eating. However, we don't have this control or confidence for **free-living populations**.

At the **population level**, food disappearance statistics can give a general picture. Food producers and distributors track food quantities. Thus, experts can note that, for example, as average annual per capita income in developing countries such as China has gone up, per capita dietary consumption of oil and beef has also increased. This kind of observation doesn't tell us, though, *who* is doing the consuming. Typically the consumption is distributed unevenly; a relatively small emerging middle class exercises greatly increased purchasing power while most people remain relatively poor.

In order to get an idea of the distribution of "right eating" in a population, the most common method is to ask a sample of people what they eat. Researchers try to obtain a representative sample (see Chapter 2: Evaluating Health Claims). Then they may ask the members of this sample to keep a food diary for a period of time, such as a week. Or they may ask the sample members to report what they ate over the last period of time (e.g., **24-hour dietary recall**.) The Canadian Community Health Survey, Cycle 2.2, of over 35,000 Canadians included a 24-hour dietary recall conducted by trained interviewers.

> Can you remember the names for these two different research methods—the one that follows people into the future and the one that asks people about the past?

Single 24-hour recalls (or even several repeated recalls) do not accurately estimate the usual intakes of *individuals*. But with **population surveys**, the objective is not to determine the nutrient adequacy of specific individuals. Instead, the relevant questions include "What proportion of the group (e.g., teen females) has usual nutrient intakes that are below requirements?" or "What is the prevalence of inadequate nutrient intakes?" (Health Canada, 2006, p. 30).

Problematically, people systematically under-report food intake (Health Canada, 2006, p. 42). Furthermore, it is not simple to adjust for under-reporting (e.g., by scaling up all the values) for a couple of reasons:

- Some types of food are more likely to be under-reported, for example, high-fat, high-sugar foods, such as cakes and cookies, versus foods that are perceived to be healthier, such as fruits, vegetables, meat, and fish (Health Canada, 2006, pp. 43, 44).
- Under-reporting is more common among some types of people, such as adults versus children or those with high body-mass index (BMI; see Chapter 8: Body Weight) versus those of "normal" weight.

Finally, we should note that assessing nutrient *intake* is different from assessing nutrient *status*. Sometimes scientists really want measures of **biomarkers**, such as serum (blood) levels of vitamin C or iron or calcium. An individual can adhere to nutritional recommendations but still have poor nutritional status due to individual differences in metabolism or to diseases that affect digestion, absorption, or utilization of certain nutrients, among other reasons.

5 The Modern North American Diet

In the past, nutritional recommendations for North Americans focused on **deficiencies** of nutrients (e.g., thiamine, riboflavin, and other B vitamins). Today's problems are **nutritional excesses**. These excesses are associated with

- Affluence
- Availability of convenience foods
- Perceived shortage of time, which has increased reliance on fast and convenience foods
- Aggressive corporate advertising

> Why do you think the author wrote *perceived* shortage of time?

The 2015 Canadian Community Health Survey asked people to recall what they ate and drank in the previous 24 hours. Responses revealed that (Statistics Canada, 2017a)

- About half (47%) of total calories consumed were carbohydrates.
- About a third of total calories consumed were fats.
- The remaining sixth of total calories came from proteins.
- On average, males consumed more total calories than females did. Male energy intake was highest from ages 14-to-18 (about 2,400 kcal daily), remained relatively constant until age 30, and then declined with advancing age. Female energy intake peaked in the 9-to-13 age range (about 1,800 kcal) and then declined a bit with age.

Almost half of Canadians reported using nutritional supplements (Statistics Canada, 2017a):

- Females were more likely to use supplements than males, with the biggest difference in the 51-to-70 age range (65% of females vs. 43% of males).
- Twenty-three percent of Canadians take at least one multivitamin supplement.

- Omega-3 fatty acids were used by 12% of Canadians.
- A third of Canadians use vitamin D supplements.

Canadian Living magazine did its own nutrition survey (Buchner, 2016), and found

- Sixty-eight percent said they "eat whole foods." A similar proportion report eating less processed food now than five years ago. Three out of four say they are willing to pay more for healthy food, while the other quarter says they cannot afford to eat as healthy as they would like to.
- Seventy-three percent said "I eat everything in moderation."
- Many take nutritional supplements: 38% take a multivitamin, 39% take omega-3, and 60% use a vitamin D supplement.
- Over half said they eat local food as much as possible.

> What is the most likely explanation for the difference in reported rates of nutritional supplement use between the Canadian Living survey and the Canadian Community Health Survey?
>
> In what ways do you think your diet is better or worse than the average Canadian's?

6 Dietary Recommendations for North Americans
6.1 *Reduce* total calorie *intake*

Excess caloric intake is a major contributor to overweight, which is associated with a number of health problems discussed in Chapter 8: Body Weight.

Unlike alcohol or other drugs, you can't choose to not eat. The key to healthy eating is to eat selectively. Choose foods that are rich in nutrients. Avoid "empty calorie" foods, such as candy, pop, and chips. The things we label "junk food" tend to be high in fats, calories, and sodium (salt), low in fibre, and deficient in some, but not all, vitamins and minerals.

For example, a Big Mac contains

541 kcal
26 g protein (about 1/3 the daily requirement)
4 mg iron (about 1/4 to 1/3 the daily requirement)
1 g sodium
31 g fat (at 9 kcal/g = 279 kcal; thus, 52% of total calories from fat)

It is wrong to call this "junk food," as it contains lots of nutrients. There is room in most diets for occasional servings of pizza, ice cream, cookies, alcohol, and so on. However, if you eat such food too often, you may have a *junk diet.*

6.2 Maintain (or reduce) protein intake

Protein is found in animal foods (such as meat, poultry, fish, eggs, milk, and other dairy products), as well as beans (especially soybeans and soybean products, such as tofu), lentils, and nuts. Some vegetables also have small amounts of protein.

6.3 Reduce ratio of saturated fat to unsaturated fat

For decades, health agencies in Canada, the USA, and elsewhere advocated limiting total fat intake. That advice has shifted to optimizing the *type* of dietary fat rather than reducing *total* fat (Mozaffarian & Ludwig, 2015). Fats in foods are made up of four different types of fatty acids: polyunsaturated, monounsaturated, saturated, and trans. **Saturated** refers to chemical bonding. The more saturated a fat is, the more solid it is at room temperature. Margarine is made from vegetable oil by partly saturating it (Health Canada, 2009).

In general, animal products are higher in saturated fat than plant products. For example, only 10% of the fats in canola oil are saturated, while butter contains about 65% saturated fat. However, palm oil and coconut oil, both from plants, are 50% and 90% saturated, respectively. These so-called tropical oils are often hidden in food products such as ice cream (read the labels). Saturated fat intake is associated with CVD and cancer.

Fish oils, especially those from large cold-water fish such as salmon and tuna, reduce risk of CVD. Experts advocate eating the fish rather than taking capsules of fish oil, because vitamin A is so concentrated in fish oil capsules that regular administration of these capsules can lead to vitamin A toxicity.

6.4 Reduce trans-fats

In trans-fats, the extra chemical bond is in the opposite position from normal. Trans-fats occur naturally at low levels in some animal-based foods, such as dairy products, beef, and lamb. Some oils, such as canola, soybean, and fish oils, can also contain small amounts of trans-fats, which are formed during the commercial processing of the oils. Trans-fats can also be formed when manufacturers process liquid oil into a semi-solid form, like shortening or margarine. Consuming either saturated or trans-fats raises blood levels of LDL cholesterol.

Trans-fat also reduces blood levels of HDL cholesterol (Health Canada, 2009). The World Health Organization (WHO) recommends that the total daily trans-fat consumption should be less than 1% of your daily energy intake (Health Canada, 2009). So, if you consume 2,400 kcal per day, less than 24 kcal should come from trans-fats. Since fats have 9 kcal per gram, this means if you eat 2,400 kcal per day, less than three grams of that should be trans-fat.

6.5 Optimize ratio of omega-6 to omega-3 fatty acids

Omega-6 and omega-3 fatty acids are both polyunsaturated fatty acids (PUFA). The evidence regarding supplementing human diets with omega-3 is somewhat mixed. Intake of omega-3 above three grams per day is not recommended, as it may increase risk of bleeding, stroke, and other disorders.

The body converts short-chain omega-3 fatty acids to longer-chain fatty acids. These conversions are slowed by omega-6 fatty acids. Thus, the ratio of omega-6 to omega-3 may be more important than the amount of omega-3. The modern Western diet is about 10:1 or higher. Recommended ratios are closer to 1:1 (i.e., less omega-6); some authors recommend 1:4, others recommend 4:1, while still others suggest something in between. The important point is that the modern Western diet seems to have way too much omega-6 relative to omega-3. Canola oil has a ratio of 2:1, which is good. Flaxseed oil is 1:3, which is even better. Soybean oil is 7:1. Corn oil is 46:1, which is very bad.

The point here is that while groups such as Health Canada and the American Heart Association have told us to "eat more polyunsaturated fatty acids," not all PUFAs are the same.

Oily cold-water fish such as sardines, herring, mackerel, and salmon—and, to a lesser extent, tuna—are the richest natural sources of omega-3 fatty acids. The American Heart Association recommends those at low risk for cardio-vascular disease eat two or more servings of this kind of fish per week. Higher intake is recommended for those at higher risk of CVD. The omega-3 benefits of this consumption are considered much greater than the potential problems of heavy metals, toxins (poisons), and carcinogens that concentrate at higher levels in the food chain. (We'll learn more about this in Section 8, when we look at vegetarian diets.)

6.6 Increase ratio of complex to simple carbohydrates

The body takes longer to digest and absorb complex carbohydrates contained in grains, cereal, pasta, and potatoes than it does to digest and absorb simple carbo-hydrates. Thus, complex carbohydrates help keep blood glucose at more constant levels. In contrast, simple carbohydrates such as sucrose (sugar) or fructose (fruit sugar) can cause a roller-coaster effect with blood sugar. Sugar consumption also increases incidence of cavities in teeth, although this appears to be less of an issue for those who get regular fluoride treatments from their dentist.

High-fructose corn syrup (HFCS) is a highly refined carbohydrate that has been processed to convert some of its glucose to fructose. HFCS has mostly replaced sucrose in the food industry. This switch resulted from a combination of factors, including duties on imported sugar and subsidies for US corn—subsidies that are politically popular in corn-growing states. Soda pop manufacturers such as Coke and Pepsi now use HFCS rather than sucrose. You won't see sugar listed as an ingredient in pop, but you *will* see high-fructose corn syrup—65 grams, representing over 20% of the total carbohydrates and over 10% of the total calories in a 2,000 kcal daily diet. HFCS has been blamed—largely based on epidemiological evidence—for the high incidence and prevalence of obesity and diabetes (see, for example, Goran, Ulijaszk, & Ventura, 2013). However, the underlying cause is more likely increased consumption of refined carbohydrates per se. "Because the composition of HFCS and sucrose is so similar, particularly on absorption by the body, it appears unlikely that HFCS contributes more to obesity or other conditions than sucrose does." (Moeller et al., 2009)

Complex carbohydrates contain more dietary fibre, and are richer sources of vitamins and minerals, than simple carbohydrates. The 2015 Dietary Guidelines Advisory Committee report noted that over 70% of the US population eats too many refined grain products (Mozaffarian & Ludwig, 2015), for example, white bread, rice, and pasta. Emphasize whole grains rather than refined grains in the diet; for example, choose brown rice rather than white rice and whole-wheat flour rather than white flour. According to the Harvard School of Public Health (Frenk, ca. 2010),

> Refining wheat creates fluffy flour that makes light, airy breads and pastries. But there's a nutritional price to be paid for refined grains. The process strips away more than half of wheat's B vitamins, 90 percent of the vitamin E, and virtually all of the fiber. It also makes the starch easily accessible to the body's starch-digesting enzymes.

On the other hand, whole grains improve lipid profile, decrease risk of CVD, lower insulin levels, decrease risk of diabetes, help prevent constipation, and may (although data are mixed on this last point) provide moderate protection against colorectal cancer (Frenk, ca. 2010).

6.7 Increase dietary fibre intake

Fibre is a carbohydrate, but humans don't have the enzymes to break these compounds down and use them for energy. Instead, in the human diet fibre functions as filler. It passes through the digestive tract without being digested. **Soluble fibre** binds cholesterol-containing compounds in the intestine, which lowers serum cholesterol levels. **Insoluble fibre** draws water into the stool in the large intestine, which creates a larger, softer stool. The increased stool bulk stimulates smooth muscle in the lining of the intestine to contract more force-fully, promoting movement of the stool through the bowel. The softer stool is easier to defecate. For these reasons, dietary fibre helps treat and prevent con-stipation. Also, populations that eat more fibre have lower incidence of colon cancer. All plant foods contain some fibre. Fruits, legumes, and oats (especially oat bran) are rich in soluble fibre. Cereals, grains (especially wheat bran), and vegetables are good sources of insoluble fibre.

6.8 Use salt and sodium in moderation

Table salt is sodium chloride. Other products (e.g., baking powder, baking soda, and club soda) also contain sodium. In addition to the salt we add to food during cooking or at the dinner table, salt is added to many prepared foods (e.g., canned soups, Kraft dinner, and ramen noodles) as a flavouring and preservative. The average Canadian adult consumes about 3,400 mg of sodium daily (almost identical to US consumption), well in excess of the recommended daily limit of 2,300 mg. A survey of 19 popular sit-down restaurants in the USA found that the average meal contained 50% more sodium than the amount recommended for a whole day (Hui, 2017).

Sodium increases blood pressure, which is a major risk factor for CVD. Salty food also appears to be a risk factor for stomach cancer. It is thought that the salt acts as an irritant to the cells lining the stomach, which may initiate or contribute to the expression of cancer-causing genetic changes in these cells.

Health Canada had planned to set limits on the sodium content of food sold to Canadians, but in 2012 it announced suspension of these plans. At the time of this writing, Health Canada is preparing a policy that would set targets for sodium in the restaurant industry. So far, the industry has strongly resisted such intensions (Hui, 2017). The onus remains on individuals to become more informed and selective consumers, for example, by reading the labels.

6.9 Ensure adequate iron intake

A deficiency of iron can result in a condition known as *anemia*, which is often accompanied by lethargy or low energy. There are two forms of iron:

- **Heme iron** from animal products
- **Non-heme iron** from plants

Non-heme iron is absorbed from the digestive system less efficiently. Clams, oysters, and organ meats such as liver, kidney, and heart are the richest dietary sources of iron. Beef is also a good source. Eggs have some iron. Commonly eaten non-heme sources include legumes (such as lentils and beans), enriched cereals and pasta, dark-coloured dried fruits, and dark green leafy vegetables. If non-heme iron is eaten with heme iron, the absorption of the non-heme iron is improved.

Iron absorption is also promoted by vitamin C, which is contained in many fresh fruits and vegetables. Coffee and tea inhibit iron absorption, so it is better to drink them an hour or more before or after a meal rather than with the meal. If you take an iron supplement, you should do it with some awareness or guidance from a health professional. Excess iron can accumulate to toxic levels over time.

6.10 Ensure adequate calcium intake

Calcium is important in forming and maintaining healthy teeth and bones, and in preventing *osteoporosis*, a condition in which the bones become more fragile. This problem is especially severe in post-menopausal females. Dairy products, such as milk and cheese, are rich sources of calcium. Osteoporosis is less common in women who drank a lot of milk as children. Calcium is present in low amounts in dark green leafy vegetables. Many nutritionists recommend a supplement of 500 to 1,000 mg of elemental calcium daily. Exercise (weight-bearing or resistance training) helps prevent osteoporosis. So does hormone replacement therapy (i.e., estrogen) for post-menopausal women. Smoking, on the other hand, promotes bone loss.

Concern has been expressed that high dietary protein intake increases the rate at which the body excretes calcium. In a review of the literature, Bonjour (2011) notes that "dietary proteins represent key nutrients for bone health and thereby function in the prevention of osteoporosis" and that "low protein intake (< 0.8 g/kg body weight/day) is often observed in patients with hip fractures." Bonjour concludes that "There is no evidence that high protein intake per se would be detrimental for bone mass and strength. Nevertheless, it appears reasonable to avoid very high protein diets (i.e. more than 2.0 g/kg body weight/day) when associated with low calcium intake (i.e. less than 600 mg/day)." The findings of Thorpe et al. (2008) add to this. In a randomized 12-month human dietary intervention, they found that the potential adverse effects of high-protein diet on calcium and bone mineral were overcome when the diet was also high in calcium from dairy products.

6.11 Increase consumption of foods containing vitamins A and C

Fruits and vegetables are rich sources of vitamins and minerals. Also, the antioxidant properties of vitamins A (beta-carotene) and C may be helpful in preventing the onset of cancer. Vegetables that are darker orange or green are higher in these vitamins. Vegetables in the cabbage family (arugula, bok choy, broccoli, broccoli sprouts, Brussels sprouts, cabbage, cauliflower, Swiss chard, collards, kale, kohlrabi, mustard greens, radishes, rutabaga, turnips, turnip greens, and watercress) are especially good sources of these antioxidants.

6.12 Eat a variety of foods

This is a good way to ensure you meet the recommended levels of vitamins and minerals, which are the so-called **trace nutrients** or **micro-nutrients**. We may also need nutrients that have not yet been identified. Eating a variety of foods is a good way to cover this possibility.

6.13 If you drink alcoholic beverages, do so in moderation

Alcohol is normally considered a *drug* rather than a *food* (see Chapter 13: Drugs), although it contains calories. A regular beer contains about 150 kcal, a glass of white wine about 100 kcal, and a shot of vodka about 120 kcal. So, four beers in a day would represent about 20% of a young adult male's daily energy requirement. These calories can easily accumulate as stored body fat over the months. Alcohol should not be consumed during pregnancy because it causes damage to the fetus.

Summary of preceding dietary recommendations for North Americans

1. Reduce total calorie intake
2. Maintain (or reduce) protein intake
3. Reduce ratio of saturated fat to unsaturated fat
4. Reduce trans-fats
5. Optimize ratio of omega-6 to omega-3 fatty acids
6. Increase ratio of complex to simple carbohydrates
7. Increase dietary fibre intake
8. Use salt and sodium in moderation
9. Ensure adequate iron intake
10. Ensure adequate calcium intake
11. Increase consumption of foods containing vitamins A and C
12. Eat a variety of foods
13. If you drink alcoholic beverages, do so in moderation

7 How Healthy are Diets of Different Cultures?

First, different cultures certainly *do* have different diets. For me, food is one of the most interesting things about different cultures, and one of my big joys in travel. By definition, I suppose, the diets of different cultures "work"—if the diet didn't meet human nutritional needs, these people, and their culture, would die.

Second, diets of different cultures have adapted to the food that was available in their local area in the time they were developing. Perhaps you have heard of the **Stone Age** or **Paleo Diet**. The Stone Age was a period in human history before the development of agriculture, so the diet had almost no grain (e.g., corn, rice, and wheat) except for what might have been gathered in the wild (e.g., wild rice). Conversely, Stone Age humans got a lot of their calories (and protein) from meat. In this way, I suppose the Inuit diet is similar; it includes lots of meat and fat. It is hard to judge the quality of these diets on the basis of the lifespan of their people. Average life expectancy at the time these diets evolved was much shorter than it is today; people lived maybe an average of 40 years (some people lived into their 60s and beyond, but not many). They died mainly because of accidents and infectious diseases.

Third, I find it curious how peoples at different places and times learned what is good to eat, what will kill you, and how to prepare food. For example, corn (maize) yields more nutritional value if it is first soaked in lime. How did people learn this hundreds of years before nutritional science?

If we review the nutritional recommendations from the section above, we see that traditional Asian and Southeast Asian diets compare quite well. Lots of rice and vegetables, fish and other seafood, maybe small amounts of meat in the form of pork, chicken, duck, and sometimes beef. Not excessive amounts of fat or calories. Overweightness is uncommon in Asia, at least among people who stick to a traditional diet and maintain a physically active lifestyle—not going to the gym but doing manual labour and walking or bicycling for transportation, as is common in rural areas. The main limitations of this diet would seem to be too much sodium (e.g., soy sauce and pickled vegetables such as kimchee) and not enough protein or calories to support optimal growth, which is why here in Canada we see Asian grandparents who are, on average, much shorter than their North American-born grandchildren.

Japanese migrants to the United States provide an interesting contrast. Second-generation Japanese people living in Hawaii have higher incidence of and mortality from heart disease than Japanese living in Japan. Follow this group for another generation and to the mainland United States, and the diet is even more Westernized and heart disease goes up further.

The same kind of analysis could be done with other diets: South Asian, Latin American, Caribbean, Mediterranean, Middle Eastern, North African, and so on.

8 Vegetarian Diets

Exactly how beneficial is it to be vegetarian? The word "exactly" is usually difficult in the field of health because much of what we know comes from studies of groups of people, and there are almost always individuals who experience different outcomes than the rest of the group. For example, vegetarian diets tend to be lower in fat, and dietary fat intake is associated with some types of cancer, so vegetarians as a group should have lower risk of these cancers; but some vegetarians will still get and die from these same cancers.

Let's look at the question more fully.

Vegetarian diets do not contain meat. But there are several versions of vegetarian diets:

- *Vegans* eat no animal products.
- *Lacto-ovo vegetarians* don't eat flesh, but they eat milk products and eggs.
- In addition, there are people who don't eat red meat but will eat fish, or perhaps fish and chicken. This is fine, but it isn't really a vegetarian diet.

From an intake point of view, here are some of the potential benefits of vegetarian diets:

- They tend to be higher in fruits and vegetables, which increases vitamin and fibre content.
- They tend to be lower in fat, especially saturated fat. However, dietary fat (more correctly, lipid) comes not just from meat but also from dairy products (especially full-fat or homo milk vs. 2%, 1%, or skim milk, as well as many cheeses and ice cream), nuts, oil used in cooking or as dressing, and avocados. Watch out especially for desserts (e.g., the cream cheese icing on carrot cake) and fried foods.
- They tend to be lower in environmental contaminants, including pesticides and heavy metals (such as lead and mercury). Such contaminants get increasingly concentrated as one moves up the food chain. For example, if an industrial operation discharges mercury-containing waste into the ocean, seaweed and algae will take up some of the mercury. Small fish that eat these will have higher levels (grams mercury per kg) than the seaweed. Larger fish that eat the small fish will have still higher levels. However, this is not to say plants are safe; the most powerful carcinogens known are found in mouldy peanuts.
- Meat and dairy products are more likely to contain pathogens, such as some strains of E. coli bacteria, which can cause gastrointestinal distress and sometimes death.
- They tend to be less expensive. Protein-rich foods such as meat or cheese cost more than beans or rice. However, processed foods are also more

expensive than simple, basic foods. For example, a pound of flour usually costs less than a frozen pizza.

- They tend to be more environmentally sustainable. More humans can be fed from the corn and soybeans grown on 100 hectares of farmland if the humans eat the beans and corn directly than if the beans and corn are used to feed cows (or chickens, pigs, etc.) and the humans then eat these animals.

- The sense of ethical correctness. This involves values, which are largely individual and subjective. That is, this is more a matter of philosophy than of nutritional science. Some vegetarians believe humans should co-exist with other animals rather than exploit them. Some vegetarians are bothered by the perceived cruel conditions under which animals are raised or caught or killed for food.

From a health-outcomes perspective, compared with non-vegetarians, vegetarians (Craig & Mangels, 2009) have

- Lower body mass index (see Chapter 8: Body Weight)
- Lower risk of death from ischemic heart disease
- Lower low-density lipoprotein cholesterol levels
- Lower rates of hypertension
- Lower rates of Type II diabetes
- Lower overall cancer rates

It seems to me that vegans would have the same benefits (and risks, as we'll see below) as vegetarians, only more so.

However, in a meat-eating society, vegetarians and especially vegans need to be attentive to what they eat in order to obtain the necessary nutrients. For example, if the family dinner is beef, potatoes, and green beans, and a vegan family member just eats the potatoes and green beans, she will likely get insufficient iron, protein, and vitamin B-12. It is much easier to get the necessary nutrients by eating small amounts of meat or animal products (e.g., stir-fried beef with broccoli, or fried rice with egg or shrimp) than by eating no animal products.

Vegetarians must take special care to get enough of certain nutrients:

- **Protein:** Vegetarian diets typically have less protein than meat-based diets, but vegetarians do appear to get enough protein without meat. This seems true even for athletes, who need more protein than non-athletes.

- **Iron:** Iron is more poorly absorbed from plant foods, so if you are only eating plant foods, you need to take in more iron in order to ensure enough gets absorbed.
- **B-12:** Supplementation is advised for vegans, especially for pregnant and lactating women.
- **Calcium:** For vegans. Vegetarians who drink milk do not have the same concern.
- **Vitamin D:** Milk is fortified with this vitamin. Vegan foods such as soymilk may be fortified. Sunlight may be enough; 15 minutes of sunlight on the face each day is enough to stimulate the body to produce enough vitamin D itself.

9 Organic Foods

Are organic foods actually better for our bodies than regular produce?

Locally grown produce is usually fresher when you buy it, so it may taste better. It is important to note that "organic" does not equate with "local." When I have the choice of organic green onions from California or non-organic local green onions, I buy the local produce. Also, just because something isn't certified as "organic" doesn't mean it isn't organic. Some small vegetable producers haven't taken the trouble and expense to get certified as organic even though they use organic methods or haven't been in production long enough (I think three years) to qualify for the "organic" certification yet.

Two US food scientists summarized the evidence (Winter & Davis, 2006) comparing organic with non-organic produce. They start by defining "organic":

Organic production can be defined as an ecological production management system that promotes and enhances biodiversity, biological cycles, and soil biological activity. It is based on minimal use of off-farm inputs and on management practices that restore, maintain, and enhance ecological harmony. US regulations require that organic foods are grown without synthetic pesticides, growth hormones, antibiotics, modern genetic engineering techniques (including genetically modified crops), chemical fertilizers, or sewage sludge.

They continue by addressing five different issues:

- **Pesticide residues:** These have been detected in both organic and non-organic produce. Four different studies found the presence of pesticide residues to be three to five times more likely in non-organic produce. However, typical human exposure to even the highest levels found were more than 1,000 times lower than levels that do not cause toxicity in animals. "Such findings suggest that typical *dietary exposure* to pesticide residues in foods poses minimal risks to humans. From a practical standpoint, the marginal benefits of reducing human exposure to pesticides in the diet through increased consumption of organic produce appear to be insignificant." However, they noted that farm workers who work with and around pesticides *are* at risk; in 2004, 828 documented cases of *occupational* pesticide illnesses were reported in California alone (Winter & Davis, 2006, p. R120).
- **Plant toxins:** Plants stressed by pest attack produce natural toxins to fight the pests. Some of these natural toxins can cause adverse health effects (e.g., throat cancer, liver damage, lung damage, gastrointestinal toxicity) in humans and other animals that eat them. Ironically, organic plants attacked by pests may have more of these natural toxins than plants treated with synthetic pesticides.
- **Nutritional content:** On this topic, the evidence is mixed; some studies show more nutrients (e.g., antioxidants such as vitamin C) in organic foods, while other studies show no difference. Furthermore, the human health outcomes of higher nutrient intake aren't well understood. For example, one study showed organic tomatoes and purée made from these tomatoes were higher in vitamin C and polyphenols (another antioxidant), but subjects who ate the organic purée did not have higher blood levels of the antioxidants than those who ate the non-organic tomatoes. Higher nutrient intake may not matter once a certain minimal intake is achieved.
- **Nitrate levels:** Organic produce had lower nitrate levels than produce grown with synthetic nitrogen fertilizers. Nitrates increase risk of certain cancers.
- **Bacterial contamination:** Organic produce tended to have higher levels of bacteria than non-organic produce—presumably bacteria from manure used to fertilize the organic crops.

What do *you* think about the preceding comparison of organic and non-organic food?

Has it changed your intention regarding purchasing organic food?

If organic food and non-organic food were exactly the same price in the store, which would you buy? Why?

10 Genetically Modified Foods

For millennia, humans have deliberately modified the characteristics of living things. One way to do this is selective breeding. Imagine, for example, that a breeder wants to produce maize (corn) with large ears. She identifies plants that have this trait, collects their seeds, and next season plants those seeds. At the end of that season, she again takes the seeds from the best plants, and so on.

Genetic engineering uses a different approach. Genes are modified artificially; for example, they are transplanted from one organism to another. Scientists have produced genetically modified corn varieties that are resistant to drought, resistant to certain herbicides (weed killers), such as Roundup, or that produce proteins of a bacteria that are poisonous to certain insect pests. Genetically modified organisms (GMOs) have improved agricultural productivity and profitability, at least for those who have access to these patent-protected organisms.

Government agencies assure the public that GMOs do not represent a risk to human health. For example, the pest-killing bacteria proteins mentioned above don't become active in the human stomach, which has a different chemistry than the insect pest stomach. However, health concerns persist on several issues:

- **Effects on non-pest insects:** The bacteria proteins kill other insects in addition to the ones that threaten the crop they were engineered to protect. What if these non-pest insects play an important, and perhaps not yet understood, role in the ecosystem?
- **Human allergies:** The immune system recognizes foreign or non-foreign material in the body by the specific shape of proteins called antigens. Antigens on the surface of pathogens normally trigger an immune response. Other antigens are not associated with infectious organisms but in some people still produce an immune-system response. For example, proteins from peanuts, wheat, plant pollen, and mould can cause itchy red eyes, runny nose, or even death in highly sensitive individuals. The World Health Organization (WHO, 2014) asserts, "No allergic effects have been found relative to GM foods currently on the market."
- **Gene transfer:** Gene transfer from the GMO to the human or to the bacteria in the human's gut "would be particularly relevant if antibiotic resistance genes, used in creating GMOs, were to be transferred. Although the probability of transfer is low, the use of technology without antibiotic resistant genes has been encouraged by a recent FAO/WHO expert panel" (WHO, 2014).
- **Outcrossing:** Combining the GMO with conventional crops or related wild species is a process called outcrossing. The genetically modified

corn can "contaminate" natural varieties of corn. This happened in the USA when GMO corn approved for animal but not human use was detected in taco shells in supermarkets. Even before GMOs, there was concern about increasing mono-culture and loss of biological diversity. In nature, diversity adds strength to ecosystems, while loss of diversity makes them more vulnerable to pressures such as climate change (see Chapter 15: Environment).

Regulations on GMOs vary among countries. The European Union seems to be the most restrictive, with no approvals granted since 1998 and 12 applications pending (WHO, 2014). The topic remains controversial.

11 Nutritional Concerns of the Developing World

The main nutritional concerns for the developing world have been

- Insufficient clean drinking water
- Insufficient food energy
- Insufficient protein

Currently, however, many developing countries have a rapidly growing middle class whose aspirations and purchasing power have created lifestyles much like those in Canada and other developed countries—motorized transportation, sedentary leisure, and more meat, oil, convenience food, calories, fat, and so on in their diet. The following section refers to the huge number of people in developing countries who remain poor.

11.1 *Water*

In many developing countries, perhaps only one-third of town dwellers have access to sufficient clean (i.e., free of pathogens) drinking water. Villagers often walk long distances to carry water from a stream or well, which increases their energy requirements. Alternatively, they boil dirty water to sterilize it. This takes fuel, which is also often in short supply. Over-cutting of trees for firewood leads to erosion. The loss of topsoil decreases soil fertility, which decreases agricultural yields, compounding the problem of food shortage.

It is estimated that 17 of the 25 main water-related diseases found in the developing world could be reduced 50% to 100% simply through provision of ample safe water. Education regarding the need to separate sewage disposal from drinking water and provision of reliable sources of drinking water (e.g., wells or pipes to carry water from remote streams) are simple, low-cost solutions to this problem.

11.2 *Energy and protein*

Inadequate energy (calories) and protein impair growth. Classic evidence in support of this phenomenon is provided by observations of Asian immigrants to North America. Children born in North America are often much taller than their parents, who grew up in China or Japan or Vietnam, because of the higher protein and calorie content in the Western diet. In addition to outright starving to death, under-nutrition can damage health in many ways. Small females have more difficulty delivering babies through the smaller birth canal, thus increasing the risk to both mother and baby. In addition, small mothers bear smaller babies, who have higher infant mortality rates, especially in countries without the sophisticated medical systems that can keep very premature or small babies alive in Canada. Targeting food supplements to mothers and children is part of the World Health Organization's strategy of providing primary (meaning basic) health care. Ironically, in many households in developing nations, the men traditionally eat first and the women eat what is left.

Under-nutrition increases susceptibility to disease. The cells that make up the immune system need energy and protein for growth and repair. It is estimated that 50% of all childhood mortality in the developing world is caused by insufficient food. For example, in Latin America 10% of childhood deaths are attributed to measles; in 60% of these cases, malnutrition is a contributing cause. Some types of diseases, in turn, contribute to malnutrition. For example, parasitic infections may destroy the intestinal wall, decreasing the ability to digest and absorb nutrients.

> Have *you* visited a poor section of a developing country such as Mexico or India or China or Nigeria?
>
> If so, how does what you experienced on that visit compare with the discussion in the preceding section?

12 Conclusion

The central nutritional issues in both the developing and industrial worlds are more social and political than scientific or technical. There is ample information on which to act. Individuals in the industrial world can take control and make better nutritional choices. It does take some effort and skill to separate fact from myth in nutritional claims and avoid the hype around "miracle foods." The key seems to lie in maintaining a sensible diet in our busy, complex, consumer-oriented modern society. In the developing world, progress seems to depend more on political changes to decrease inequities and on social and economic development to improve the general standard of living. There is, however, considerable scope for action at the community level with small-scale agricultural innovations to increase the local food supply.

Study Questions

1. What is the difference between "digestion" and "metabolism"?
2a. What are the six categories of essential nutrients?
2b. Which two of these are normally the main source of energy?
3. In a single short sentence, describe the general opinion expressed in this chapter regarding how to meet one's nutritional needs.
4. What four factors are implicated in the excesses in the modern North American diet—that is, what are the social causes of these excesses?
5. According to the 2015 Canadian Health Measures Study, how are Canadians in general doing with each of the following:
    - Protein
    - Fats
    - Carbohydrates
6a. Name six things the dietary guidelines for North Americans recommend reducing in the typical diet.
6b. Name six things these guidelines recommend increasing in the typical diet.
7. Identify the main functions and the richest sources of each of the following:
    - Protein
    - Carbohydrate
    - Fat
    - Calcium
    - Iron
    - Fibre
8a. What is the difference between a vegetarian and a vegan?
8b. Discuss the benefits and the potential problems associated with vegetarian diets.
9a. What are "organic" foods? That is, what is different about the way organic food is produced compared with non-organic food?
9b. According to the Winter & Davis report, how do organic foods compare with non-organic foods?
10. What are the three main nutritional issues for poor people living in developing countries?
11. To what social and political issues does the author refer in the conclusion to this chapter?

Glossary

amino acids—the building blocks of proteins
anemia—low blood levels or tissue stores of iron

calorie—a unit of energy; specifically, the amount of energy required to raise one kilogram of water by one degree C

carcinogen—a cancer-causing substance

diet—food and drink regularly provided and consumed

digestion—the process by which the foods and beverages we consume are broken down

lacto-ovo vegetarians—people who choose not to eat flesh but will eat milk products and eggs

metabolism—the complex set of chemical changes in living cells that provides energy and material for vital processes

nutrition—the act or process of nourishing or being nourished

osteoporosis—a condition in which bone density is decreased; the bones become more fragile and more easily fractured

toxin—poison; fatal when consumed in large enough amounts

vegans—people who choose to eat no animal products

Additional Resources

Health Canada (2011) Eating Well With Canada's Food Guide.
http://www.hc-sc.gc.ca/fn-an/food-guide-aliment/index-eng.php

USDA (United States Department of Agriculture), National Agricultural Library Dietary Reference Intakes (2010 values) http://www.iom.edu/Activities/ Nutrition/SummaryDRIs/~/media/Files/Activity%20 Files/Nutrition/ DRIs/5_Summary%20Table%20Tables%201-4.pdf
These eight pages of tables specify values for people at different stages of life: infancy, youth, pregnancy, lactation, older age, etc.

Food-A-Pedia
https://www.supertracker.usda.gov/foodapedia.aspx
This interactive calculator gives you the nutritional content of thousands of different food items that you either type in or select from a list.

References

Bonjour, J. P. (2011). Protein intake and bone health. International Journal for Vitamin and Nutritional Research. 81(2–3), 134–142.

Buchner J. (2016). Results from the Canadian Living Nutrition Survey. Canadian Living. Retrieved May 4, 2018 from http://www.canadianliving.com/health/nutrition/ article/results-from-the-2015-canadian-living-nutrition-survey

Craig, W. J., Mangels, A. R. (2009). Position of the American Dietetic Association: vegetarian diets. Journal of the American Dietetic Association. 109(7), 1266–1282.

Frenk, D. J. (ca. 2010). Health gains from whole grains. Harvard School of Public Health. Retrieved February 22, 2013 from http://www.hsph.harvard.edu/nutrition- source/ health-gains-from-whole-grains/

Goran, M. I., Ulijaszek, S. J., Ventura, E. E. (2013). High fructose corn syrup and diabetes prevalence: A global perspective. Global Public Health. 8(1):55064.

Health Canada. (2006). Canadian community health survey cycle 2.2, nutrition (2004) a guide to accessing and interpreting the data. Ottawa, ON: Office of Nutrition Policy and Promotion Health, Products and Food Branch. Retrieved July 29, 2014 from http://www.hc-sc.gc.ca/fn-an/surveill/nutrition/commun/cchs_guide_escc-eng.php. Health Canada. (February 2, 2009). General questions and answers on trans fat. Retrieved July 29, 2014 from http://www.hc-sc.gc.ca/fn-an/nutrition/gras-trans-fats/tfa-age_question-eng.php

Hui A. (2017). As Canadians consume 'harmful' levels of sodium, officials urge chefs to limit salt but face resistance. The Globe and Mail. Retrieved May 4, 2018 from https://www.theglobeandmail.com/news/national/salt-sodium-health-canada-guide-liberal-restaurant-industry/article37023811/

Moeller, S. M., Fryhofer, S. A., Osbahr, A. J. III, Robinowitz, C. B. (2009). The effects of high fructose syrup. Journal of the American College of Nutrition. 28(6):619-626.

Mozaffarian, D., Ludwig, D. S. (2015). The 2015 US Dietary Guidelines: Lifting the Ban on Total Dietary Fat. Journal of the American Medical Association. 33(24):2421-2422.

Statistics Canada. (2017a). Health Fact Sheets: Nutrient intakes from food, 2015. Retrieved May 4, 2018 from http://www.statcan.gc.ca/pub/82-625-x/2017001/article/14830-eng.htm. Statistics Canada. (2017b). Canadian Community Health Survey – Nutrition: nutrient intakes from food and nutritional supplements. Retrieved May 4, 2018 from http://www.statcan.gc.ca/daily-quotidien/170620/dq170620b-eng.htm

Thorpe, M. P., Jacobsen, E. H., Layman, D. K., He, X., Kris-Etheron, P. M., Evans, P. M. (2008). A diet high in protein, dairy, and calcium attenuates bone loss over twelve months of weight loss and maintenance relative to a conventional high-carbohydrate diet in adults. Journal of Nutrition. 138(6), 1096–1100.

USDA. (January 31, 2011). USDA and HHS announce new dietary guidelines to help Americans make healthier food choices and confront obesity epidemic. (News Release). Washington, DC: United States Department of Agriculture. Retrieved July 29, 2014 from http://www.fns.usda.gov/pressrelease/2011/004011

USDA. (2010). Dietary guidelines for Americans: Executive summary. Washington, DC: United States Department of Agriculture). Retrieved February 27, 2013 from http://www.cnpp.usda.gov/publications/dietaryguidelines/2010/policydoc/execsumm.pdf

Winter, C. K., Davis, S. F. (2006). Organic foods. Journal of Food Science. 71(9), R117–R124. Institute of Food Technologists, The Society for Food Science and Technology. Scientific Status Summary.

World Health Organization. (2014). 20 questions on genetically modified foods. Retrieved May 19, 2014 from http://www.who.int/foodsafety/publications/biotech/20questions/en

8 Body Weight and Weight Management

Learning Objectives

By the time you have finished this chapter you should be able to

- Differentiate between "overweightness," "overfatness," and "obesity"
- State the overall prevalence of obesity or overweight in North America and trends in prevalence
- Identify subgroups at higher risk of being overweight or obese
- Describe the methods of determining ideal weight and the limitations of each
- Explain the problems associated with unsound weight-loss diets
- Discuss the three main eating disorders
- Summarize the guidelines for sensible weight control
- Discuss the health consequences of excess body weight from a holistic perspective
- Outline a broad strategy to address the health problems associated with body weight

1 Overview

Body weight and weight control are major health concerns today, and not just in industrial nations but, increasingly, in the growing middle and upper classes of developing countries. This is a complex health concern because both medical and social issues are involved. There is also an incredible amount of information and misinformation regarding obesity and weight control, and it is often difficult to separate facts and half-truths from blatant manipulations of emotions and pocketbooks.

2 Definitions of *Overweight, Overfat,* and *Obese*

The definitions of "overweight," "overfat," and "obese" all derive from the concept of an **ideal weight**. A person is considered *overweight* if he exceeds this ideal, or criterion, **weight**. Similarly, if a person exceeds her recommended percentage of body **fat** by a certain margin, she is considered to be *overfat. Obesity* is "a large excess" above overfatness.

It is possible to be overweight without being overfat. Professional football players, weightlifters, bodybuilders, and other individuals who are very muscular often exceed ideal weight recommendations but have a low percentage of body fat. On the other hand, it is also possible to be overfat without being overweight.

A number of years ago, I measured the body fat levels of a group of Vancouver office workers as part of an employee fitness program. Most of the female staff were close to their ideal weight, but carried an "excess" (I'm using quotation marks because the whole notion of what is considered excessive is subjective) of 2 to 5 kg (about 5 to 10 lb.) of body fat. These females had maintained their body weights by careful dieting, but they were mostly sedentary, so their muscles had shrunk. Consequently, they looked good in clothes, and they felt satisfied when they stepped on the scales, but they had too much body fat and not enough muscle.

3 Methods of Determining *Ideal Weight*

3.1 Height-weight tables

Life insurance companies have published tables that show "ideal weight" for males and females of various heights and frame sizes. Perhaps the best-known height-weight tables are those produced by the Metropolitan Life Insurance Company in the United States. This company first published its tables in 1942 and issued updated tables in 1959 and again in 1983. The 1983 edition revised the ideal weights upward for most categories.

Life insurance companies are interested in assessing statistical risk so that the company can determine how much to charge for life insurance premiums. A client pays a yearly or monthly premium to the life insurance company, similar to the premium that a person pays for automobile insurance. When the policyholder dies, the life insurance company pays a lump sum to the family or estate of the policyholder. If the amount that the average policyholder pays to the company during his lifetime (plus the money the company makes on investing this money) is less than the average settlement the company pays to the survivors, the company loses money. Therefore, life insurance companies are interested in predicting how long a person will live, and they have determined that longevity is related to body weight.

Sample height-weight tables are available online at http://www.ideal-weight-charts.com/healthy-weight-chart.html. A footnote to the tables explains that people were measured wearing shoes with 1-in. heels and street clothing weighing 3 lb. for females and 5 lb. for males, presumably because this is quick and easy for the person making the measurement. Therefore, to find your ideal weight from these tables, measure your height without shoes and add one inch. For example, a female who measures 5'4" (163 cm) tall in bare feet (5'5" or 165 cm in shoes) and who has a "medium frame" should weigh 127–141 lb. (58–64 kg) while wearing indoor clothing, or 124–138 lb. (56–63 kg) without clothing.

There are a number of problems with height-weight tables, the most glaring of which is that they don't consider differences in **body composition**; that is, they don't look at body fat, just body weight. Thus, a person who is muscular but lean may be classified as overweight by these tables.

> According to these tables, for your height, how much should *you* weigh — remember that these tables give height in shoes and weight in indoor clothing?
>
> How does this compare with your actual weight? What do you think? Do the tables correctly classify *your* "ideal weight"?

3.2 *Body mass index (BMI)*

Another approach to "ideal weight" is the ***body mass index***, which equals (body mass in kg)/ (height in metres)^2.

Body mass index is commonly used in studies because it's based on data that are easy to obtain—height and **body mass** (weight). Many studies that use BMI are based on **self-reported** height and weight; that is, the respondents give their height and weight rather than having these measured by a research assistant. BMI calculated from self-reported data is, on average, lower than that calculated from **measured data**; people tend to under-report their weight or over-report their height. This finding has important implications for research, and indicates that studies where the respondents are seen in person will tend to be more accurate than those that collect data by mail, telephone, or Internet.

BMI classifications for ideal weight, underweight, overweight, and obese are based on **epidemiological data**, which, you will remember from Chapter 2: Evaluating Health Claims, refers to observational studies of populations rather than controlled scientific experiments. These classifications are presented as ranges (CDC, 2015):

Underweight	BMI less than 18.5
Normal or healthy weight	BMI 18.5 to 24.9
Overweight	BMI 25.0 to 29.9
Obese	BMI 30.0 or higher

In other words, this won't give a precise "most healthy" weight for an individual. For a height of 178 cm, (5'10") the "normal or healthy" BMI range corresponds to weights of between 59 and 79 kg (129 and 174 lb.). This is a *large range*.

> What is *your* BMI? Does it fall within the "healthy" zone?
>
> To calculate your BMI, measure your height in metres (1 m= 100 cm; 1 inch = 2.54 cm). For example, 5'10" = 178 cm = 1.78 m.
>
> Now, square this (i.e., multiply it by itself). For example, 1.78 × 1.78 = 3.17.
>
> Now, divide that into your body weight in kilograms (1 kg = 2.2 lb.). For example, 165 lb. = 75 kg, so 75 ÷ 3.17 = 23.7 BMI.

A limitation of BMI is that it says nothing about body composition, like how much of the weight is muscle versus fat. It also doesn't indicate the distribution of body fat. **Abdominal obesity,** or excess fat carried around the waist (also known as an apple-shaped body), is associated with greater health risks than excess fat on the hips and thighs (a pear-shaped body). Also, excess fat around the internal organs (heart, kidneys, liver, etc.) poses more health risk than excess fat under the skin.

> *Is there a more accurate way than BMI to determine if you are overweight?*

Yes.

First, let's consider the issue of *overweight*—overweight relative to what?

From a medical point of view, "overweight" means a weight at which risk of disease and premature death is increased. There are significant health risks associated with overweight. "Both overweight and obesity ... contribute to heart disease, hypertension, diabetes, and some cancers as well as psychosocial and economic difficulties" (Donnelly et al., 2009).

"Obesity is a significant risk factor for and contributor to increased morbidity and mortality, most importantly from cardiovascular disease (CVD) and diabetes, but also from cancer and chronic diseases, including osteoarthritis, liver and kidney disease, sleep apnea [this means difficulty breathing], and depression" (Pi-Sunyer, 2009).

Other criteria of "overweight" are more **subjective,** such as the weight at which you feel you look good and feel good about yourself. You probably already have a sense of what that weight is for you. For me, overweight means (a) my pants fit too tightly at the waist and I need to let my belt out a notch, (b) I don't like the way my belly sticks out when I see a photograph of myself, or (c) my wife says, "You're getting fat."

Now, let's look at some other methods of determining "ideal weight."

3.3 *Waist circumference (girth)*

A World Health Organization report (2011) gives a thorough discussion of waist circumference and BMI as predictors of CVD, other diseases, and all-cause mortality (Figure 8.1). "It has been suggested that waist circumference, waist-hip ratio, and waist-height ratio, which reflect abdominal adiposity, are superior to BMI in predicting CVD risk" (WHO, p. 15). The report concludes that waist circumference and waist-hip ratio are similarly accurate predictors of abdominal obesity. Because measuring hip circumference is technically more difficult than measuring the waist, waist circumference alone is a more practical measure than waist-hip ratio (WHO, p. 26).

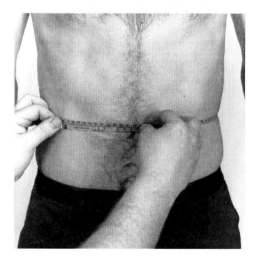

Figure 8.1. Location for measurement of waist circumference.

Waist circumference tells us something about the amount of fat around a person's middle, including the fat below the skin and the fat deeper in the abdomen. For example, I measured a middle-aged man's waist girth as 112 cm (44 in.), which is 18 cm above the recommended upper limit of 94 cm. His abdominal skinfold thickness measured 8 cm, or about four times the thickness for a "healthy" person. Even so, his subcutaneous fat only accounted for 8 of the 18 cm of excess waist girth. Presumably, the other 10 cm of extra girth consisted of fat deposits around his internal organs. I have seen MRI images of a person with a large abdomen. An MRI is like an X-ray, but it shows many different tissues while X-rays only show bone. The MRI showed this deep fat as fist-sized white lumps inside the abdomen.

The WHO report also notes, "The evidence with regard to anthropometric measures—in particular, waist circumference or waist-hip ratio measures and all-cause mortality—is predominantly from white European and American adults ..." (WHO, p. 16). "Chinese and South Asian men and women display a greater amount of visceral adipose tissue for a given waist circumference than Europeans" (WHO, p. 10). The same is true for East Asians (p. 10). Conversely, African populations have less visceral adipose tissue for a given waist circumference (WHO, p. 10).

Diabetes Canada (2018) gives the following criteria for waist circumference (values above these cut-points represent increased risk):

Women	> 80 cm
Europid men	> 94 cm
Asian or South Asian men	> 90 cm

> What is *your* waist circumference?
> How does this compare with the cut-points presented above?
> Remember, 1 in. = 2.54 cm. For example, 34 in. = 86 cm. This is below the 94 cm upper limit for "Europid" men.

There are other, potentially more accurate ways of determining body density or body composition. I will briefly describe a few here.

3.4 Skinfold thickness

The thickness of pinches of skin and fat lying under the skin can be measured quite reliably and objectively with special sensitive spring-loaded calipers that look like large pliers (Figure 8.2). These reflect changes in weight gain or loss due to exercise and diet. Various equations have been developed to predict body density from skinfolds measured at six or so sites around the body. One limitation of the skinfold method is that the fat under the skin is only part of the total fat. There are also fat deposits around the heart, kidneys, and abdominal organs.

3.5 Body density by hydrostatic weighing

Density is the mass of an object relative to its volume. Mass is easy to measure with a weighing scale. You can measure volume by submerging the object in a container of water (you need a container about the size of a telephone booth to

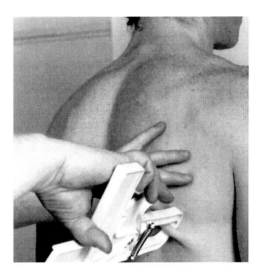

Figure 8.2. Clinician measuring skinfold thickness over the scapula (shoulder blade). Note how the left hand grasps and controls the skinfold as the right hand holds the caliper.

do this with a person). The volume of water displaced (pushed upward) equals the volume of the object. The body density of a population can be correlated with mortality (or with success in athletic performance, such as gymnastics).

3.6 Whole body electrical impedance

This measures the resistance to the flow of a mild electrical current through the body. This method is based on the low electrical conductance of body fat compared with other tissues because fat has a low water content. So a person who conducts electricity poorly is inferred to have a higher percentage of body fat. Estimated body fat percentages for a population can be correlated with mortality, among other things.

3.7 Dual-energy X-ray absorptiometry (DXA)

DXA aims two X-ray beams of different energies at the patient's or subject's body. It is primarily used to measure bone density. It can also be used to measure body fat content. I think the accuracy of this method for estimating body fat is similar to the hydrostatic weighing method described above.

3.8 CAT scan or MRI

Computed axial tomography (CAT, also called computed tomography, or CT) and magnetic resonance imaging (MRI) are widely used imaging methods for diagnosis of fractures or tumours. CT or MRI can also be used to produce a picture of a two-dimensional "slice" through the subject's abdomen. Special computer software then calculates the areas of subcutaneous and abdominal fat deposits and estimates the total mass of these deposits. See, for example, Shen et al. (2007) and Mourtzakis et al. (2008).

4 Prevalence of Obesity

Prevalence of obesity is high and apparently increasing. According to Wei et al. (2007) the age-standardized prevalence proportion of obesity in Canada has increased from 10% in 1970 to 23% in 2004. Statistics Canada (2011) compared obesity rates in Canada with those in the USA. A total of *24% of Canadians* were considered obese (BMI 30.0 or higher) compared with *34% of Americans*. There was no real difference between male and female obesity rates in Canada, but in the USA women were more likely than men to be obese (36% vs. 33%).

Note that the preceding figures do not include those who are "overweight" (BMI 25.0 to 29.9). When overweight people are counted with those who are obese, the resulting prevalence is higher.

Using the body mass index criteria presented earlier in this chapter, Statistics Canada concluded that in 2015, 27% of Canadian adults were "obese." An additional 35% of Canadian adults were "overweight." The good news is that reported levels of obesity in Canadian children and youth dropped from 13% in 2004 to 12% in 2015 (Vogel, 2017). The use of BMI probably underestimates the size of the problem. An estimated 85% of men, 69% of women, 48% of boys, and 44% of girls were "overfat" (Vogel, 2017).

5 Causes of Obesity

In Chapter 7: Nutrition, you read about the following aspects of modern society that contribute to excess body weight:

- Affluence
- High food availability
- Advertising
- Perceived shortage of time

Metabolic factors, such as malfunctions of the thyroid gland, which regulates metabolic rate, are responsible for less than 2% of all cases of obesity.

The hormone **leptin** plays an important role in regulating energy intake and expenditure. Leptin acts on the brain to inhibit appetite. Blood levels of leptin are proportional to body fat content. However, fasting for a day lowers leptin levels, even though body fat levels do not change much in that time. A very small number of humans have a genetic disorder that causes them to be unable to synthesize leptin, causing them to experience chronic hunger, eat enormous amounts, and become huge. Logically, treatment of obese people with external doses of leptin should suppress appetite and eating, and therefore reduce body fat. However, so far this has only been shown to work with very high leptin doses and for very obese people.

There is clearly some **family factor** in obesity. Children of obese parents are more likely to be obese as adults than are children of normal-weight parents. This may be partly caused by learned eating behaviours.

Think about the way *your* family eats, or the way they ate when you lived with them.

List several of your current eating behaviours that you developed during this period. For example,

a) Do you always have a set mealtime, such as dinner at 6:00 p.m.?

b) Do you have to eat all of your vegetables before you can have dessert?

c) Do you eat at the dining room table, or in the living room in front of the television?

d) Do you serve plates in the kitchen and then bring them to the table, or are the serving bowls placed on the dining room table?

e) Do you eat in your bedroom?

The ***set point theory*** says that each individual's body weight or percent body fat is maintained within quite narrow limits around a point, called the *set point*. For example, in one study, prison volunteers were fed up to 8,000 kcal/day. The average adult male probably requires about 2,700 kcal to meet all of his energy requirements. So 8,000 kcal is a lot of food. Some of the subjects in this study gained weight on this diet, but others did not gain any weight. Furthermore, those who didn't gain weight showed an increased **metabolic rate**. These results were interpreted as evidence that the bodies of those who didn't gain weight maintained a set percentage of body fat by automatically increasing the rate at which the calories in the food they ate were converted to body heat.

Energy balance obviously plays a role in weight gain and loss. Energy balance compares the number of kcal of energy consumed in a day with the number of kcal of energy expended in muscular activity and basic metabolic processes (Figure 8.3). Energy requirements are higher for larger people, more active people, and during growth periods such as childhood, adolescence, and pregnancy. Average adult females and males need about 2,200 and 2,700 kcal per day, respectively.

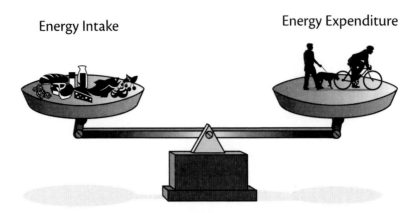

Energy Intake   Energy Expenditure

Figure 8.3. If the energy consumed in food exceeds the energy expended in metabolism and physical activity, theoretically a person will gain weight. Conversely, weight loss will (theoretically) occur if energy expenditure exceeds energy consumption.

One kg of body fat stores about 7,700 kcal. Therefore, if you consumed 100 kcal (equivalent to about 15 ml, or one tablespoon, of butter) more than you need each day, in 77 days, you would gain one kilogram of fat. This equals 4.7 kg (about 10 lb.) per year.

The energy balance concept makes a lot of sense, but it is obviously an over-simplification of reality. You probably know two people who are the same sex, age, size, and activity level, but one can eat anything she wants without gaining weight, while the other has to eat very carefully to avoid weight gain.

In Chapter 6: Physical Activity, you read about the increasingly inactive life of those living in North America and other industrialized parts of the world.

Psychological and cultural factors appear to play an important role in the onset of obesity. Food has powerful psychosocial meaning. Food represents love, happiness, and security. When guests come, we offer them food and drink. Birthdays and holidays are celebrated with food—often special foods and larger quantities. Food consoles us when we feel bored, depressed, sad, or lonely. A coffee and doughnut provide a break from the routine at work. So, we eat not just to satisfy our physical needs but other needs as well.

Cohen (2008) argues that the prevalence of overweight in North America today is not due to some recent change in humans' genetic makeup, or a failure of self-control, but rather to several combined influences, including

- "Hard-wired," **intrinsic responses**, such as seeing food, seeing other people eat, being unable to accurately judge calorie content or portion size, inherently preferring sweets and fats, and so on

- An environment loaded with **eating cues**
- **High availability and affordability** of food, especially fast food, 24/7
- **Aggressive advertising** by food and beverage companies

6 Social Issues Regarding Obesity

A review by Puhl & Heuer (2009) concluded that "fatism" is alive and well. For example,

> Obese people were much more likely than normal-weight people to report employment discrimination: being the target of derogatory humour from coworkers, not being hired, not being promoted, and being fired.
>
> More than half of doctors surveyed had viewed their obese patients as awkward, unattractive, ugly, and non-compliant. A third of these physicians also labeled obese patients as weak-willed, sloppy, and lazy. Some studies have shown that obese people on average achieve lower educational levels, e.g., being less likely to advance from high school to college. There is some evidence that educators may be biased against obese students as early as elementary school.
>
> In another study, college students indicated that they would prefer a hypothetical sexual partner that was in a wheelchair, missing an arm, had mental illness, or had a history of sexually transmissible infection rather than an obese person.

Each of the many studies compiled in the Puhl & Heuer review has its limitations. However, collectively this is such a large body of evidence that it seems highly likely it speaks to a real phenomenon—society is prejudiced against obese people.

Not surprisingly, attitudes toward body size and weight, whether one's own or others', varies among socio-cultural groups.

In an international study of over 4,000 women and over 3,000 men from 41 sites in 26 countries, subjects were shown a series of nine line drawings of women's bodies arranged and numbered from one (smallest) to nine (largest). Men were asked to select the line drawing they perceived as the most physically attractive (yes, the study has an inherent heterosexual bias). Women were asked to select the line drawing that (a) they perceived as the most physically attractive to men of their own age, (b) they thought most closely approximated their current body, and (c) they would most like to possess (Swami et al., 2010). Prominent findings of this study were

- Body dissatisfaction and desire for thinness were commonplace in high-socioeconomic settings (SES) across world regions.
- In two countries where both a high-SES and a low-SES site were sampled (Malaysia and South Africa), heavier bodies were preferred in the low-SES sites.
- Men across all world regions except East Asia selected a significantly heavier figure as being most physically attractive compared to what women believed was most attractive to men.

A different survey of over 4,000 German adults age 25 to 74 reported that women (48%) were more likely than men (33%) to be dissatisfied with their body weight. Among respondents of normal weight, the odds of being dissatisfied were similar across socioeconomic groups for both sexes. However, among "pre-obese" and obese men, the probability of body weight dissatisfaction was associated with socioeconomic status. This socioeconomic-dissatisfaction association was less evident for obese and "pre-obese" women (Lengerke & Mielck, 2012).

From another part of the world, Israel, in a survey of almost 1,400 Jewish and Arab women aged 21 years or older, 39% of the Jewish women reported body weight dissatisfaction, compared with only 29% of Arab women. Among older overweight-obese respondents, Arab women were less likely to be dissatisfied with their body weight than Jewish women. However, this difference between Arab and Jewish women was not observed among younger normal-weight respondents (Niskar et al., 2009).

> Is this surprising? Why or why not?
> What about *you?* How do you feel about *your* body weight, size, and shape?

It will be interesting to see how this issue unfolds. It is easier to sustain social prejudice against visible minorities. A single fat child is an easy target for school bullies. As mentioned above, Puhl & Heuer (2009) report that obesity can be a barrier to educational advancement. However, they note "in schools where female obesity was more prevalent, obese students had the same chance of attending college as nonobese students" (p. 949). In other words, when obese people are less of a minority, there seems to be less prejudice against them. Epidemiologists tell us the prevalence of obesity is increasing, among children as well as adults. As obesity becomes the "new normal," will social prejudice toward obese people decrease?

Why are we so obsessed with image?

Humans are social animals. As I understand it, humans in all societies modify their appearance with clothing, headgear, body marking, jewellery, and other accessories. These signify to others our place in society: rank, kinship, age, marital status, and so on. So it is natural for humans to care about their image.

In some societies (e.g., Pacific Islanders) being large and fat is a mark of affluence and high status. Perhaps the implication is that one becomes fat through abundant food and minimal work, both of which require wealth.

Modern Western society has equated thinness with affluence: "you can never be too rich or too thin."

One could also suggest that we are so obsessed because we are somewhat insecure and disconnected from the happiness and self-esteem that come from feeling loved and accepted, feeling we belong, and having satisfying social relationships. Maybe some of this is a consequence of materialism. Corporate advertising plays on this by implying that if you had a new car, new clothes, a new hairstyle, a thinner body, *then* you would be happier. Such happiness tends to be superficial and temporary. So, we buy more things.

In my opinion, positive responses to the obsession with body image are to

- Help people to feel more accepting of themselves and other people
- Focus less on body size, shape, or weight and more on healthy behaviours such as healthy eating (regular, balanced meals) and physical activity as integral parts of daily living

7 Unsound Weight-Loss Dieting

Fad diets have long been a popular method of weight reduction. The belief is that some special food or combination of foods will magically help you lose weight. Every issue of every women's magazine seems to contain a new diet secret. If there were a secret, don't you think it would be well known by now? The reason for the continued stream of new fad diets is that none of them work. You should be suspicious of unrealistic claims such as "Lose 10 pounds in 7 days," "Eat anything you want and still lose weight," or "Get rid of ugly fat painlessly by eating just these few foods." These promises are usually empty.

There are problems with fad diets:

- Most of these fad diets are simply a **disguise for a low-calorie diet**. Single-food diets such as the hard-boiled egg diet are boring, so people tend to eat less.
- Some fad diets are successful at inducing a rapid weight loss initially because they promote a **loss of body water** by increased urination. This water is readily replaced. Anyway, weight reduction should focus on loss of excess body fat, not water.
- Fad diets are usually **not nutritionally balanced**. They usually do not contain enough servings from all of the four food groups.
- Fad diets often involve **too severe a reduction in caloric intake**. Approximately 1,200 kcal of energy are required per day simply to meet minimal metabolic requirements. Canada's Guidelines for Healthy Eating recommends a minimum of 1,800 kcal per day.
- Prolonged or repeated strict dieting can actually **lower the basal metabolic rate**, which means the individual may gain weight despite a marked reduction in caloric intake. A small minority of people can diet successfully, but most people have poor long-term success.
- Fad diets cannot be maintained for the **long term**. If people stay on the diet for a number of weeks, they may become nutritionally deficient. On the other hand, once people stop eating according to the fad diet, they usually resume their previous eating habits and regain the weight they lost.

> Have *you* tried any of the preceding diet strategies to lose weight? How did that work for you?

8 Eating Disorders

With eating disorders, *food is not the issue*. The abnormal eating behaviour may be a way of dealing with uncomfortable emotions, including the shame and anger associated with sexual abuse, low self-esteem, or a desire to feel control over some aspect of life. Though people with eating disorders are often above-average performers in school, they are also often insecure and depend upon others for approval. Eating disorders affect all ethnic groups, and are more common among LGBTQ people. Eating disorders have the highest mortality rate of any mental illness (ANAD, 2018). Treatment of eating disorders should be interdisciplinary, addressing medical, psychological, and familial issues.

8.1 Anorexia nervosa (AN)

This eating disorder is characterized by

- Inability to maintain body weight within 15% of ideal weight
- Intense fear of getting fat
- Distorted body image such that the individual thinks she is fat even when she is extremely skinny
- Denial or lack of insight into the cause and seriousness of the weight loss

Anorexia means "lack of appetite," while **nervosa** classifies this as a psychiatric disorder rather than a physical problem with the digestive system. Weight loss is often very extreme and affects virtually all organ systems.

Incidence rates of AN are highest among females aged 15 to 19, who make up approximately 40% of all cases (Smink, van Hoeken & Hoek, 2012). Lifetime prevalence of AN is slightly less than 1% among females (ANAD, 2018). **Lifetime prevalence** is a little different than prevalence. **Prevalence** expresses what portion of a population *have* a disorder. *Lifetime* prevalence means "have the disorder now, or used to have it, or will have it at some time in their lifetime." Anorexia is much less common among males (Duckworth & Freedman, 2013a). However, "many recent community-based studies have found that AN is more common among males than previously thought" (Smink, van Hoeken & Hoek, 2012).

AN can cause fatigue, insomnia, hair loss, cessation of menstruation, intolerance to cold, constipation, osteoporosis, low blood pressure, fainting, and irregular heartbeat (Mayo Clinic, 2012). It can also interfere with normal adjustment to pubertal development, and can lead to social isolation, family conflict, depression, or alcoholism.

Mortality risk is elevated for *all* eating disorders, especially AN. One in five individuals with AN who died had committed suicide (Smink, van Hoeken & Hoek, 2012; ANAD, 2018). "Anorexia nervosa has the highest mortality rate of any psychiatric illness, both due to the complications of malnutrition and the high rate of suicide in this population" (Duckworth & Freedman, 2013a).

8.2 Bulimia nervosa (BN)

This disorder features episodes of **binge eating** followed by **purging** with self-induced vomiting or laxatives. **Bulimia** comes from the Greek word for "great hunger." During a binge, the person feels out of control and usually continues binging until he runs out of food, is interrupted by someone, or develops abdominal discomfort. After the binge, the individual feels physically and emotionally drained, ashamed and disgusted with herself, and fearful of weight gain from what she has eaten.

Bulimia seems to be more common than anorexia. BN is harder to detect than AN because the bulimic individual usually conceals his eating behaviour and gets enough food between purges to maintain a fairly normal weight (Duckworth & Freedman, 2013b). The National Association of Anorexia Nervosa and Associated Disorders (2018) estimates lifetime prevalence of BN among US women at 1.5%. Prevalence of BN may be as high as 3%; most of these people are female, but at least 10% are male (Duckworth & Freedman, 2013b).

The medical risks of BN are less serious than for AN, but are not trivial:

- Stomach acid in vomit can erode tooth enamel.
- There can be damage to the stomach or the esophagus, the tube that connects the mouth with the stomach.
- Dehydration and disturbed body electrolyte (salt) balance can cause irregular heartbeat and even death (Duckworth & Freedman, 2013b).

Smink, van Hoeken, & Hoek (2012) report that, in the studies they reviewed, suicide accounted for 23% of deaths in BN patients.

8.3 Purging disorder and binge eating disorder (BED)

Lifetime prevalence of binge eating disorder (BED) in Americans is 2.8%. More than half of patients with BED also have an anxiety disorder (ANAD, 2018). (We will learn more about this in Chapter 9: Mental Health.) BED may be relatively common among adolescents, and compared with other eating disorders, it is more common among males and older individuals. "BED is often seen in obese individuals, but is distinct from obesity per se regarding levels of psychopathology, weight and shape concerns and quality of life. BED aggregates strongly in families independently of obesity, which may reflect genetic influences" (Smink, van Hoeken & Hoek, 2012, pp. 407 and 412).

9 Guidelines for Sound Weight Control

Safe, sensible, effective long-term weight control involves four elements (Figure 8.4, next page).

9.1 Physical activity

The obvious benefit of increased physical activity is increased **caloric expenditure**, which helps tip the energy balance equation in favour of a caloric deficit. The rate at which exercise "burns up" calories depends on the type and intensity of exercise and on the subject's body mass; 500 kcal/hour is a reasonable average figure.

> It is likely that any increase in physical activity (PA) has the potential for weight loss; however, it seems that PA <150 min·wk⁻¹ results in

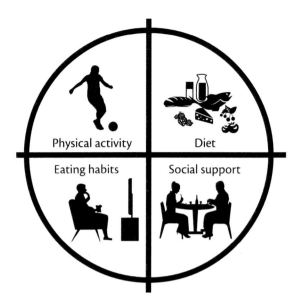

Figure 8.4. The four keys to long-term control of body weight.

> minimal weight loss compared to controls, PA >150 min·wk⁻¹ results in modest weight loss of ~2–3 kg, and PA between 225 and 420 min·wk⁻¹ results in 5- to 7.5-kg weight loss. Thus, a dose effect is apparent for PA and weight loss, and higher doses are capable of providing 3% or greater weight loss from initial weight. (Donnelly et al., 2009)

There are several other benefits in addition to the calories expended during exercise:

- **Metabolic rate** remains elevated for many hours after exercise, causing a further expenditure of energy.
- Exercise helps to **maintain muscle mass**, ensuring most of the weight lost will be fat loss. Approximately half of the weight lost as a result of caloric restriction in the absence of increased physical activity is a loss of muscle mass. Since muscle is a very metabolically active tissue, muscular people expend more energy per day from their resting metabolism.
- Exercise can **improve the appearance** of one's figure by toning and firming muscle. Untrained people who begin an exercise program often report no change in body weight for a number of weeks, presumably because they are losing body fat but also adding muscle. However, because muscle is denser than fat, body *size* will decrease although

body *weight* doesn't. One loses centimetres instead of kilograms, and centimetres are more related to appearance than kilograms are.

• Exercise helps **relieve depression and anxiety**, which are emotions that factor significantly into overeating.

Regularity is key. As you read in Chapter 6: Physical Activity, "activity" can include many things besides going to the gym to lift weights, ride the exercise bicycle, or do aerobics classes. For example, it can include walking the dog, hiking, dancing, playing Frisbee, shooting a basketball, washing the car, climbing stairs rather than taking the elevator, playing with kids, and so on. Choose activities you enjoy, because you are more likely to stick with them than if you choose things you don't like but think you *should* do because they are "good for you."

The **duration** of an activity is more important than intensity when weight reduction is the goal. Ideally, be active at a moderate pace of an hour or more. This does not have to be all in one sustained period. Periods as short as ten minutes each, accumulated over the day, works almost as well for weight loss.

Resistance training (RT) alone will *not* promote clinically significant weight loss. It may or may not promote fat loss; studies seem evenly split on this issue. When combined with aerobic exercise, RT may lead to greater weight loss than aerobic exercise alone. RT combined with caloric reduction (i.e., dieting) is effective for weight loss, mainly due to the effect of the dieting (Donnelly et al., 2009).

Overweight people should be encouraged to be active, and large people can do most of the same activities as those of normal weight. Large people may be self-conscious about their bodies, and it may help to have a large instructor.

The emphasis should be on **increased work capacity**, improved muscle tone, and feeling better, not weight loss.

9.2 Diet

According to the American College of Sports Medicine, physical activity alone has a modest effect on weight loss unless the volume of activity is quite high. Virtually all experts recommend combining physical activity with diet for weight control (Donnelly et al., 2009).

> **Which foods are typically the best to obtain leanness?**

This question seems a bit misguided. In my opinion, it is more useful to think of the *overall diet* than specific foods. Despite what some magazine covers promote—"I lost 10 pounds in 10 days on the grapefruit diet" or "Five foods to avoid if you want to lose belly fat"—I don't think there are any "magic" foods for weight loss.

So, thinking in terms of diet, the way to obtain leanness is through

- **An overall deficit in calories.** There should be fewer calories of food energy coming in than the number of calories the body uses.
- **A modest deficit in caloric intake** rather than a drastic deficit. Caloric intake should be at least 1,200 kcal/day.

    A moderate reduction in caloric intake can be sustained over a period of time. This is better than a drastic reduction for a week or two followed by a resumption of previous eating patterns. A sensible plan is to reduce intake by up to 500 kcal (this will be a reduction of about 15% or 20% from the calories you are currently eating if you are maintaining weight). A 500kcal/day reduction should, theoretically, result in a loss of about 0.4 kg (about one pound) of body fat per week.

    A drastic reduction in caloric intake is more likely to trigger changes in metabolism that cause the body to become more conservative in energy expenditure. Drastic dieting is also more likely to produce feelings of hunger, deprivation, and craving, which make one more likely to binge eat.
- **Regular meals.** Eating three or four times a day is preferred to skipping meals and eating a single larger meal, which may promote energy storage in the form of body fat. Some sources recommend eating four of five smaller meals throughout the day rather than three larger meals. Regular meals also reduce variations in blood levels of glucose and fatty acids, thus keeping energy levels high and suppressing appetite. Those who refrain from eating all day are more likely to overeat and actually consume more calories in a day.
- **A balanced diet.** A diet with a variety of foods is better than a diet that focuses on a few foods (e.g., grapefruit or hard-boiled eggs) or that eliminates certain categories of foods (e.g., a very low-carbohydrate diet).

    For the most part, eliminate empty-calorie or low-nutrient-density foods, such as snack foods (candy, chocolate, chips, sugared beverages), sugar and cream in coffee or tea, butter on toast, and alcohol. You notice I use the phrase, "for the most part." A diet that includes some "treats," such as an occasional pizza, ice cream, or piece of chocolate cake, is one you will more likely stick with than a more rigid diet that completely eliminates such foods.

- **Lower-fat food options**. Choose skim milk rather than whole (homo) milk, and cottage cheese rather than cheddar cheese; cut fat from meat before cooking it; skin chicken; eat toast dry rather than buttered; use mustard rather than mayonnaise on sandwiches; eat pickles for snacks instead of peanuts; use lemon juice rather than oil on salads.
- **Lower-fat cooking methods**. Microwave, steam, roast, or broil rather than frying or deep-frying (e.g., boiled eggs, broiled fish, and roasted chicken).
- **Eating lots of fruits and vegetables**. These are good sources of many vitamins and minerals. Many vegetables are also high in fibre, which contributes to a sensation of fullness. This is especially true of lettuce and celery, which are very low in calories.
- **Conscious eating habits,** as outlined in Section 9.3.

9.3 Eating habits

Developing conscious eating habits means not only changing the *content* of your diet but also the *way* you eat. Behaviours such as eating at your desk while working, eating in the car while driving, and eating while watching television may cause you to eat more than you need or want to. Habit is a main factor in determining what, when, and where we eat. You may find it interesting to keep a record for a week of all of the different locations and situations in which you eat, to raise awareness of unconscious, habitual eating behaviours.

- **Use smaller plates.** The same portion of food on a small plate may appear larger than on a larger plate.
- **When you eat, pay attention to your eating.** Don't watch TV or read during meals. It is easy to overeat when you are eating unconsciously.
- **Eat slowly.** Chew each bite thoroughly, and put your utensils down between bites. It takes about 20 minutes for the sensation of fullness to offset appetite.
- **Take a break after a meal.** Do something else for a while, such as going for a short walk. This will give time for your food to register as fullness in your stomach and to elevate your blood sugar level.
- **Try to be sensitive to the cues** in your environment that you associate with eating and overeating, and change your environment to remove unwanted eating cues.
- **Make healthy eating convenient.** Put cookies in closed containers in the cupboard, and leave cut vegetables, such as carrots and celery, in plain view inside the refrigerator.

- **Serve in the kitchen** and put leftovers away right after the meal is finished. Leaving serving plates on the dinner table is an open invitation to take unwanted second helpings.
- **Don't go shopping while hungry.** It is a dangerous habit. The hungry shopper is more vulnerable to advertising and more likely to come home with expensive, high-calorie snack foods—and is also likely to eat some of these on the way home!

9.4 Social support

When you are working toward a goal, it can help to get support from friends, family members, or others working with issues similar to yours. Support can come as encouragement ("You're doing great!"), advice ("Here's something that worked for me"), help in problem-solving ("In what situations do you feel most vulnerable? Why do you think that is? How does it feel when you ...?"), or just empathetic listening when you are feeling discouraged or frustrated.

Support groups for dieters, such as the well-known Weight Watchers organization, typically meet regularly to discuss members' problems and to share their successes. Group members may be asked to "weigh in" at each meeting, with prizes awarded to those who have lost the most weight in a certain time period. Between meetings, members who have difficulty following their diet plan are encouraged to telephone other members for support.

10 Conclusion

Many factors influence eating behaviours, energy consumption, energy expenditure, and weight gain. Most cases of obesity are *not* caused by metabolic or glandular dysfunction. There is apparently a genetic factor that influences body fatness. This genetic factor may act through a set point for percentage body fat, through growth of fat cells during critical growth periods, and through factors influencing metabolic rate. On the other hand, there is also clearly an environmental factor in obesity. Eating and activity behaviours are learned, often from other family members. These behaviours are culturally influenced and psychologically reinforced, and they may become habitual.

A large minority of North Americans are obese and, consequently, at increased risk of medical problems. Weight loss is possible with a combined approach of exercise, change in diet, change in eating behaviours, and group support.

However, many standards for "ideal weight" are arbitrary and subjective, not based on increased health risk. "Ideal weight" does not account for differences in body composition, and body composition is difficult to assess with validity. Many forms of weight loss are unhealthy. Most people experience poor long-term success with weight-loss programs. Therefore, *prevention* of obesity, particularly in small children and adolescents, through diet and regular physical activity seems important.

There is considerable stress associated with the constant desire to lose weight, and with failure at weight loss. Rather than trying to estimate people's percentage of body fat and advise them of how much fat they need to lose, the efforts of health professionals might be better spent in attempting to

- Change the prejudices against the obese through education
- Help women deal effectively in a society that places undue importance on beauty
- Focus on healthy eating and active living rather than on weight loss itself

Study Questions

1. Explain the difference between "overweight," "overfat," and "obese."
2a. Discuss the concept of "ideal weight."
2b. Describe the different methods of determining ideal weight, and discuss the limitations of each.
3a. What is the trend in prevalence of obesity in North America?
3b. What is the current estimated prevalence of obesity in Canada and in the United States?
3c. How do prevalence estimates derived from self-reported height and weight compare with estimates obtained from directly measured height and weight?
4. Discuss the multiple factors that contribute to obesity and overweight.
5a. State the energy balance equation.
5b. How many kcal excess is associated with a gain of 1 kg of body fat?
5c. Suggest why the equation correctly predicts weight gain or loss for some people but not others.
6. Describe the limitations and problems associated with unsound weight-loss dieting.
7a. Explain the difference between anorexia nervosa and bulimia.
7b. Outline the health risks associated with each.
7c. Explain what is known about the causes of these eating disorders.
8. What are the four key ingredients for sensible weight loss or weight control?
9a. Discuss the advantages of physical activity with respect to weight control.
9b. Give an exercise prescription for weight control. Include type, frequency, intensity, and duration of exercise.
10a. What rate of weight loss (pounds per week) is considered realistic and healthy?

10b. What dietary suggestions would you give a person who is trying to lose weight?

11. Outline the health consequences of being overweight in North America. Use a holistic definition of health; that is, include the physical, psychological, and social consequences. Differentiate between problems associated with obesity and those associated with moderate overweightness.

Glossary

abdominal obesity—excess fat carried around the waist (the apple-shaped body), which is associated with greater health risks than excess fat on the hips and thighs (the pear-shaped body)

anorexia nervosa—an eating disorder that consists of an intense fear of getting fat, a distorted body image such that the individual thinks she is fat even when she is extremely skinny, and a lack of insight into the cause and seriousness of the weight loss

body mass index—a simple ratio of weight for height; equals (body mass in kg)/(height in metres)^2

bulimia nervosa—an eating disorder that features episodes of binge eating followed by purging with self-induced vomiting or laxatives

obesity—a "gross excess" (often 20% or 30% in excess) of body weight or body fat

overfat—the state of exceeding one's recommended percentage of body fat by a certain margin

overweight—the state of exceeding one's criterion weight by a certain percent (e.g., 10%) or amount (e.g., 5 kg)

set point theory—the set point theory postulates that each individual's body weight or percent body fat is maintained within quite narrow limits around a point, called the set point

Additional Resources

Vancouver Coastal Health Eating Disorders Program
   2750 East Hastings Street, Vancouver
   V5K 1Z9
   Tel: 604-675-2531
   http://vch.ca/403/7676/?program_id=13776

Kelty Resource Centre
   BC Mental Health & Addiction Services
   PHSA Research & Networks
   Mental Health Building 2
   BC Children's Hospital

Room P3-302 - 4500 Oak Street

Mail box # 69

Vancouver, BC v6H 3N1

604-875-2084

604-875-3688

1-800-665-1822

keltycentre@bcmhs.ca

http://www.bcmhas.ca/keltyresourcecentre

For help with eating disorders, contact the Kelty Resource Centre—a provincial resource centre for children, youth, and their families with mental health and addiction concerns, including people of all ages struggling with eating disorders or related issues.

References

ANAD (National Association of Anorexia Nervosa and Associated Disorders). (2018). Eating Disorder Statistics. Retrieved May 4, 2018 from http://www.anad.org/education-and-awareness/about-eating-disorders/eating-disorders-statistics/

CDC (Centres for Disease Control and Prevention). (2015). Assessing Your Weight. Retrieved May 4, 2018 from https://www.cdc.gov/healthyweight/assessing/index.html

Cohen, D. A. (2008). Neurophysiological pathways to obesity: Below awareness and beyond individual control. *Diabetes.* 57, 1768–1773.

Diabetes Canada. (2018). Waist circumference. Retrieved May 4, 2018 from https://www.diabetes.ca/diabetes-and-you/healthy-living-resources/weight-management/waist-circumference

Donnelly, J. E., Blair, S. N., Jakicic, J., Manore, M. M., Rankin, J. W., Smith, B. K. (2009). Appropriate physical activity intervention strategies for weight loss and prevention of weight regain for adults. *Medicine and Science in Sports and Exercise.* 41(2), 459 –471.

Duckworth, K., Freedman, J. L. (January, 2013a). *Anorexia nervosa.* National Alliance on Mental Illness. Retrieved April 22, 2014 from http://www.nami.org/Content/ContentGroups/Helpline1/Anorexia_Nervosa.htm

Duckworth, K., Freedman, J. L. (January, 2013b). *Bulimia nervosa.* National Alliance on Mental Illness. Retrieved April 22, 2014 from http://www.nami.org/Content/Navigation-Menu/Inform_Yourself/About_Mental_Illness/By_Illness/Bulimia_Nervosa.htm

Katzmarzyk, P. T. & Mason, C. (2006). Prevalence of class I, II and III obesity in Canada. *Canadian Medical Association Journal.* 174(2),156–157.

Lear, S. A., James, P. T., Ko, G. T., et al. (2010). Appropriateness of waist circumference and waist to hip ratio cutoffs for different ethnic groups. *European Journal of Clinical Nutrition.* 64(1), 42–61.

Lengerke, T., Mielck, A. (2012). Body weight dissatisfaction by socioeconomic status among obese, probese and normal weight women and men: results of the cross-sectional KORA Augsburg S4 population survey. *BMC Public Health.* 12:342.

Mayo Clinic. (January 5, 2012). Anorexia nervosa: Symptoms. Retrieved March 1, 2013 from http://www.mayoclinic.com/health/anorexia/DS00606/DSECTION=symptoms

Mourtzakis, M., Prado, C. M., Lieffers, J. R., Reiman, T., McCargar, L. J., Baracos, V. E. (2008). A practical and precise approach to quantification of body composition in cancer patients using computed tomography images acquired during routine care. *Applied Physiology, Nutrition, and Metabolism.* 33:997–1006.

Niskar, A., Baron-Epel, O., Garty-Sandalon, N., Keinan-Boker, L. (2009). Body weight dissatisfaction among Israeli Jewish and Arab women with normal or overweight-obese body mass index. *Preventing Chronic Disease.* 6(2), A51. Retrieved April 22, 2014 from http://www.cdc.gov/PCD/issues/2009/apr/08_0118.htm

Pi-Sunyer, A. (2009). The medical risks of obesity. *Postgraduate Medicine.* 121(6):21-33.

Puhl, R., Heuer, C. A. (2009). The stigma of obesity: A review and update. *Obesity.* 17, 941–964.

Shen, W., Punyanitya, M., Chen, J., Gallagher, D., Albu, J., Pi-Sunyer, X., Lewis, C. E., Grunfeld, C., Heymsfield, S. B., Heshka, S. (2007). Visceral adipose tissue: relationships between single slice areas at different locations and obesity-related health risks. *International Journal of Obesity.* 31(5), 763–769.

Smink, F. R. E., van Hoeken, D., Hoek, H. W. (2012). Epidemiology of eating disorders: Incidence, prevalence, and mortality rates. *Current Psychiatry Reports.* 14, 406–414.

Statistics Canada. (June 21, 2011). Adult obesity prevalence in Canada and the United States. Retrieved March 1, 2013 from http://www.statcan.gc.ca/pub/82-625-x/2011001/article/11411-eng.htm

Swami, V., Frederick, D. A., Aavik, T., et al. (2010). The Attractive Female Body Weight and Female Body Dissatisfaction in 26 Countries Across 10 World Regions: Results of the International Body Project I. *Personality and Social Psychology Bulletin* 36(3), 309–325.

Vogel, L. (2017). Overweight or overfat? Many Canadians are both. *Canadian Medical Association Journal.* 189(37):E1202-E1203. Retrieved January 9, 2018 from http://www.cmaj.ca/content/189/37/E1202

Wei, L., Morrison, H., de Groh, M., Waters, C., DesMeules, M., Jones-McLean, E., Ugnat, A-M., Desjardins, S., Lim, M., Mao, Y. (2007) The burden of adult obesity in Canada. *Chronic Diseases in Canada.* 27(4), 135–144. Retrieved April 1, 2008 from http://www.phac-aspc.gc.ca/publicat/cdic-mcc/27-4/index.html

WHO. (2011). Waist circumference and waist-hip ratio: Report of a World Health Organization expert consultation, Geneva, December 8–11. Retrieved January 21, 2013 from http://whqlibdoc.who.int/publications/2011/9789241501491_eng.pdf. The authors of this report credit Professor Scott Lear from SFU's School of Kinesiology with "substantial support and inputs."

Zilberter, T. (December 20, 2011). Carbohydrate-biased control of energy metabolism: the darker side of the selfish brain. *Frontiers in Neuroenergetics.* Volume 3, Article 8, pp. 1–4.

9 Mental Health

Learning Objectives

By the time you have finished this chapter you should be able to

- Describe the qualities of "self-actualized" people
- Outline the process of growing up psychologically
- Explain the role of defence mechanisms in psychological health
- Describe the key features of common psychological disorders
- Discuss suicide, including the epidemiology, risk factors, and prevention
- Differentiate stress from distress
- List different types of stressors
- Explain the general adaptation syndrome model of stress
- Summarize recommendations regarding stress management
- Identify changes you can make that will help you sleep better
- Summarize current research on gratitude and mental health

1 Overview

Recently, Western thinkers have recognized the connection between the mind and body. The body is not just a life-support system that carries around our brain. Poor blood flow to parts of the brain (e.g., because of atherosclerosis) affects the way we think and feel. The pain caused by physical injury interferes with concentration and relaxation. Nutritional deficiencies or substance use can impair the functioning of the mind. On the other hand, through the autonomic nervous system (ANS), thoughts and feelings are reflected physically. Muscles around blood vessels tense and relax, altering blood flow, nutrient supply, and temperature of different regions. Glands secrete hormones that alter metabolism. A positive mental attitude can enhance immune system activity, while anger and tension can suppress it. So, developing optimal mental wellness should be just as much a priority as maintaining a healthy body weight and good aerobic fitness.

2 Mental Health

Much literature focuses on mental *illness*. It is harder to define mental *wellness*. It is more than being "normal," because this just means being close to average. If everyone were the same, life would be very boring. Diversity in the way people think and act makes society more interesting, richer, and more powerful. Abraham Maslow looked into mental wellness by studying a group of successful people who seemed to be living their lives to the fullest. He called these *self-actualized* people—people who had fully realized their mental and emotional potential in life.

Maslow found his group of self-actualized people shared certain qualities:

- They had a realistic but positive self-image and self-esteem.
- They largely accepted themselves and others for who they were.
- They were autonomous, meaning they acted on the basis of their own values and feelings, rather than bending to peer pressure or trying to fit someone else's ideal.
- They responded to life in a genuine and spontaneous way.
- They were capable of intimacy, willing to be vulnerable and expose their thoughts and feelings to others.
- They were creative, playful, and embraced change.

The path to self-actualization starts in childhood. Having a stable environment with consistent parenting, feeling safe and protected, and being loved and respected all help build a strong foundation for psychological health. Infants believe the world revolves around them and others exist solely to satisfy their needs. As we grow up, we realize others have feelings and rights too, and we learn to cooperate and share.

Throughout childhood, we are quite dependent on our parents. As we mature through adolescence, we develop our own identity, built around our core values and beliefs, which may differ from our parents' values and beliefs. This process of *individuating* and separating from our parents is one of the major challenges of the teenage years.

Honest communication is central to asserting our own wishes and needs. It is also the way we gain an understanding of and appreciation for others. Sometimes we don't get what we want. For example, maybe we have secret sexual feelings for our high school English teacher. We know we can't act on these feelings. Various psychological *defence mechanisms* may come into play to protect us:

- We may fantasize that our love object has feelings for us, even though nothing the person has said or done would indicate this.
- We may repress our feelings, refusing to acknowledge them consciously.
- We may sublimate, which means we channel these unacceptable urges into socially acceptable activities, such as sports or studying.

Such defence mechanisms can help us cope in the short term. However, they are obstacles to achieving ultimate resolution of the conflict.

3 Psychological Disorders
3.1 Schizophrenia

Schizophrenia is characterized by disordered thinking. This may cause the individual to seem confused, not make sense when he is talking, act inappropriately, have visual or auditory hallucinations (e.g., see things that are not really there, hear voices ordering him to do something), or have delusions, such as being persecuted, being invulnerable, or having a personal mission to save the world (NIMH, 2013c).

Schizophrenia usually starts in the late teens to early adulthood, although it is increasingly being recognized in childhood (NIMH, 2013c). Schizophrenia is one of the most devastating mental disorders. Medical authorities used to think that bad parenting was the cause of schizophrenia. Now, it is recognized as a developmental brain disorder. Even with the best of current treatments, most people with schizophrenia never fully recover. They are often unable to hold a job or take care of themselves (NIMH, 2013c).

There are two common stereotypes about schizophrenia that are incorrect:

- **Multiple personalities:** It is true that some people with schizophrenia think and behave as if two or more different people or personalities were living within their body. However, this is extremely rare. Most psychiatrists will never encounter a case of multiple personality.
- **Serial violence:** It is true that people with schizophrenia can behave in bizarre and unpredictable ways. Sometimes they *are* violent. When this happens, it is almost never premeditated, but rather is the result of acting out against something they've seen or heard incorrectly (e.g., they may think a caregiver is actually an enemy agent sent to imprison them). Psychopathic killers are extremely rare.

3.2 Depression

Mood and anxiety disorders are the most common mental illnesses in Canada, with an estimated prevalence of over 11% (Mental Health Commission of Canada, 2012). Depression is the most common ***mood disorder.*** Most people have felt depressed at some time. Clinical depression, known as **major depressive disorder,** is more restricted. As defined by the *Diagnostic and Statistical Manual of Mental Disorders* (APA, 2013), the diagnosis of depression requires that five or more of the following symptoms be present during the same two-week period and represent a change from previous functioning. At least one of the symptoms must be either depressed mood or loss of interest or pleasure.

- **Depressed mood most of the day**, nearly every day. In children and adolescents, this can be irritable mood.
- **Markedly diminished interest or pleasure** in all, or almost all, activities most of the day, nearly every day.
- **Significant weight loss** when not dieting, or weight gain (e.g., a change of more than 5% of body weight in a month), or decrease or increase in appetite nearly every day. Note: In children, this can be failure to make expected weight gains.
- **Insomnia or hypersomnia** (i.e., being unable to sleep or sleeping a lot, respectively) nearly every day.
- **Psychomotor agitation or retardation** nearly every day.
- **Fatigue or loss of energy** nearly every day.
- **Feelings of worthlessness** or excessive or inappropriate guilt nearly every day.
- **Diminished ability to think or concentrate**, or indecisiveness, nearly every day.
- **Recurrent thoughts of death** (not just fear of dying), recurrent suicidal ideation without a specific plan, or a suicide attempt or a specific plan for committing suicide.

In addition, the diagnosis of depression requires that the symptoms

- **Cause clinically significant distress** or impairment in social, occupational, or other important areas of functioning.
- **Are not due to the direct physiological effects of a drug** or a general medical condition.
- **Persist for longer than two months** or are characterized by marked functional impairment, morbid preoccupation with worthlessness, suicidal ideation, psychotic symptoms, or psychomotor retardation.

Many people with depression also have anxiety. Clinicians generally regard such anxiety as a good sign, because it means the individual hasn't simply accepted her depressed mood.

It is now understood that many people with depression have lower brain levels of a ***neurotransmitter*** called serotonin. Neurotransmitters are chemicals that are produced naturally by the body and released from nerve cells, which change the excitability of different regions of the brain. One class of drugs used to treat depression (e.g., Paxil, Effexor) works by increasing serotonin levels at the connections between brain cells.

> Do *you* know someone who has had serious (clinical) depression? What did they do about this (i.e., how did they manage it)? How did this work for them?
>
> (Section 5 of this chapter outlines treatment for mental health problems. The Additional Resources section may also be useful.)

3.3 *Bipolar disorder*

People with this disorder (formerly called **manic depression**) experience dramatic mood swings between the manic and depressive states. As described above for depression, the depressive phase is characterized by intense sadness or despair, loss of interest in activities formerly enjoyed, loss of energy, disturbance of sleep (too much or too little) and appetite (increase or decrease), difficulty concentrating, and thoughts of death or suicide (APA, 2014a).

By contrast, the manic phase presents as (APA, 2014a)

- **Abnormally and persistently elevated**, expansive, or irritable mood
- **Inflated self-esteem** or grandiosity
- **Decreased need for sleep**
- **More active and talkative** than usual; possibly agitated.
- **Excessive involvement in pleasurable activities** that have a high potential for painful consequences (e.g., engaging in unrestrained buying sprees, sexual indiscretions, or foolish business investments)

If untreated, bipolar disorder can severely damage relationships, work, and school. The good news is that it's highly treatable, through a combination of psychotherapy and medications called **mood stabilizers** (APA, 2014a).

3.4 *Anxiety disorders*

There are many potential causes of anxiety disorders. Family history and genetics predispose some people to getting an anxiety disorder. Increased stress and inadequate coping mechanisms to deal with that stress may also contribute to anxiety. Anxiety symptoms can result from a variety of factors, including having had a traumatic experience, having to face major decisions in one's life, or having developed a more fearful perspective on life.

3.4.1 Generalized anxiety disorder (GAD)

This condition is much more than the normal anxiety people experience day to day. It's chronic and exaggerated worry and tension, even though nothing seems to provoke it. People with GAD can't seem to shake their concerns, even though they usually realize their anxiety is more intense than the situation warrants.

People with GAD seem unable to relax. They often have trouble falling or staying asleep. Their worries are accompanied by physical symptoms, especially rapid pulse, irregular heartbeat, trembling, restlessness, muscle tension, sweating, dry mouth, stomach complaints, numbness, difficulty concentrating, dizziness, and headaches. GAD can also cause sleep disorders (IQWiG, 2011).

3.4.2 Panic attack

A *panic attack* is a specific period of intense fear or discomfort. During a panic attack, the person may experience rapid and strong heart rate, sweating, weakness, faintness, or dizziness. The hands may tingle or feel numb. The person may feel flushed or chilled, have chest pain or smothering sensations, a sense of unreality, or fear of impending doom or loss of control. The individual may genuinely believe he's having a heart attack or stroke, is losing his mind, or is on the verge of death (NIMH, 2013a).

3.4.3 Panic disorder

People with *panic disorder* have feelings of terror that strike suddenly and repeatedly with no warning. Not everyone who experiences panic attacks will develop panic disorder; many people have one attack but never have another. In panic disorder, the attacks occur repeatedly and unpredictably. Many people with panic disorder develop intense anxiety between episodes, worrying when and where the next one will strike. It is important for those with panic disorder to seek treatment. Untreated, the disorder can become very disabling (NIMH, 2013a).

3.4.4 Social anxiety disorder

Social anxiety disorder (also known as *social phobia*) is an intense fear of becoming humiliated in social situations, specifically of embarrassing oneself in front of other people. Social phobia often begins around early adolescence or even younger. The most common social phobia is a fear of public speaking.

This disorder is not the same as shyness. Shy people can be very uneasy around others, but they don't experience the extreme anxiety in anticipating a social situation, and they don't necessarily avoid circumstances that make them feel self-conscious. In contrast, people with social phobia aren't necessarily shy at all. They can be completely at ease with people most of the time, but particular situations, such as walking down an aisle in public or making a speech, can give them intense anxiety. Social phobia can be quite disabling, interfering with career or social relationships.

People with social phobia are aware their feelings are irrational. Still, they experience dread before facing the feared situation, and they may go out of their way to avoid it. Even if they manage to confront what they fear, they usually feel very anxious beforehand and are intensely uncomfortable throughout. Afterward, the unpleasant feelings may linger, as they worry about how they may have been judged or what others may have thought or observed about them.

3.4.5 Other phobias

Many people experience specific phobias—intense, irrational fears of certain things or situations, such as dogs, closed-in places, and heights.

> Do *you* know someone with a specific phobia?
>   If so, how does this affect her life?

3.4.6 Obsessive-compulsive disorder

People with obsessive-compulsive disorder (OCD) experience persistent, unwanted thoughts. The sufferer recognizes these persistent images are a product of his own mind and are excessive or unreasonable, but he cannot stop these images by logic or reasoning. Instead, these thoughts lead to *compulsions* (urges to do something to lessen discomfort) and *rituals*, such as cleaning for hours or repeatedly checking to insure the door is locked. The **obsessions** and **rituals** significantly interfere with the person's routine, making it difficult to work or to have a normal social life or relationships (NIMH, 2013b).

4 Suicide

4.1 Epidemiology

Over 4,000 Canadians kill themselves every year, which makes suicide the ninth leading cause of death nationally (Statistics Canada, 2015). Because suicide rates for Canadian males are consistently higher than for females (about 18 vs. 6 per 100,000 population, respectively) (Statistics Canada, 2018), suicide ranks as the seventh leading cause of death for males and the 11th for females (Statistics Canada, 2015).

Suicide rates are higher than the national average in certain demographic subgroups:

- **Canadian First Nations youth.** Suicide rates are 5 to 7 times higher for First Nations youth than for non-Indigenous youth. Inuit youth suicide rates are 11 times the national average (Government of Canada, Indigenous Services, 2018).
- **Gays and lesbians.** Males are six times more likely and females twice as likely to attempt suicide compared with their heterosexual counterparts.
- **Those in custody**, including jail and prison.
- **Those who have attempted suicide** before.
- **Older people**, ages 45 to 59 (Statistics Canada, 2018).
- **Adolescents.** Suicide is the second leading cause of death in Canadians age 15 to 24 (Health Canada, 2016). Cheung & Dewa (2006) report that depression and suicidality are common in adolescents, with lifetime prevalence rates of over 7% for depression and over 13% for suicidality. Females seem more affected: 11% of females had depression (vs. 4% for male) and 18% of females had suicidality (9% males). Male adolescents, however, consistently have higher rates of *completed* suicides, a finding attributed to the male tendency to choose more lethal means (e.g., hanging and firearms vs. pills).

> Although suicide rates are highest for older Canadians, suicide ranks higher as a cause of death among younger Canadians; it is the second leading cause of death among those age 15 to 24, while it is only the ninth most-common cause of death overall.
>
> How do you account for this apparent discrepancy?
>
> What do you think is the leading cause of death for Canadians age 15 to 24?

4.2 Risk factors

Cohesion in society decreases suicide, while social disorganization promotes it. There is some evidence that suicide is correlated with unemployment. Mental disorders, particularly mood disorders, and especially **depression**, are associated with suicide. Some 30% to 70% of those who complete suicide had depression. **Substance abuse** is the other major risk factor. Poor relations with parents and a stressful life event, such as death of a parent or breakup of a relationship, also increase risk of suicide.

4.3 Prevention

A number of strategies at the community and national level can help prevent suicide:

- **Improve societal conditions**, including unemployment, prejudice, and marginalization.
- **Implement school-based programs** to improve coping and life skills.
- **Decrease availability and lethality of means of suicide**, such as firearms and lethal doses of prescription drugs.
- **Provide general education** to decrease the sense of shame or disgrace associated with seeking treatment, especially in males, for whom seeking help in time of crisis may be seen as a weakness.
- **Target interventions to high-risk groups**, such as older males during the year following the death of their spouse.
- **Fund crisis and suicide prevention centres** (see the Additional Resources section at the end of this chapter).

> *What should you do if you are concerned a person might be suicidal?*

- Express concern; show love and caring.
- Encourage them to talk.
- Ask them direct questions, such as "Are you thinking about suicide?"
- Encourage them to get professional help.
- If the person is in immediate danger, don't leave her alone.
- In an emergency, call the Crisis Centre (see Additional Resources near the end of this chapter).
- At most universities or workplaces, contact the Health, Career, and Counselling Services (see Additional Resources).

5 Treatment for Mental Health Problems

Psychological disorders can have a medical cause or component. A thorough **medical exam** is often indicated before beginning psychological or psychiatric care.

Hospitalization is indicated in the acute phase of schizophrenia or other serious disorders, with regular follow-up care after discharge. In British Columbia, the closure of hospitals has caused many mentally ill people to be discharged into the community.

Medication is a primary treatment option for depression, bipolar disorder, and schizophrenia. Some medications work right way, while others take weeks of regular use to become effective. Often the individual must continue taking medication regularly even after symptoms improve. Compliance is an issue in the outpatient population. Many medications have side effects, such as drowsiness, weight gain, and interference with sexual functioning. Once a person has been taking his medications long enough for the symptoms of the psychological disorder to subside, it is tempting to discontinue the medication because of these side effects. This usually causes the symptoms of the psychological disorder to return.

Electroconvulsive therapy (ECT) is electric shock given to the brain to cause seizure. ECT is often effective in severe depression, catatonic schizophrenia (a rare type in which the patient appears to be awake but makes no voluntary movement), and in some cases of *mania* when other treatments are unsuccessful. ECT is not used as much these days, even though the modern procedure is much safer than earlier approaches. "Much of the stigma attached to ECT is based on early treatments in which high doses of electricity were administered without anesthesia, leading to memory loss, fractured bones and other serious side effects" (Mayo Clinic Staff, 2012).

Education can help patients and those close to them understand the effects of the disorder and how to cope.

Balanced nutrition, regular physical activity, and **adequate rest** are good self-care strategies to help restore and to maintain mental health.

Self-help groups are groups in which patients and families support each other. Self-help groups are also discussed in Chapter 8: Weight Management and Chapter 13: Drugs.

Professional therapy or counselling can be done individually, with groups of patients, or with the patient and his family. There are many different philosophies and styles of so-called talk therapy. Before starting a therapeutic relationship with a mental health professional, it is useful to learn a little about the professional's background, philosophy, and therapeutic style (see the Additional Resources section near the end of this chapter). It is also important that you feel comfortable working with that particular person, a feeling that may take more than one session to establish.

6 Stress

One of the first people to study stress scientifically was Dr. Hans Selye (born Vienna 1907; died Montreal 1982). Dr. Selye defined *stress* as any event or situation that disrupts the body's normal homeostasis and precipitates changes directed at re-establishing this homeostasis (Selye, 1956). *Homeostasis* is the state of dynamic equilibrium or balance that the body normally maintains. For example, homeostasis includes the regulation, within fairly narrow limits, of body core temperature, blood levels of oxygen and acidity, and cellular concentrations of salts. This allows optimal functioning of the human organism.

6.1 General adaptation syndrome

Humans experience many different *stressors*, or things that cause stress. These stressors include

- **Psychological stressors:** anxiety, fear, excitement, or even joy
- **Physiological stressors:** pain, cold, exercise, hunger, trauma
- **Environmental stressors:** pollution, noise, poverty, and prejudice

Dr. Selye labelled the body's response to stress the **general adaptation syndrome**, or GAS. A *syndrome* is a group of symptoms that commonly occur together and that may be diagnostic for a certain condition. The term "general adaptation" suggests this group of symptoms is the typical way that the body responds to any stressor, regardless of the nature of the particular stressor.

The general adaptation syndrome starts with the **alarm stage**, which features activation of part of the *autonomic nervous system* (ANS). The ANS is responsible for "housekeeping" duties, such as circulation, respiration, digestion, and metabolism. Fortunately, we do not have to consciously will our heart to beat. If we did, our mind would be fully occupied with just staying alive—and what would happen when we fall asleep? The ANS spares higher centres in the brain for reasoning, memory, creativity, and so on. In the alarm stage, there is an increase in

- Heart rate and blood pressure
- Rate and depth of respiration
- Skeletal muscle tension
- Blood levels of glucose and fatty acids, fuels for muscular work
- The rate at which blood clots

In addition,
- Blood is shifted away from the gut and into the skeletal muscles.
- Digestion slows.
- The **adrenal glands** (which rest on top of each kidney) secrete **epinephrine** (adrenaline) and **norepinephrine**. These hormones circulate throughout the body in the blood and add to the stimulating effect of the nervous system.

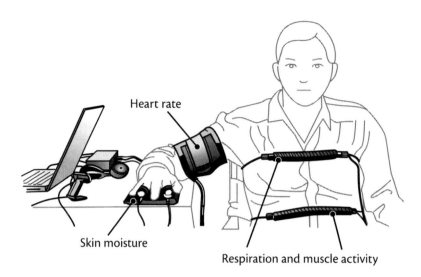

Heart rate

Skin moisture

Respiration and muscle activity

Figure 9.1. The polygraph, or "lie detector," measures a number of physiological responses that change when one is stressed, such as when lying.

It may help you remember the alarm stage if you think of the polygraph, or "lie detector" (Figure 9.1). This machine has been designed to detect small changes in a number of the physiological responses that occur during the alarm stage. The polygraph records heart rate, breathing rate and depth, sweatiness of the palms, and so on. When people lie, their bodies often betray them with involuntary physiological signs.

The alarm stage has sometimes been called the **flight-or-fight response**. When our prehistoric ancestors were confronted by danger, they could either fight or run away. Modern life is more complicated. For example, if your boss dumps a load of work on your desk an hour before the end of work on Friday, you may want to run away or punch her, but neither of these responses would be considered socially correct. Instead, you probably grit your teeth and say "Yes, ma'am," even though physiologically you are aroused.

Repeated or prolonged exposure to a stressor triggers the responses of the second stage of the general adaptation syndrome, the stage of **resistance**. In the resistance stage, a hormone called **cortisol** is secreted in increased amounts by the adrenal glands. Dr. Selye noted that laboratory animals exposed to prolonged stress had enlarged adrenal glands. The elevated cortisol inhibits the release of substances that cause inflammation. Prolonged elevations in cortisol levels cause a number of undesirable effects, including reduced synthesis of protein, connective tissue and bone, weakened immune system, and delayed wound healing.

It is incorrect to think of this stage as a successful resolution of the stress, or as psychological coping with the stressor. The stress has *not* gone away. On the surface, behaviour may suggest that the stressor is no longer having an effect on the body. However, chemical changes are taking place in the body during this stage. These changes may lead to breakdown and illness.

If the stress is too great for too long, the final stage of exhaustion sets in. In this stage, the body reserves are used up and the body is more susceptible to disease. Cardiovascular disease, colds and other infections, headaches, digestive problems, insomnia, and back pain all may be caused or worsened by excessive stress.

6.2 Stress or distress

Some authors discuss stress in terms of "good stress" and "bad stress." Selye focused more on the similar way in which the body processes stressors. He felt it was the *sum total* of all the recent stressors that determines whether you are over-stressed (which is bad, and is thus called *distress*), under-stressed (which is also *distress*), or optimal (*eustress*) (Selye, 1975).

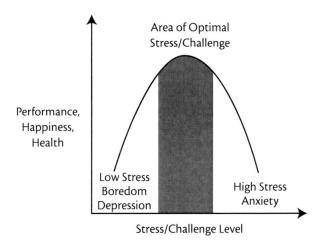

Figure 9.2. The relationship between stress and health. Above and below an optimal level of stress, health suffers. The optimal level varies among people.

Dr. Selye emphasized that stress is not necessarily bad. We need a certain amount of stress to function optimally and, in fact, to stay alive. The right amount of stress helps us perform better. On the other hand, too much stress (distress) causes us to perform worse and may compromise our health (Figure 9.2). When you are very angry, your heart races, your hands shake, your voice trembles, and it is very difficult to think or speak clearly. Perhaps you have seen an athlete "choke" in competition because he was over-aroused. Maybe you have studied hard for an examination and know the material well, but do poorly because you are so nervous you can't think clearly or you forget to answer some of the questions. These are examples of overstress or distress.

The responses of human bone to physical stresses are another example of the principle of eustress. Under-loading of bone, such as experienced by astronauts who temporarily live in conditions of reduced gravity, or by sick people who have to stay in bed, causes bone to lose some of the minerals that make it strong. Less extreme conditions, such as the sedentary lifestyle of many North Americans, produce a similar effect. On the other hand, the excessive stress imposed by the fitness instructor who teaches 20 exercise classes a week can cause painful and disabling stress fractures in the legs. A balance between activity and rest provides optimal conditions for development and maintenance of strong, normally formed bone.

The key is to manage our stress at reasonable levels, neither too low nor too high. The optimal stress level is an individual thing. Some people would find a routine desk job distressing because it's too boring or over-stimulating, while it might be just right for someone else.

> How about *you?*
>   a) What are the major stressors in your life currently?
>   b) What are you doing to manage your stress at reasonable levels?
> Suggest additional ways you could:
>   a) Remove yourself from stressors
>   b) Change stressors
>   c) Change your response to stressors

6.3 Stress management

There are three main approaches to stress management:

- Change the stressor
- Remove yourself from the stressor
- Change your response to the stressor

There are many specific stress management strategies. The trick is to know your own style and pick what will work for you. Strategies include

Know yourself. Be aware of your current stress level. Identify the major stressors in your life. Recognize your own optimal stress level. The goal is not to *remove* stress but to *optimize* it.

Plan life changes for stable times. Some life changes, such as the death of a spouse or a serious illness, may be unavoidable. However, other life changes, such as moving to a new residence, accepting a new job or a promotion, or taking a holiday, can be scheduled. If you have already had a lot of change in your life recently, it makes sense to delay a move until the end of the semester, stay in your present job for another year, or plan to stay home rather than going to Thailand for Christmas.

Develop communication skills. Stress is often the result of poor or insufficient communication with others. Communication can help identify the source of the problem and arrive at a solution. Also, it may be helpful to "let off steam" by talking to someone you trust. It is beyond the scope of this course to teach you the principles of effective communication, but you may find one of the many self-help books or adult education courses that deal with communication to be helpful.

Practise time management. Plan ahead. Set priorities. Schedule appointments and deadlines on a day-timer or calendar. Delegate rather than trying to do everything yourself. Set realistic expectations. Avoid over-committing yourself. There is only so much time in the day. Choosing to sleep less may be an option in the short run, but it will soon wear you down. If you're going to take on a new activity, something else will probably have to go. If you feel overloaded, remember that you have the right to change your mind. Ask yourself three questions:

- Does this need to be done at all?
- Does this need to be done now?
- Could this be done differently?

Be aware of how often you use the words "should," "must," and "have to." Actually, these are almost all choices. We say "I *should* do my homework" or "I *should* leave now," but what we really mean is "I choose to do my homework because I know that if I don't, I won't get a good grade, and good grades are important to me." You may think this is just a matter of wording. Actually, it is a small but powerful shift in thinking that puts you in control of your life.

Be more flexible. Relax your standards. Let the grass grow and the dust collect in the corners of the kitchen for another week.

Cultivate relationships. People who have close ties to their friends and family tend to be better off physically and psychologically than loners (House, Landis, & Umberson, 1988; Seeman, 1996). Don't hide in your apartment feeling sorry for yourself. Reach out to others. Ask for help when you need it. Offer your time to help others. Happy people tend to focus their attention on other people's needs instead of their own (Thomas, 1994).

Be happy with what you have. "Once people have met the basic needs of food, clothing, shelter, and human rights, happiness relies largely on things unrelated to money, such as meaningful activities and enriching relationships" (Thomas, 1994).

Consider new work. If your job is a constant source of stress for you, maybe you will be better off somewhere else. After all, you can't buy health—or happiness. Even so, it often takes courage and faith in the future to leave something that is known, even when it is making you sick.

Learn to like yourself. Every day do something that you really enjoy. Take time for hobbies and leisure activities.

Cultivate your sense of humour. Smile. Laugh.

Be optimistic. Don't worry about things that you can't change. Spend more time living in the present. Much unconstructive energy is spent in regret for things that happened in the past and fear of things that might happen in the future.

Listen to nice music. For centuries people have used music to relax. Slow, gentle, harmonic music affects brain waves in a positive way.

Exercise. Exercise removes you from the stressful environment, perhaps taking your mind off the problem or giving you time to think about the problem. Exercise with a partner provides the opportunity to talk about what's bothering you. After 30 minutes or so of sustained exercise, blood levels of **endorphins** increase. These chemicals produced by the body are similar in structure and function to the drug morphine, and have been credited with the "high" or euphoric feeling produced by exercise. Competitive sports such as squash or golf may not be good choices for stress relief if the competition makes you tense or frustrated.

Take a hot bath or get a massage. Hot baths and massage help promote muscle relaxation. The warmth is calming. The touch of a caring person is calming. Notice how a distraught child settles down when her mother holds her and strokes her forehead.

Practise relaxation training. Breathe deeply. Techniques include yoga, transcendental meditation, biofeedback, hypnosis, and autogenic training. All are designed to promote awareness, help let go of tension, and develop harmony between mind and body.

Have faith. Religion offers social support, long-term hope, and a sense of purpose in life. It is gratifying to believe that there is a higher power, an order to the universe, perhaps some kind of life after death, and a plan for humankind that we may never know or need to know.

Use drugs. Alcohol works quickly and relatively safely if it is consumed in moderate amounts. Many people take a drink or two after work to help them relax. A number of **medications** intended to relieve some symptoms of stress (e.g., anxiety and depression) are available over the counter or through prescription. Doctors commonly prescribe Valium (diazepam), Librium, and Atavin for the relief of anxiety. Drugs have a valid role in the treatment of stress reactions. However, drugs do not change the situation that caused the stress. Also, there are health risks with drug use. Because they are potentially addictive, drugs are probably best used for *temporary* relief of stress symptoms. An individual who continues to use alcohol or other drugs to deal with stress symptoms may over time become chemically dependent, which adds more problems to the already existing ones.

Rest when you are tired. Many people take a "coffee break" every couple of hours while working or studying. A break may be very useful, but habitual use of coffee (or tea or other stimulants) to elevate energy may be harmful. Usually the appropriate response to a sense of tiredness is to rest. It is unrealistic to expect the body to perform at high levels continually. Often when you are tired from working at an activity for a period of time, it is most helpful to change posture (get up and move if you have been seated, sit and elevate your feet if you have been standing or walking) and change the nature of the activity (for example, if you have been reading, it may help to vacuum the living room or wash the dishes; if you have been gardening, it may be nice to sit and watch the birds or read a book). Beverages are also often refreshing—a glass of water is usually a better choice than a cup of coffee.

Sleep. Sleep provides us shelter and recovery from the cares of the day. There are probably few things as truly refreshing as a good night's sleep. Of course, some people find it hard to get a good sleep when they feel anxious, while other people tend to oversleep when they are distressed.

Turn off the television. Television news is stressful. Wolfgang Luthe, the late physician who helped developed autogenic training, termed TV news "brain pollution" (Luthe, 1980). The television networks may have an interest in informing the public, but they are also concerned about attracting viewers and selling commercial time. If it bleeds, as they say, it leads, meaning that stories about death and violence are usually put as the lead story because they have the most power to grab people's attention (Skene, 1995).

A headless human body pulled out of the woods, an automobile crumpled under a truck, victims of war, earthquake, and famine. These are horrifying images, and we *should* be horrified. The problem is that this human suffering is brought into our living rooms, and there is little we can do to relieve it. These images continue to be processed in our unconscious mind long after we shut off the TV, and this can cause sleep disturbances (Luthe, 1980). And if we *don't* feel disturbed by these images, what does that say about our humanity? That we have become so exposed that we are desensitized; we have normalized the abnormal.

Besides, TV news may not be that informative anyway.

> But the problem with pictures is the essential problem of television news: while they stimulate and entertain, they do little to inform. Although more than three quarters of the population say the tube is their primary source of news and information, research shows that by the end of an average evening news show they won't be capable of remembering the content of the first three stories. Two hours after the show is over, they will have forgotten 90 per cent of the news they watched and will not be able to recall the basic details of a single story. Yet they will have formed an opinion on the story with the most emotional impact, usually the one with the most graphic pictures. (Skene, 1995, pp. 48–49)

The point is, one simple way to reduce exposure to stress is to turn off the TV news.

7 Sleep
7.1 What is sleep?
In some ways, the body rests when it sleeps. We become relatively insensitive to sensory stimuli, as if part of the brain shuts off. Other parts of the brain become more active. Total brain energy consumption decreases by only 5% to 10%. Once asleep, voluntary movement ceases, although people do move around, sometimes quite vigorously.

7.2 Why do we sleep?
We don't know. Staying still to reduce exposure to predators? A wakeful, sedentary condition would be better than sleep, with its reduced sensitivity to sensory stimuli. Sleep's value goes beyond energy conservation. Hibernating animals have to come out of hibernation in order to sleep, so for them sleep actually wastes energy. Sleep seems to have something to do with repair and recovery of body systems (e.g., the immune, musculoskeletal, and nervous systems). One sleep expert said that after 50 years in the field, the only definite reason he knew why we sleep is that we become sleepy (Max, 2010).

We may need sleep in order to dream. Scientists still do not know much about why or how we dream. Sigmund Freud, "the father of psychoanalysis," argued that dreams give access to unconscious repressed conflicts. In the 1950s, scientists learned that dream frequency is higher during a stage of sleep in which the eyes move rapidly, called **rapid eye movement (REM)** sleep, than during other stages of sleep (Figure 9.3). Many people reportedly experience their most vivid dreams during REM sleep. The best method currently available to determine dream content is to wake the sleeper and ask him (National Sleep Foundation, 2013).

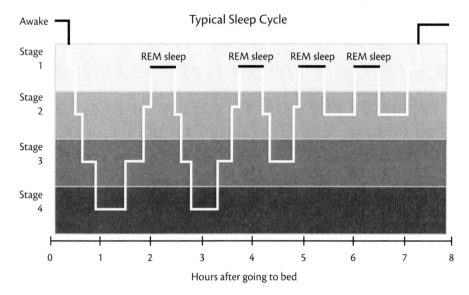

Figure 9.3. A typical night of human sleep. The sleeper descends to deeper and deeper stages of sleep, and then ascends to a light stage of sleep associated with rapid eye movements (REM). This cycle repeats a number of times over the night.

7.3 How much sleep do we need?

The average young adult needs about eight or nine hours of sleep, but there are individual differences. The best indication you need more sleep is how rested or sleepy you feel during the day.

7.4 What happens if we don't get enough sleep?

Sleep deficiency causes fatigue and irritability. Memory, learning, reaction time, processing time, and attention all suffer, and there is a greater tendency to persevere with ineffective solutions. Performance decreases and susceptibility to errors and accidents increases (Durmer & Dinges, 2005; NIH, 2012).

Yang et al. (2014) trained mice to walk atop a rotating rod, which activated cells in the motor cortex region of the brain. These same cells became active during later deep sleep. Two groups of mice trained for an hour, after which one group slept while the other group was kept awake. The sleeping mice formed more **dendritic spines**, which are physical connections between other brain cells. Disrupting their deep sleep prevented dendritic spine growth.

This study showed that not only sleep but learning causes *physical* changes in the brain. These changes occur in specific regions in response to specific learning; for example, when the mice ran forward on the rod, it resulted in spine growth on different dendritic branches than when they ran backwards on the rod.

Extra training did not compensate for lack of sleep. Mice that did an hour of training and then slept were compared with mice that trained for three hours and were then deprived of sleep. The mice that were allowed to sleep *still* formed more brain connections than those that trained more.

7.5 What can you do to get better sleep?

Healthy sleeping habits can be developed just as with healthy eating and healthy exercise. A good start is to take a look at your lifestyle and sleep environment. Then pick one or a few simple, small changes you can make. Put these into action, and keep with it until it becomes routine (APA, 2014b). For example,

- **Set a routine.** The body's "biological clock" can more easily adjust to an earlier bedtime if you regularly go to bed at the same time. If you stay up late on the nights when you don't have an early class the next morning, this makes it harder to fall asleep earlier on the nights when you retire early.
- **Exercise.** This helps many people manage stress, and stress is a major barrier to falling asleep. But in the minutes and hours after exercise, the body is still activated: heart rate, breathing rate, body temperature, and nervous activity remain elevated. So, exercise earlier in the day, maybe before dinner, unless the exercise is quite gentle, such as yoga or tai chi.
- **Don't drink caffeinated beverages.** The caffeine in beverages such as coffee, tea, or colas is a stimulant. The nicotine in tobacco products is also a stimulant. This probably accounts at least partly for the poorer sleep experienced by smokers.
- **What about alcohol?** Yes, alcohol is a central nervous system depressant, which is essentially the opposite of a stimulant. Low doses of alcohol (e.g., one beer or equivalent) can aid relaxation and sleep. The problem with recommending alcohol as a sleep aid is that "experienced" drinkers tend to feel *stimulated* after a drink rather than sedated, and moderate

and higher doses (two or more drinks) interfere with the phase of sleep that is most refreshing.

- **Don't drink a lot of fluids of any kind before bed.** While you are asleep, the blood continues to circulate, the kidney filters blood, and urine accumulates in the bladder. When the bladder fills past a certain level, it signals the need to urinate, which will eventually wake you—unless you sleep so soundly you miss these signals and wet the bed!
- **Create a dark, cool, reasonably quiet sleeping environment.** Earplugs can help block noise from traffic, roommates, and so on. Blinds, curtains, and sleep masks reduce light levels.
- **Avoid mentally stimulating activities before sleep.** In the period before sleep, say the hour before going to bed, take a warm bath, listen to relaxing music, have your partner give you a relaxing massage, or read a novel (preferably one without too much suspense or violence).
- **Use the bed only for sleeping.** Do not use it for other things, such as studying, watching television, or even reading. The only exception would be making love, if that is part of your lifestyle.

If you have difficulty sleeping because of acute distress, such as grief related to the death of a loved one, your physician may prescribe a short course (a week or two) of **sleep medication**. However, if your sleep difficulty persists, you should probably discuss this with your health care provider and investigate other solutions. Some sleep medications are addictive, while others become less effective if taken chronically.

> How much sleep do *you* think you need?
>   How much sleep do you get?
>   How rested do you feel upon waking?
>   What interferes with the quality and quantity of your sleep?
>   Propose three simple, specific things that you could do in the near future that would improve your sleep.

8 Gratitude

The last decade has seen much research into the relationship between mental health and gratitude. Gratitude is the state of being grateful. Grateful means "feeling or showing an appreciation for something done or received" (Oxford Dictionaries, 2018). Some studies report that gratitude is associated with fewer depressive symptoms (e.g., Lambert at al., 2012; Cheng, Tsui and Lam, 2015). Another study found that among patients admitted for acute coronary symptoms (ACS), levels of *optimism* at intake were significantly associated with higher levels of physical activity six months later, and with lower rates of readmission. In this study, gratitude was minimally associated with post-ACS outcomes (Huffman et al., 2016).

Gratitude **journaling** is a common research intervention; that is, subjects in the experimental group are asked to write down things for which they feel grateful. Jackowska et al. (2016) reported that a group of young females who did gratitude journaling for two weeks experienced increased feelings of well-being and optimism, better sleep quality, and lower blood pressure compared with counterparts who journaled about everyday events or got no treatment. Redwine et al. (2016) randomly assigned older (average age 65) patients with heart disease to a journaling intervention or a control group that received treatment as usual. After eight weeks, the experimental group showed increased gratitude scores and decreased levels of **inflammatory biomarkers**, that is, blood levels of chemicals associated with inflammation, which is a typical physiological response to injury or trauma. Wong et al. (2018) randomly assigned adults seeking university-based psychotherapy services to one of three conditions: psychotherapy only (the control group), psychotherapy plus expressive writing, and psychotherapy plus gratitude writing. The "gratitude" participants wrote letters expressing gratitude to others, while the "expressive writing" group wrote about their thoughts and feelings around stressful experiences. Four weeks after the writing intervention, the "gratitude" subjects reported significantly better mental health than the other two groups; these differences were still present 12 weeks post-writing.

Henning et al. (2017) noted that self-reported gratitude intensity correlated with activity in distinct regions of the brain (the medial pre-frontal cortex) associated with social reward and moral cognition. They proposed that gratitude improves health by reducing physiological stress and by producing **reward**— both personal and social—in its place. They suggest that the μ-opioid receptor system mediates these effects. Receptors are sites on the surface of cells to which chemicals can bind. Nerve cells have receptors for opioids and other molecules. When opioid drugs such as heroin and morphine bind to brain cells, they induce euphoria (a feeling of great well-being) and block pain. Human nerve cells *make* three different kinds of opioids. The opioid system has an important role in pain, emotion, stress responses, and the rewarding effects of food, sex, and psychoactive drugs. We will explore these terms and concepts in Chapter 13: Drugs.

9 Conclusion

Mental wellness is central to enjoying life to the fullest. Many people suffer from disabling mental health problems. To some extent, everyone's quality of life is from time to time affected by feelings of depression or stress. Mental health problems are common, and they are often treatable. Unfortunately, social stigmas around mental health can inhibit discussion and seeking help. Many people with mental health problems have not had a proper diagnosis, and rely on self-medication, such as with alcohol or cannabis, to try to manage unpleasant thoughts and feelings.

It can be a tricky to find the right amount of stimulation that allows your life to flow in a happy, energetic, and peaceful way. Good mental health starts in early childhood. However, even those who did not have the best childhood can develop the attitude and skills needed for mental wellness. Stress is an unavoidable and essential part of life. However, overstress or distress erodes our health and may cause a variety of ills. For optimal wellness, we should manage our stress at optimal levels. This balancing of stress can be achieved through knowing yourself and understanding the stressors in your life, then taking control of these stressors and your responses to stress.

Study Questions

1. What qualities did Abraham Maslow observe as typical in self-actualized (mentally healthy) people?
2a. Give several examples of psychological defence mechanisms.
2b. Should these be encouraged or discouraged? Explain.
3a. What is the most common mood disorder?
3b. List at least five of the criteria for a clinical diagnosis of this disorder.
4. What is the current name for the mood disorder that used to be called "manic depression"?
5. Describe briefly how someone with generalized anxiety disorder experiences life.
6a. What is the difference between panic attack and panic disorder?
6b. What is the most common social phobia?
6c. What is the difference between shyness and social phobia?
7. Explain the role of compulsions and rituals in obsessive-compulsive disorder.
8a. How would someone with schizophrenia experience the world?
8b. What are the two main incorrect stereotypes regarding schizophrenia?
9a. In Canada, what demographic groups have higher suicide than the national average?
9b. What are the two biggest risk factors for suicide?
9c. State at least four things you could do to help someone you think might be considering suicide.

10. Describe briefly some of the elements that are useful for treating psychological disorders.

11. Show that you understand the concept of "stressor" by listing at least six different stressors.

12. Is stress bad for health? Explain, using the concepts of "eustress" and "distress."

13a. Explain why Selye called the response to stress the "general adaptation syndrome."

13b. Explain the three stages in the general adaptation syndrome.

14a. What are the three main approaches to stress management?

14b. List 10 things a person can do to more effectively manage stress.

15a. Why do humans sleep?

15b. What is the best indication of whether or not you are getting enough sleep?

15c. Give at least six recommendations that could help a person sleep better.

16a. What is the main research intervention used in studies of gratitude?

16b. What effects does gratitude seem to have on mental health?

Glossary

autonomic nervous system—the ANS is responsible for "housekeeping" duties, such as circulation, respiration, digestion, and metabolism; although it can be altered by the conscious mind, it functions automatically on its own

bipolar disorder—formerly called "manic depression," this disorder features mood swings between the manic and depressive states

compulsions—urges to do something to lessen discomfort, usually caused by an obsession

defence mechanisms—psychological responses that help us protect ourselves (our egos, actually) when we don't get what we want

depression—a chronic state of a depressed mood, or markedly diminished interest or pleasure in all, or almost all, activities, in combination with a number of other features that include fatigue, feelings of worthlessness, inability to concentrate, and so on

distress—a state in which your stress level is not optimal but instead is too low or too high

eustress—a state in which your stress level is optimal

generalized anxiety disorder—chronic and exaggerated worry and tension, even though nothing seems to provoke it

homeostasis—the state of dynamic equilibrium or balance that the body normally maintains

individuating—the process of forming one's own identity, separate from one's parents

mania—a hyper-elevated mood which in many ways is the opposite of depression

mood disorders—a group of psychological disorders that feature problems with one's mood or "feeling state"; depression is a mood disorder, as is mania

neurotransmitter—chemicals that are produced naturally by the body, are released from brain cells, and change the excitability of different regions of the brain

obsessions—constant, intrusive, unwanted thoughts that cause distressing emotions such as anxiety or disgust

panic attack—a specific period of intense fear or discomfort

panic disorder—people with panic disorder have feelings of terror that strike suddenly and repeatedly with no warning

rituals—things people do in response to a compulsion; in the most severe cases, a constant repetition of rituals may fill the day, making a normal routine impossible

schizophrenia—a major form of mental illness characterized by disordered thinking, which may cause the individual to seem confused, to jump from topic to topic in conversation, or to have delusions

self-actualized—the highest state on Maslow's hierarchy of needs; a state of fully becoming oneself psychologically

social phobia—an intense fear of being humiliated in social situations, specifically of embarrassing yourself in front of other people

stress—any event or situation that disrupts the body's normal homeostasis and precipitates changes directed at re-establishing this homeostasis

stressor—something (either inside or outside of the body) that causes a stress response

syndrome—a group of symptoms that commonly occur together and that may be diagnostic for a certain condition

Additional Resources

Canadian Association of Suicide Prevention
http://www.suicideprevention.ca/

Canadian Counseling and Psychotherapy Association (CCPA)
http://www.ccpa-accp.ca/en//
The counselling profession in Canada is not regulated by law except in the provinces of Quebec, Ontario, and Nova Scotia. The CCPA established a credentialing service for its members in 1986. Only counsellors who are certified by the CCPA are permitted to use the protected title Canadian Certified Counselor or the abbreviation CCC.

Canadian Mental Health Association
http://www.cmha.ca

Canadian Professional Counsellors Association (CPCA)

http://www.cpca-rpc.ca/

This non-profit society has listings of counsellors in your area.

Crisis Centre of BC

Tel: 604-872-3311 or toll-free at 1-800-784-2433 (free, confidential, 24/7)

Simon Fraser University Health & Counselling

778-782-4615 (9:00 a.m. to 4:30 p.m.)

http://www.sfu.ca/students/health/

Free (for students currently registered in classes or Co-op), confidential counselling (individual, couples, family, group). Suicide prevention training. Workshops. Audio, print, and video materials.

References

APA. (2013). *Diagnostic and statistical manual of mental disorders DSM-5. 5th ed.* Arlington, VA: American Psychiatric Association. Retrieved April 23, 2014 from http://www.psychiatryonline.com

APA. (2014a). Bipolar disorder. American Psychiatric Association Retrieved April 23, 2014 from http://www.psychiatry.org/bipolar-disorder

APA. (2014b). Why sleep is important and what happens when you don't get enough. American Psychiatric Association. Retrieved May 10, 2014 from http://www.apa.org/topics/sleep/why.aspx

Cheng, S. T., Tsui, P. K., Lam, J. H. (2015). Improving mental health in health care practitioners: randomized controlled trial of a gratitude intervention. *Journal of Consulting and Clinical Psychology.* 83(1):177-186.

Cheung, A. H., Dewa, C. S. (2006). Canadian community health survey: Major depressive disorder and suicidality in adolescents. *Healthcare Policy.* 2(2), 76–89.

Durmer, J. S., Dinges, D. F. (2005). Neurocognitive Consequences of Sleep Deprivation *Seminars in Neurology.* 25(1), 117–129. Retrieved September 27, 2012 from http://www.med.upenn.edu/uep/user_documents/dfd3.pdf

Government of Canada, Indigenous Health. (2018). Suicide Prevention. Retrieved May 18, 2018 from https://www.canada.ca/en/indigenous-services-canada/services/first-nations-inuit-health/health-promotion/suicide-prevention.html

Health Canada. (2016). Suicide in Canada. Retrieved May 18, 2018 from https://www.canada.ca/en/public-health/services/suicide-prevention/suicide-canada.html

Henning, M., Fox, G. R., Kaplan, J., Damasio, H., Damasio, A. (2017). A Potential Role for mu-Opioids in Mediating the Positive Effects of Gratitude. Frontiers in Psychology. 8:868.

House, J. S., Landis, K. R. & Umberson, D. (1988). Social relationships and health. Science, 241(4865), 540-545.

Huffman, J. C., Beale, E. E., Celano, C. M., Beach, S. R., Belcher, A. M., Moore, S. V., Motiwala, S. R., Gandhi, P. U., Gaggin, H. K., Januzzi, J. L. (2016). Effects of optimism and gratitude on physical activity, biomarkers, and readmissions after an acute coronary syndrome: The Gratitude Research in Acute Coronary Events Study. Circulation: Cardiovascular Quality and Outcomes. 9(1):55-63.

IQWiG. (September 27, 2011). *Fact sheet: Generalized anxiety disorder.* Institute for Quality and Efficiency in Health Care, National Library of Medicine. Retrieved April 23, 2014 from https://www.ncbi.nlm.nih.gov/pubmedhealth/PMH0016272/

Jackowska, M., Brown, J., Ronaldson, A., Steptoe, A. (2016). The impact of a brief gratitude intervention on subjective well-being, biology and sleep. Journal of Health Psychology. 21(10):2207-2217.

Lambert, N. M., Fincham, F. D., Stillman, T. F. (2012). Gratitude and depressive symptoms: The role of positive reframing and positive emotion. Cognition and Emotion. 26(4) Retrieved February 15, 2018 from http://www.tandfonline.com.proxy.lib.sfu.ca/doi/full/10.1080/02699931.2011.595393?scroll=top&needAccess=true

Luthe, W. (1980). Personal communication.

Maslow, A. (1970). *Motivation and Personality* (2nd ed.) New York: Harper & Row.

Mayo Clinic Staff. (October 25, 2012). *Electroconvulsive therapy (ECT)* Retrieved May 10, 2014 from http://www.mayoclinic.org/tests-procedures/electroconvulsive-therapy/basics/definition/PRC-20014161

Max, D. T. (May 2010). The secrets of sleep. *National Geographic Magazine.* Retrieved May, 10, 2014 from http://ngm.nationalgeographic.com/2010/05/sleep/max-text

Mental Health Commission of Canada. (2012). Making the Case for Investing in Mental Health in Canada. Retrieved May 18, 2018 from https://www.mentalhealthcommission.ca/sites/default/files/2016-06/Investing_in_Mental_Health_FINAL_Version_ENG.pdf

National Sleep Foundation. (2013). *Dreams and sleep.* Retrieved May 10, 2014 from http://sleepfoundation.org/sleep-topics/dream-and-sleep/

NIH. (February 22, 2012). *What are sleep deprivation and deficiency?* National Heart Lung and Blood Institute, National Institute for Health, US Department of Health and Human Services. Retrieved September 27, 2012 from http://www.nhlbi.nih.gov/health/health-topics/topics/sdd/why.htm

NIMH. (2013a). *Panic disorder: When fear overwhelms.* NIH Publication No. TR 10-4679. US Department of Health and Human Services, National Institutes of Health, National Institute of Mental Health. Retrieved April 23, 2014 from http://www.nimh.nih.gov/health/publications/panic-disorder-when-fear-overwhelms/index.shtml

NIMH. (2013b). *Obsessive-compulsive disorder.* Retrieved April 23, 2014 from http://www.report.nih.gov/NIHfactsheets/ViewFactSheet.aspx?csid=54&key=O

NIMH. (2013c). *Schizophrenia.* US Department of Health and Human Services, National Institutes of Health, National Institute of Mental Health. Retrieved April 23, 2014 from http://www.report.nih.gov/NIHfactsheets/ViewFactSheet.aspx?csid=67&key=S

Oxford Dictionaries. (2018). Grateful. Oxford University Press. Retrieved May 20, 2018 from https://en.oxforddictionaries.com/definition/grateful

Redwine, L. A., Henry, B. L., Pung, M. A., Wilson, K., Chinh, K., Knight, B., Jain, S., Rutledge, T., Greenberg, B., Maisel, A., Mills, P. J. (2016). Psychosomatic Medicine. 78(6):667-676.

Seeman, T. E. (1996). Social ties and health: the benefits of social integration. *Annals of Epidemiology, 6*(5), 442-451.

Selye, H. (1956). *The stress of life*. New York: McGraw Hill.

Selye, H. (1975). Confusion and controversy in the stress field. *Journal of Human Stress*. 1(2), 37−44.

Skene, W. (1995, September). Six o'clock low: BCTV captures a larger share of the local news market than any other station on the continent. *Vancouver Magazine, 28*(5), 44−51.

Statistics Canada. (2015). *Deaths and causes of death, 2015*. Retrieved May 1, 2018 from http://www.statcan.gc.ca/daily-quotidien/180223/dq180223c-eng.htm

Statistics Canada. (February 23, 2018). Suicides and suicide rate, by sex and age group. Retrieved May 18, 2018 from https://www.statcan.gc.ca/tables-tableaux/sum-som/l01/cst01/hlth66a-eng.htm

Thomas, J. (1994, January 11). How to be happy. *Your Health*. (pp 45-46).

Wong, Y. J, Owen, J., Gabana, N. O. T., Brown, J. W., McInnis, S., Toth, P. (2018). Does gratitude writing improve the mental health of psychotherapy clients? Evidence from a randomized controlled trial. *Psychotherapy Research*. 28(2). Retrieved February 15, 2018 from http://www.tandfonline.com.proxy.lib.sfu.ca/doi/full/10.1080/105033 07.2016.1169332?scroll=top&needAccess=true

Yang, G., Sau Wan Lai, C., Cichon, J., Ma, L., Li, W., Gan, W-B. (2014). Sleep promotes branch-specific formation of dendritic spines after learning. *Science*. 344(6188), 1173−1178.

10 Intimate Relationships and Human Sexuality

Learning Objectives

By the time you have finished this chapter you should be able to

- Outline the health benefits of intimate relationships
- Describe the features typical of intimate relationships
- Summarize the normal human sexual response
- Describe the basic anatomy and physiology of human sexual reproduction
- Define the concept of healthy sex
- Differentiate healthy from unhealthy variations in normal sexual behaviour
- Discuss the effects of pornography on health at the individual and societal levels
- Suggest reasons why people practise unhealthy sex, and offer strategies to improve this situation

1 Overview

The area of human sexuality is sensitive and complex. Health issues, both physical and emotional, are mixed in with moral and religious beliefs, such as the belief that a person should wait until marriage before having sexual intercourse. The point of view expressed in this text is outlined below. Not all people share this point of view, and other points of view are also okay.

- Human sexual behaviour is normal, healthy, and an integral part of intimate relationships.
- There is a range of normal variations in sexual behaviour.

- Individuals should be free to make informed personal choices in this area and to have those choices respected, as long as they do not violate the rights of other people.
- Healthy sexual expression happens in the context of respect, caring, sharing, and communication.

Canada has become increasingly pluralistic, which means diverse ethnic, racial, religious, and social groups retain and develop their traditional cultures and beliefs within the confines of the broader common society. Accordingly, expressions of sexuality and relationship status have become increasingly diverse. Although some Canadians assert that the only "proper" sexual relations are between a man and a woman in a monogamous (exclusive) marriage, the reality is that many Canadians live in different situations: unmarried couples who are sexually active, in a committed relationship, and perhaps living together *(cohabitating);* single people who are sexually active with more than one partner; **straight** people (heterosexuals), who are attracted to members of the opposite sex; people who are attracted to members of the same sex (homosexuals) and identify as **gay** (males) or **lesbian** (females); **bisexuals**, who feel attraction to both sexes; **transgender** people, whose gender identity is different from the sex they were assigned at birth. Lesbian, gay, bisexual, and transgender people collectively—as a political movement that has pressed for greater acceptance by mainstream society—have labelled themselves with the abbreviation **LGBTQ**.

> What about *you?* What do you consider to be the appropriate place for sexual activity in human relationships?
>
> For example, should people wait until they are married to have intercourse?
>
> What about "recreational sex," where sex is something consenting adults do for fun without expecting they will have an ongoing relationship?

2 Intimate Relationships

The ability to form and maintain intimate relationships is important for both physical and emotional wellness. Marriage is the traditional form of such relationships. Married people have, in general, lower mortality rates than their unmarried (never-married, widowed, divorced, or separated) counterparts.

A **meta-analysis** (a study that combines and re-analyzes data from other studies) of over 500 million individuals calculated that compared with currently married individuals, never-married (single) people have on average a 24% increased risk of mortality. The authors reported "hazard ratios have been modestly increasing over time for both genders, but have done so somewhat more rapidly for women" (Roelfs et. al, 2011).

An analysis of over 200,000 cancer deaths in Norway over a 40-year period (1970–2007) showed that all categories of unmarried people had significantly more cancer mortality than married people (Kravdal & Syse, 2011). The authors offered a number of possible explanations for the benefits of marriage with respect to cancer survival (p. 8):

- **Support:** Having a spouse may provide a built-in source of support.
- **Children:** Raising children appears to have a positive effect on cancer survival, "probably because children induce a healthier lifestyle and (especially if they are adults) may provide support during treatment and later."
- **Selection:** "Healthy individuals are probably more likely to enter and remain in a marriage than the less healthy, although there are also studies indicating a negative health selection into marriage."
- **Values:** "Individuals who are engaged in religious activities, for instance, appear more prone to avoid risky health behaviors. In addition, they are less likely to divorce their spouses."

The Norway data may actually underestimate the benefit of marriage on cancer survival. People cohabitating were counted as "unmarried." However, if cohabitation confers some of the same benefits on health as marriage, the decision to classify them as unmarried would have improved cancer survival rates for that group.

In their analysis of over 190,000 Americans, Liu and Reczek (2012) found that

- Divorced, widowed, and never-married *white men* had higher mortality rates than cohabitating white men.
- Never-married *black men* had higher mortality rates than cohabitating black men.
- Mortality rates of non-married white and black *women* were not different from those of their cohabitating counterparts.
- Mortality rates of *married* white men and women were lower than their *cohabitating* counterparts.

The Liu and Reczek findings seem to show that:
   a) Marriage is better than cohabiting (at least, reduces mortality rates).
   b) Cohabiting is better than being divorced, widowed, or never married for men.
   c) The same is not true for women.
How would you explain part (a)?
What might explain part (c)?

Healthy and fulfilling intimate relationships, whether marriage or not, share many of the same features:

- **Love, sex, and commitment:** Falling in love is easy. It has been argued that this is not real love but instead a temporary, sex-linked, erotic experience. Real love takes work, discipline, and the willingness to extend oneself for someone else (Peck, 1978).
- **Mutual trust and affection:** Each partner is an emotional resource for the other, giving and receiving support.
- **Realistic expectations:** Partners need to be tolerant of each other's imperfections and the ups and downs in the relationship.
- **Open communication:** Partners share their expectations and feelings and have effective ways of handling conflict. Conflict is inevitable, and attempts to avoid conflict are unhealthy. The key is being assertive regarding your own needs and wants, being open to hearing the other person's position, and working to resolve the conflict.
- **Mutual respect:** Partners have the right to be themselves, to be valued for who they are, and to grow and change.
- **Egalitarian roles:** Partners share duties and responsibilities both inside and outside the home. This does not mean each person does half of the cooking, washes the dishes half of the time, cuts the lawn every other week, and so on. Some specialization of labour according to individual interests and abilities makes sense. North American surveys suggest women still take most of the responsibility for home and children even when they work outside the house.
- **Balance of individual and joint interests and activities:** It is rare that partners enjoy doing all the same things, and it is probably unhealthy to want to spend every minute of the day together.
- **Agreement on religious and ethical values:** When people select partners for long-term relationships, they tend to choose people like themselves:

people who live in the same geographical area, have similar interests, values, beliefs, socio-economic backgrounds, levels of education, and degrees of physical attractiveness.

> Think about *your* current or previous intimate relationship.
>   How does it compare with the preceding list of features typical of successful intimate relationships?

*Is it normal to **not** have a boyfriend or girlfriend?*

This question raises the "*normal* versus *typical*" discussion. That is, if most people do something, we can say it is typical to do this. However, that doesn't mean someone who doesn't do it isn't normal, as in, they are bad or wrong or they *should* be doing it (whatever "it" is). For example, many teens are eager to get their driving license when they are old enough, but some teens have no interest in this and are content to walk, bike, bus, or get rides with friends.

Adolescents typically become interested in dating. Dating has a social element (e.g., spending time and doing things together), but usually we think of "boyfriend" or "girlfriend" as an exclusive social and sexual relationship with one other person. It often also has a sexual element, which may be just kissing, or may go further.

It is typical for teens and young adults to want a boy/girlfriend, and many are successful in forming such relationships. I don't know what percentage is unsuccessful in finding a partner. Some people don't want a boy/girlfriend, maybe because they prefer to date more freely or because they are too busy with school or work to want to spend the time and emotional energy intimate relationships require.

3 What Is *Love?*

We use the word "love" in many different ways: "I love to ski," "I love ice cream," "I love you," are examples, and so is "making love." A sense of passion is conveyed in some of these uses of the word. Often at the beginning of a new intimate relationship there is a powerful passion, a "high" you feel when talking to or being with your loved one and a sense of longing when you are apart. Sexual feelings are often quite intense at this stage. Often this passion lessens after a number of months. When the passion fades, you may drift apart from your lover, or the relationship may deepen into something else, a type of love based on caring and commitment. This caring nature of love is probably what we mean when we say "I love you" to a special friend or pet.

In his classic book, *The Road Less Traveled: A New Psychology of Love, Traditional Values, and Spiritual Growth,* Peck (1978) defined love as "The will to extend one's self for the purpose of nurturing one's own or another's spiritual growth." Thus, love is seen as an act of the *will* rather than an act of *desire*. "Real love" is different than "falling in love." Falling is love is not an act of will. It is a temporary collapse of ego boundaries and a temporary escape from the loneliness of individual identities. When we become one with our beloved, we are no longer alone. On the other hand, real love is a choice, involves effort, and maintains ego boundaries. According to Peck, "falling in love" is a "biological trick" whose purpose is to tempt us into marriage and having children, which ensures the survival of the species. Perhaps most fundamentally, Peck writes, we are incapable of loving another unless we first love ourselves, a point of view with widespread support among health professionals.

> Have *you* ever been "in love"?
>   How did that feel?
>   How did your feelings change with time in that relationship?

4 Human Genital Anatomy

Ova (eggs) are stored in a woman's *ovaries* (Figure 10.1). Starting in adolescence, each month one (or more) ovum develops, and then is released from the ovary into the abdominal cavity near the opening of the **oviduct** (Fallopian tube), an event known as **ovulation**. The ovum almost always drifts into and down the oviduct. The ovum takes about two days to travel the length of the oviduct. If fertilization occurs, it usually happens in the oviduct. If fertilization does not occur, the ovum drifts on through the uterus and vagina and is expelled. The woman usually does not observe this, as the unfertilized ovum is less than 10% of the size of the head of a pin.

From adolescence until late middle age, women menstruate about once a month (the textbook *menstrual cycle* is 28 days long). This cycle involves rising and falling levels of various hormones that stimulate development of the ova and prepare the lining of the uterus. The uterine lining thickens and small blood vessels multiply beneath its surface, which readies the uterus to protect and nourish a fertilized ovum. The *uterus* (womb) is where the fetus will stay for the duration of pregnancy. The onset of menstrual bleeding is labelled as Day 1 of the cycle; ovulation occurs at about Day 14. If a fertilized ovum implants on the uterine wall, hormonal signals maintain the thickened uterine lining for the duration of the pregnancy and block further menstruation. Thus, missing

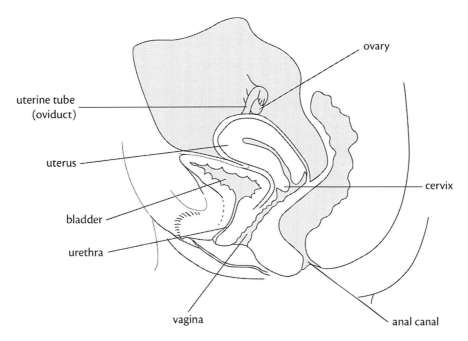

Figure 10.1. Human female genital anatomy; this diagram shows a cross section through the abdomen and pelvis.
Source: Health Awareness Connection (2000) *Young people's guide to sexually transmitted diseases (STD's) and AID/HIV disease.* Brookline, MA: Health Awareness Connection.

a period may mean the woman is pregnant, although stress, heavy exercise, under-nutrition, and other things can also stop menstruation. Menstrual bleeding typically lasts three to five days, with the heaviest flow on the first days. Shedding of the thickened uterine lining causes the bleeding.

Why do some high-performance athletes stop menstruating?

A posting to the website of The Center for Young Women's Health speaks to this:

> Most girls who play sports have regular menstrual periods, and girls who are very active may skip a few periods. However, some girls who train really hard may skip *many* menstrual periods, or they may get their period at a late age, especially if they've lost weight or developed an eating disorder. Girls may begin to skip periods if they are not getting proper nutrition, or if there is too much stress on their body from sports. This stress lowers estrogen levels, which may cause skipped periods. Low estrogen levels and a lack

of menstrual periods can lead to low bone mass and stress fractures (small cracks) in your bones. (CYWH, 2010)

The *vagina* is a corrugated, tube-like organ that runs from the *cervix* (opening of the uterus) to the outside. Muscular walls allow the vagina to change size considerably, they can among other things, adapt to penises of various thicknesses and dilating sufficiently to accommodate the newborn during delivery. The *labia* are folds of skin that cover the opening of the vagina. There are two layers of labia, inner and outer. The *clitoris*, a small sensitive organ, is located at the most forward end of the labia, under a hood of skin. The **urethra**, the tube that carries urine from the bladder, exits between the clitoris and the vagina.

Sperm are produced in the male **testes** and then stored in the coiled tubes called the **epididymides** (singular **epididymis**) that sit on top of each *testicle* (Figure 10.2). The testicles hang in the pouch-like **scrotum**. This keeps the testicles outside of the abdomen, where sperm production would be inhibited by the higher internal temperature. The testicles also produce testosterone, the hormone responsible for the development of male secondary sex characteristics, such as a hairy chest, a deeper voice, and larger muscles.

The urethra carries urine from the bladder through the **penis**. A tube called the *vas deferens* connects the epididymis with the **urethra**. That is, unlike in the female, where the urinary tract and the genitals are separated, in the male they share the same tube for part of their length. Fortunately, it is impossible to urinate and ejaculate at the same time, because a reflex closes off the male bladder at orgasm. Several glands (including the **prostate gland**) produce the fluids that make up the major portion of the semen. These glands each connect with the vas deferens. The *foreskin*, a flap of skin, covers the *glans* (the end of the penis).

At orgasm, about a teaspoon (5 ml) of semen, containing 100 million or more sperm, is ejaculated. The sperm swim with whip-like movements of their long, slender tails. Providing there is no barrier (e.g., a condom or a diaphragm), they swim from the cervix up through the uterus and into the oviduct (Fallopian tube). Most sperm die along the way. Hours later, the remaining sperm (several thousand of them) cluster around the much larger ovum. Eventually, the ovum actively takes in a single sperm that has bound to it. This triggers the formation of a thick barrier around the ovum, which denies access to any other sperm. Thus, fertilization involves the union of a single ovum with a single sperm. The genetic material from the sperm combines with the genetic material in the ovum. Over the nine months of pregnancy, the fertilized ovum subsequently divides repeatedly to form the trillions of different cells that form the brain, muscles, bones, and other tissues.

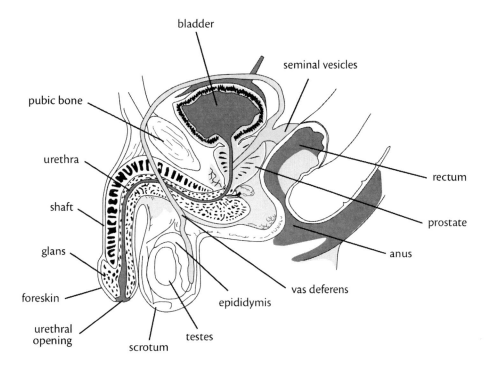

Figure 10.2. Human male genital anatomy; this diagram shows a cross section through the abdomen and pelvis.
Source: Health Awareness Connection (2000) *Young people's guide to sexually transmitted diseases (STD's) and AID/HIV disease.* Brookline, MA: Health Awareness Connection.

> ### Is it better to have sex with a circumcised or uncircumcised man?

This is a tricky question. First, health educators try to avoid the term "better," as it implies a value judgment. Instead, we prefer the approach of explaining, and then encouraging individuals to make an informed decision about what is best for them in their circumstances.

In sub-Saharan Africa, the answer seems to be clearly "Yes, sex with a circumcised man is much safer than sex with an uncircumcised man." In this part of the world, male circumcision reduces HIV infection substantially. It also reduces incidence of HSV-2 (herpes simplex virus, type 2) and HPV (human papilloma virus). The health benefit of circumcision in other parts of the world, especially industrial nations, is less clear.

In a small percentage of newborns, circumcision is indicated for medical reasons. Otherwise, the decision to circumcise or not is influenced by religious, cultural, and social reasons. Circumcision is common in Muslim and Jewish societies. Prevalence of circumcision varies worldwide. Prevalence is generally high in the Middle East, the United States, South Korea, and parts of Southeast Asia and Africa. Prevalence of circumcision is low in Europe, Central Asia, Latin America, and parts of Southern Africa.

An estimated 75% to 90% of men in the USA are circumcised (WHO, 2007). For 40 years, the American Academy of Pediatrics repeatedly stated there were insufficient data to recommend routine circumcision. In 2012, the Academy took a new position:

> "Evaluation of current evidence indicates that the health benefits of newborn male circumcision outweigh the risks and that the procedure's benefits justify access to this procedure for families who choose it. Specific benefits identified included prevention of urinary tract infections, penile cancer, and transmission of some sexually transmitted infections, including HIV" (*Pediatrics* 2012).

The Canadian Paediatric Society (2018) takes a somewhat different position.

> "While there may be a benefit for some boys in high-risk populations and circumstances where the procedure could be considered for disease reduction or treatment, the Canadian Paediatric Society does not recommend the routine circumcision of every newborn male" (Sorokan, Finlay and Jefferies, 2015). Circumcision rates in Canada have declined since the 1970s and may currently be 30% to 40% (WHO, 2007, pp. 11–12).

There are medical complications of circumcision. These consist mainly of bleeding, infection, and removal of too much or too little foreskin. The complication rate is less than 2% for newborns and higher for older children. There is currently some opposition to circumcision on the grounds that the parents and the doctor make the decision, the procedure causes pain, and the infant or child getting circumcised is unable to exercise informed consent.

What about *you?*

If you are a man, are you circumcised or uncircumcised? How do you feel about that?

If you have had sex with a man, does it make a difference to your sexual experience whether your partner has been circumcised?

5 Human Sexual Response

(Note: The material for the rest of this chapter comes primarily from *Human Sexual Response* by Masters & Johnson, 1970, and *Human Sexuality* by Masters, Johnson & Kolodny, 1988, unless otherwise cited.)

William Masters and Virginia Johnson were pioneers in research on human sexual responses. In 1957, Masters (a gynecologist) hired Johnson (a psychologist) as a research assistant. They conducted studies in which almost 700 male and female volunteers masturbated and had intercourse in the laboratory while being observed and measured. A total of 2,500 male and 10,000 female orgasms were documented. Heart rate, blood pressure, skeletal muscle tension, skin colour, and temperature were recorded. Changes in size of the penis and clitoris were measured. Masters and Johnson's results, published in the book *Human Sexual Response* in 1966, showed four stages in the sexual response (Figure 10.3):

- **In the excitement stage**, breast size increases and the nipples become erect. The penis becomes erect, lengthening and thickening due to trapping of blood in spongy tissues. The skin of the scrotum tenses and thickens, and the testes are drawn in toward the body. The vaginal labia expand and flatten out to spread away from the vaginal opening, and the vagina begins to lubricate. The clitoris enlarges, also due to engorgement with blood (although the clitoris is smaller than the penis, it increases proportionally more in size). The uterus pulls up and away from the vagina.

- **In the plateau stage**, the breast enlarges further, the **areolae** (the circles around the nipples) fill with blood and darken, and a "sex flush" generally appears on the breasts. The clitoris pulls back under a flap or hood of skin. The labia turn bright red. Muscles in the wall of the vagina contract, producing a grasping effect on the penis. The glans penis (the head of the penis) darkens in colour. The testes increase in size and are fully elevated.

- **At orgasm**, contractions in the vas deferens, urethra, penis, and other structures force semen out of the penis. The vagina also contracts rhythmically. Expulsion of fluids from the vagina can occur, although this is not typical. In both genders, the **rectal sphincter** (the circular muscle at the anus) contracts. Orgasm is usually associated with a profound feeling of well-being, which may be perceived as a sense of warmth and fullness centred in the pelvic area.

- **The resolution stage** features a return to the pre-aroused state. The sex flush disappears. Breasts, nipples, and areolae return to normal size. The clitoris and labia return to their pre-aroused size and position. The penis becomes soft. The scrotum thins and the testes descend. The uterus descends to its normal position.

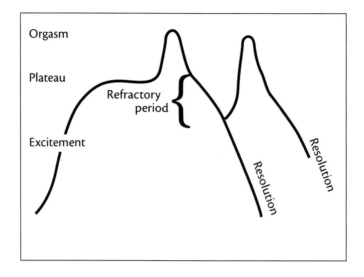

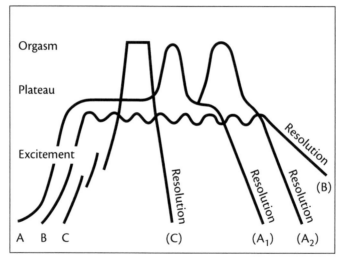

Figure 10.3. Normal human sexual response. Top panel shows male. Bottom panel shows that there are several variations in the female response.

Source: Levy MR, Dignan M & Shirreffs JH (1992) *Life & Health. Targeting Wellness* (p 207) New York: McGraw-Hill.

Most males experience a ***refractory period*** following orgasm, during which they cannot achieve another orgasm. This period varies from several minutes to several hours. In older men, the refractory period may be 24 hours or longer.

Note that sexual excitement affects not only the genital areas but the whole body, including skeletal muscle tension, breathing rate, heart rate, and blood pressure. This should remind you of the chapter on stress and of the general adaptation syndrome (GAS). The sexual response mirrors the alarm stage of the GAS, which should not be surprising, as sexual excitement is another example of a stressor.

Figure 10.3 shows the similarity between male and female sexual responses. There are also differences:

- Males typically experience a **refractory period**, while females don't.
- Females may experience a prolonged, or **status**, **orgasm**.
- The female resolution stage may be **longer**.
- Males may be more quickly and easily aroused by **visual stimuli**.

However, the general similarities between the two sexes are much greater than the differences. There are also large *individual* differences in sexual preferences. The message here is for partners to communicate and, within the context of respecting personal boundaries, try different forms of sexual pleasuring.

In intercourse, the female's clitoris receives some indirect stimulation as the thrusting penis tugs on the skin around the clitoris, and also from her partner's pubic bone. She may, however, value additional manual clitoral stimulation both before and during intercourse. "Women are in an interesting predicament anatomically. The vagina is where the penis enters and where the fusion of the partners' bodies occurs. In a psychological sense, the vagina is where the woman perceives the relationships of sex. Yet the vagina and the penis may not be comparable organs. The erotic potential of the penis is more comparable to that of the clitoris" (Byer & Shainberg, 1994, p. 208). This is not surprising, as the clitoris and the penis come from the same structure. In early fetal life, the male and female external genitalia are identical. Later in fetal development, one structure becomes the male penis or the female clitoris, while another tissue becomes the female labia or, in the male, closes over to form the scrotum.

What is the right age to have sex?

The idea of "right" and "wrong" involves value judgments, which we usually try to avoid in health education. Instead, we support options and informed choice.

Sex spans a large range of activities. I assume the person asking the question meant **sexual intercourse**. Here is what comes to mind when I think of an answer to this question:

From a biological point of view, the onset of puberty (around age 11 or 12 for girls and a year or so later for boys) typically signals the onset of sexual readiness. Blood levels of sexual hormones increase; this triggers development of secondary sex characteristics, such as breasts and hips in females, more prominent testicles in males, and pubic hair in both sexes. The physiological changes in puberty also typically evoke an interest in sex, expressed through flirting, kissing, dating, and so on. Some parts of the world celebrate puberty ritually, and young people begin marriage and intercourse (not always in that order) shortly thereafter.

The norm in modern Western culture is a prolonged adolescence. Young people are considered too young to drive until age 16 or so, too young to vote until age 18, too young to purchase alcohol legally until age 19, and so on. That is, our culture considers youth unable to make informed, responsible decisions until their later teens. The same applies to consent for sexual activity.

In Canada, the legal **age of consent** for sexual intercourse is 16 if the other partner is an adult (if the youth is 14 or 15, Canadian law allows sex with a partner who is less than five years older). In other words, our laws imply that younger teens are not emotionally or intellectually mature enough to be trusted with such important decisions.

It seems logical to me to provide pre-teens with the facts, at home or at school. This information would include basic reproductive anatomy and physiology, human sexual response, contraception, disease, and safer sex practices. Also, it makes sense to help these youth develop self-esteem, self-confidence, assertiveness, and communication skills, so they can make better choices about if, when, how, and with whom to have sex.

At the other end of the lifespan, there is no age that is inherently "too old" to have sex.

Older men typically have a longer refractory period (the interval after one orgasm before they can have another orgasm). The refractory period in a 20-year-old may be 10 minutes, while for a 60-year-old it might be 48 hours. Some older men experience **impotence**, an inability to maintain a firm enough erection for long enough to achieve orgasm. Impotence can be caused by a number of different things: acute or chronic alcohol consumption, recreational or prescription drug side effects, atherosclerosis, anxiety, and dysfunctional relationships, among many other things.

Older women typically experience thinning and drying of the vaginal walls. They may need supplementary lubrication or longer foreplay before the vagina is moist enough for pleasant penetration.

6 Variations in Sexual Behaviour

Typically, sex involves kissing, touching, and intercourse. However, a number of variations are considered healthy and acceptable. **Healthy sex** occurs between consenting adults who treat each other in a caring and respectful way. Within these boundaries, a wide range of behaviours can be sexually exciting and pleasing. The key is communicating with your partner, and possibly experimenting with various positions and techniques, to find the type and amount of sexual activity satisfying for both partners.

6.1 Rape

Sexual assault is *unhealthy* because it violates the requirement for consent. Even within a marriage, it is *not* okay for one partner to force the other to do something she doesn't want to do.

6.2 Sex with children

Sex involving children is also *unhealthy* and is almost universally condemned. The key issues here are inability to properly give consent if one is too young, and exploitation due to an imbalance in power between adult and child. Sexual exploitation of children is a growing concern here in Canada, and elsewhere. For example, there is a growing practice of selling children in the developing world (e.g., India and Thailand) to "sex tourists" from within these countries and from Europe and North America.

6.3 Masturbation

There is nothing inherently unhealthy about masturbation or other variations described in the rest of Section 6.

Masturbation means stimulating oneself (usually the genitals) for erotic pleasure. Masturbation is common: 92% to 97% of males and 72% to 78% of females report masturbating. Males begin masturbating earlier, and do it more frequently than females. Single or divorced people masturbate more than their married counterparts, although well over half of married people masturbate regularly. Some cultural shame is attached to masturbation, and consequently there is some secrecy, guilt, and anxiety around it. However, health experts consider masturbation harmless, unless it is used consistently instead of what could be more rewarding interpersonal encounters. Masturbation of one's partner is an option with a very low risk of disease or pregnancy, although this risk increases if the ejaculate falls near the female genitals.

> ### Can masturbation hurt?

Yes, but it shouldn't if it is done right.

Technically, masturbation means using one's hand to stimulate one-self or someone else sexually. A somewhat broader definition includes physical stimulation with something other than the mouth/tongue or genitals. This broader definition includes things like inserting penis-shaped objects such as carrots or dildos (rubber artificial penises) into the vagina or anus; inserting the penis into a milk bottle or a hole cut in a watermelon; or allowing pressured water (such as from a bathtub tap) to flow over the clitoris.

It seems there are two main kinds of physical hurt masturbation could cause: **friction** and **puncture**. Rubbing the skin, especially rapidly and repeatedly, or if the skin is dry, causes friction. If you do too much of this to your clitoris or penis, the skin will become irritated and red, and will feel like a rash or a mild sunburn.

Penetration seems more dangerous. The anus and vagina can adapt to accommodate objects quite large in diameter. I have seen photos of an anus dilated to over three centimetres in diameter (i.e., large enough to accommodate a cucumber). Accounts of **fisting** (inserting the hand into the rectum or vagina to the level of the wrist or further, and then pumping with an in-and-out motion) are not uncommon for both homosexual and heterosexual males and females. However, this kind of accommodation takes time (probably building up to larger and larger objects gradually over weeks and months) and lots of lubrication. Inserting something that is too large, with too much force, or without enough lubrication can tear tissues and cause bleed-ing that might need surgical repair.

Another risk of penetration is losing the object into the body cavity and being unable to retrieve it. I have seen three X-ray images from hospital emergency rooms that show (a) a golf ball, (b) a light bulb, and (c) a spray can of underarm deodorant lodged in people's rectums. People had put these things into themselves for the purpose of sexual stimulation, and then couldn't get them out. Not fun! I assume the objects were recovered by sedating the patient, stretching the anus with surgical spreaders, and then sewing up any resulting damage.

6.4 Oral sex

Cunnilingus (the stimulation of the female genitals with the lips and tongue) and *fellatio* (the stimulation of the penis with the mouth) are common forms of sexual expression. Various surveys have reported that 60% to 95% of couples practise oral sex. It may be used as part of foreplay (i.e., stimulation leading to intercourse) or it may be carried on to orgasm. Cunnilingus may be more comfortable for the recipient than manual stimulation, because the tongue is moister and softer than the hand. If fellatio is continued to orgasm, a condom can help protect the receptive partner from potential pathogens in the semen. **Dental dams** (thin sheets of rubber about 10 cm, or 4 inches, square, which are used to cover part of a patient's mouth during some dental procedures) can provide similar protection of the female genitalia.

6.5 Anal intercourse

Both homosexual and heterosexual couples have anal intercourse. There are no biological differences between the male and female anus. Because of the anus's association with excrement, some people consider anal sex to be a "turn-off." On the other hand, the anus and lower end of the rectum have many sensory endings. This explains why the receptive partner can learn to enjoy this practice. Anal sex is reportedly popular in cultures that place a high value on female virginity at marriage.

The anus adapts to repeated penetration. In one of the more remarkable examples of biological adaptation, over time the anus can relax and enlarge enough to receive an adult's closed fist and forearm. The anus has little natural lubrication, so it should be well lubricated, as should anything inserted into it, and the anus itself should be manually dilated before insertion. Forcing anything into the anus can cause injury.

Also, bacteria and other organisms are normally present within the anus. Anything that has been inserted into the anus can cause infections if subsequently inserted into the vagina. Thus, the object should be thoroughly washed before insertion into the vagina, or a lubricated condom should be used and removed before vaginal intercourse.

6.6 Homosexuality

Homosexuality means sex with a person of the same gender. An important distinction should be made between **sexual behaviour** and **sexual orientation.** The percent of the population who report having sex with a person of the same sex is consistently higher than those who identify themselves as being homosexual, gay, lesbian, or bisexual. In 1948 and 1953, Alfred Kinsey reported on the sexual behaviour of the human male and female, respectively. These books came to be known collectively as *The Kinsey Reports* (Kinsey, Pomeroy, & Martin, 1948; Kinsey et al., 1953). Based on in-depth, face-to-face interviews with 5,300 white males and 5,940 white females, he concluded that 37% of the males and 13% of the females had at least some overt homosexual experience of orgasm (either their own or their partner's orgasm). Ten percent of the males and 2% to 6% of the females were considered "more or less exclusively homosexual." Four percent of males and 1% to 3% of females had been exclusively homosexual since the end of adolescence.

Many subsequent surveys have attempted to estimate the prevalence of homosexuality in North American youth and young adults. It is difficult to establish prevalence of homosexuality because many people are hesitant to answer sexual surveys, and because of differences in samples and case definitions used (e.g., "engaging in sexual behaviour with a person of the same sex" vs. "being attracted to people of the same sex.") Whatever the exact figure, it is a sizeable minority.

Before 1980, the American Psychiatric Association classified homosexuality as a mental illness. Many therapists attempted to help their gay and lesbian patients revert to a "normal" sexual orientation. Now, homosexuality is considered by health experts to be a normal variation. Evidence is mounting that homosexuality (at least in males) is biologically determined, perhaps by low blood levels of testosterone and other male hormones during fetal and early infant brain development. This makes an even stronger case for helping gay and lesbian individuals accept their sexual identity rather than trying to "convert" them. There is also a need to help them deal with their parents, friends, and coworkers, and at the societal level to decrease prejudice against homosexual people.

> Think of the variations of sexual expression described in Sections 6.3 to 6.6.
>
> Are there some you find particularly unappealing? How does the philosophy of this chapter encourage you to think about your feeling?

7 Commercial Sex

Commercial sex workers include prostitutes, escorts, exotic dancers, massage parlour workers, and actors in adult movies. The consumers of this sex are overwhelmingly male, while both males and females act as providers. Prostitution is illegal in all of the US states except for Nevada. In Canada, prostitution per se (i.e., having sex for money) is not illegal. It *was* illegal to operate a brothel, to earn a living working for a prostitute (e.g., as a driver or bodyguard), and to communicate in public about prostitution. In 2013 the Canadian Supreme Court struck down those laws because they violated sex workers' right to "life, liberty and security of the person" as guaranteed under the Canadian Charter of Rights and Freedoms.

A year later the federal government brought in new legislation (Bill C-36) that criminalizes those who buy sex, as well as making it illegal to benefit from the sale of sexual services or to communicate for the sale of sexual services; sex workers can still advertise their services, but places that run these ads—newspapers, websites, and so on—are illegal. The expressed intent of the new laws was to discourage prostitution by reducing demand for it. The Canadian Civil Liberties Association (2015) says Bill C-36 has created several civil liberties issues, including that "prohibiting the purchase of sex and communication in public regarding that purchase may endanger the security of prostitutes, as those seeking to purchase sexual services may be motivated to meet in more secluded areas to avoid criminal sanction." Advocates for sex workers have raised the same concerns:

> Targeting clients is just as bad as targeting sex workers, the advocates said. Their premise is that sex work should not be criminalized, neither for receivers, nor providers of sexual services.... All of the advocates said the law would create dangerous conditions for sex workers, pushing them into alleyways and industrial sectors to escape police surveillance and to protect their clients and income. (Stevenson, 2014)

There are a number of thorny issues involved with commercial sex. Some people have labelled commercial sex a "victimless" crime—a legitimate exchange of money for services among consenting adults. Some sex workers choose this work to support children, pay for student tuition, or supplement income from another job. It has been argued that it is safer for both provider and consumer for this exchange to occur in licensed and inspected brothels than in back alleys, automobiles, and rented hotel rooms.

There are strong religious and moral objections to all forms of commercial sex, in which it is argued that sex outside of marriage, or at least outside a loving intimate relationship, is wrong. There is also the concern that the growing social acceptance of commercial sex (e.g., strippers in pubs, X-rated video shops in suburban malls) objectifies and degrades women in general and undermines healthy intimate relationships.

There is a strong association between sex work and substance abuse. Money to purchase drugs may be the initial motive to start this work, and the drugs help suppress feelings of shame and disgust, and so allow people to continue doing it. Finally, people may be forced into commercial sex by actual or threatened physical abuse by pimps or boyfriends. In this case, the "consenting adults" argument falls apart, and it is no longer a victimless arrangement.

What's *your* opinion?
  a) Should the Canadian law around commercial sex stay as it is?
  b) Should prostitution itself be made illegal?
  c) Should people who purchase sex from prostitutes be prosecuted?
  d) Should prostitution be more legitimized within society, with special places designated as "red light" districts, licensing, and periodic health inspections?

8 Pornography

Pornography, the description or depiction of sexual acts for the purpose of sexual pleasure, has existed for millennia. Archaeologists have discovered images of sexual scenes from ancient Egypt, China, Greece, and elsewhere. The publications of *Moll Flanders* (1722) and *Fanny Hill* (1748) are literary landmarks. The 20th century saw the rise of the film industry; pornographic films were mainly an underground phenomenon until they began screening at X-rated movie theatres in the 1970s. Such films became more widely distributed on videotape in the 1980s. Today, the Internet seems to be the main platform for the distribution and consumption of pornography.

Is pornography **obscene?** Canadian law states that "In order for a work or material to qualify as 'obscene,' the exploitation of sex must not only be its dominant characteristic, but such exploitation must be 'undue.' " Discussing the **undue exploitation of sex,** the Canadian Supreme Court ruled that

> The portrayal of sex coupled with **violence** will almost always constitute the undue exploitation of sex. Explicit sex which is **degrading** or **dehumanizing** may be undue if the risk of harm is substantial. Explicit sex that is not violent and neither degrading nor dehumanizing is generally tolerated in our society and will not qualify as the undue exploitation of sex unless it employs **children** in its production. (Supreme Court of Canada, 1992; bold added)

Child pornography shows a person who *is* or *is depicted as being* under the age of eighteen years and is engaged in or is depicted as engaged in explicit sexual activity.

It seems impossible to get an accurate figure for how many or what type of people consume pornography (porn). It does seem clear that consumption is widespread and that porn is a multi-billion-dollar industry. Traditionally, porn has targeted males; however, a sizeable portion of females also identify as consumers (Hess, 2013; Winter, 2013; Borreli, 2015). Porn is a highly charged issue. Most of the debate and research has focused on the *negative* effects: porn is evil, destroys the minds and souls of those who consume it, tears at the social and moral fabric of the family and society, and leads to depression, social isolation, objectification of humans (especially females), adultery, loss of interest in normal sex, and sexual violence (Abel, 2013; The Family and Christian Guide to Movie Reviews, no date; Fight the New Drug, 2018). Others assert that porn per se is not a problem, and that porn can actually *improve* personal and relationship wellness (Ley, Prause and Finn, 2014).

Remember what Chapter 9: Mental Health said about **fantasies:** these and other defence mechanisms can help people cope in the short term, but are obstacles to achieving ultimate resolution of conflict. For example, a person who has been unable to find opportunities for sexual fulfillment with another person might find some solace in porn. However, staying home and watching or reading porn isn't going to resolve the loneliness issue.

What about porn **addiction?** According to the holistic model, it is probably unhealthy to do *anything* to the extent that it interferes with balance physically, mentally, emotionally, socially, and so on. The scientific evidence on pornography addiction is mixed. For example, one study found that compared with normal controls, those with "compulsive sexual behaviour" had *greater* activity in certain brain areas following exposure to sexual cues (Voon et al., 2014). These authors suggested that addiction to sex, porn, and/or Internet use may all be manifestations of addictive behaviour similar to drug addiction (Love et al., 2015; Brand et al., 2016). Another study reported that in frequent porn viewers, a part of the brain was smaller and *less active* than in those who viewed less porn (Kuhn & Gallinat, 2014). By contrast, in a third study, brain activity in subjects shown erotic imagery was the *same* in sex addicts as in normal people. It was level of sexual desire (libido)—not porn addiction—that associated with brain activity (Ley, 2013).

The *Diagnostic and Statistical Manual of Mental Disorders* (DSM-5) has diagnostic categories for various substance use disorders (alcohol, tobacco, cannabis, etc.). It also has a new category called "behavioral addictions," in which it includes "gambling disorder." The DSM-5, however, contains no diagnosis called "pornography addiction." We explore the emotionally charged concept of addiction more in Chapter 13: Drugs.

In 1969, Denmark became the first country in the world to legalize porn (Denmark made child porn illegal in 1980 and sex with animals illegal in 2015).

Kutchinsky (1973) suggested that the subsequent decline of sex crimes in Denmark is a result of the legalization of porn—the so-called **Danish experiment.** The same author subsequently compared statistics from Denmark with three other countries where pornography was relatively accessible. He concluded,

> In sum, the aggregate data on rape and other violent or sexual offences from four countries where pornography has become widely and easily available during the period we have dealt with would seem to exclude, beyond any reasonable doubt, that this availability has had any detrimental effects in the form of increased sexual violence. (Kutchinsky, 1991)

As you learned in Chapter 2: Evaluating Health Claims, just because two things are *associated* does not mean that one *causes* the other. Perhaps rape and child abuse were declining *anyway*, for example, due to lower social tolerance of these acts. Some people (e.g., Net Nanny, 2009) claim that the rape statistics featured in this association were reported incorrectly and that rape actually *increased* in Denmark after 1970. This underscores the difficulty of determining what is and isn't true about pornography.

Three other health concerns deserve mention.

- Porn films often show unprotected sex, so pornographic actors are likely particularly vulnerable to sexually transmitted infections (Lubben, 2008).
- Porn is almost always produced and consumed as entertainment, not as sex education. The actors' physiques, their stamina, the size of their sex organs, the sex acts they are pretending to enjoy, etc. portray a very unrealistic and often unhealthy view of sexual intimacy (Clark-Flory, 2014).
- Some people spend a lot of time consuming porn. This might reasonably be considered a waste of time by those who identify lack of time as a barrier to physical activity, preparing healthy meals, studying, relaxing, and so on.

9 Sexual Health Promotion

Many youths and young adults practise unhealthy forms of sex, despite having ample information regarding the risks, and despite knowing how to practise safer sex. This contradiction has been explained several ways:

- Young people tend to be egocentric and perceive themselves as invulnerable.

- They may have trouble visualizing the consequences. The same factor explains why fear of lung cancer is not a strong motivation for young people to quit smoking.
- If the knowledge is to influence their decision-making and subsequent behaviour effectively, individuals must learn to believe it is *their own behaviour*, and not that of others, that puts them at risk of contracting AIDS and other STDs.

There are a number of risk factors associated with unsafe sexual behaviours.

- **Earlier age of first coitus:** Those who have intercourse the first time at a young age are at increased risk of unsafe sexual behaviours.
- **Substance use:** Use of alcohol or other drugs increases risk.
- **Male gender:** Males are at greater risk of unsafe sexual behaviours than females.
- **Peers as the main source of sex information:** When peers are young people's main source of information, and when young people have sexually active peers, they are more likely to become sexually active themselves, and their age increases their risk for unsafe behaviours.
- **Television:** Young people who get a lot of their information about sex from television are at increased risk of unsafe sexual behaviours.

Parents and older siblings can act as healthy role models, countering the effects of the above risk factors on younger children in the family. Young people, especially women, who adhere to a religious faith, are at reduced risk of participating in unsafe sexual practices.

Optimal sexual health can be promoted by lifelong sex education, starting in elementary school, before children have become sexually active and when they are more open to these messages. Public health nurses and family physicians can help reinforce these messages. Those with significant risk factors can be targeted for extra help.

10 Conclusion

Accepting one's sexual identity, forming meaningful intimate relationships, and learning how to behave responsibly around sex are among the most important health goals of adolescence and young adulthood. The greater freedom in modern society offers opportunities for a variety of living and loving arrangements. At the same time, it creates many new temptations and pressures. Sexual health education can help young people make informed choices. Such programs will be more effective if they are tailored to the needs and motivations of particular subgroups, and deal with values, beliefs, and communication skills as well as basic biological information.

Study Questions

1. What four points of view does the author articulate in the Overview of this chapter?

2. Give four plausible explanations for the observation that married people have lower mortality rates than their non-married counterparts.

3. What features do most intimate relationships share?

4a. How does Peck define "love"?

4b. Peck says rather than being an act of desire, love is an act of what?

4c. Peck says "we are incapable of loving another unless" we do what first?

5. You should be able to identify these anatomical structures on a diagram:
   - Penis
   - Urethra
   - Glans
   - Scrotum
   - Testicle (testes is the plural form)
   - Prostate gland
   - Vas deferens
   - Foreskin
   - Labia
   - Clitoris
   - Vagina
   - Cervix
   - Uterus
   - Ovary

6. Describe the process of conception, starting with the ovum (egg) and sperm and continuing to implantation of the fertilized ovum on the wall of the uterus.

7a. What is circumcision?

7b. What is the medical health value of circumcision?

8a. List the four stages in the normal human sexual response.

8b. Draw a diagram showing the change in sexual tension with time. Show the typical male and female responses as separate lines on the same graph.

8c. Describe the physiological changes typical of each stage.

9. Discuss variations (healthy and unhealthy) of sexual behaviour.

10. Discuss the legal, social, and ethical issues around commercial sex (sex for money).

11. What health effects have been linked with regular viewing of pornography?

12a. Describe in several sentences the concept of "healthy sex."

12b. Suggest several reasons why many Canadian youths and young adults practise unhealthy sex.

12c. What characteristics are more common in those who practise unsafe sex?

Glossary

cervix—the bottom (outer end) of the uterus, where it joins with the vagina

clitoris—a small, sensitive part of the female genitalia located at the forward end of the labia

cohabitation—living together, usually implying the absence of a formal union such as marriage

cunnilingus—oral sex on a woman

fellatio—oral sex on a man

foreskin—a flap of skin that covers the end of the penis

glans—the end of the penis

labia—folds of skin that cover the opening of the vagina

menstrual cycle—a complex series of coordinated events that happens about once a month in fertile females; a number of hormones play a role in regulation of this cycle, the most obvious feature of which is bleeding from the uterus, which is normally counted as Day 1 of the cycle

ova (singular = ovum)—ova are "eggs," the female reproductive cells; if fertilized, an ovum may develop into a fetus

ovaries—the part of the female reproductive system where ova (eggs) are produced; females normally have two ovaries

ovulation—an event in which one or more ova are released from the ovaries; this occurs about once a month in fertile females

refractory period—a part of the resolution stage in males; during this stage, it is not possible to achieve another orgasm

uterus—the womb, a hollow organ that is part of the female reproductive system; if an ovum (egg) is fertilized, it may implant into the wall of the uterus, where it may develop into a fetus

vagina—part of the female genitalia, this corrugated, tube-like organ runs from the outside of the body (where it is flanked by the labia) to the cervix

sperm—the male reproductive cells; if a sperm successfully fertilizes an ovum, that ovum may develop into a fetus

testicle—the part of the male genitalia in which sperm are produced; males normally have two

vas deferens—the tube that connects the epididymis with the urethra; it carries sperm and seminal fluid out through the penis

References

Abel, I. (June 7, 2013). Was I actually 'addicted' to Internet pornography? *The Atlantic.* Retrieved May 22, 2018 from https://www.theatlantic.com/health/archive/2013/06/was-i-actually-addicted-to-internet-pornography/276619/

American Academy of Pediatrics. (2012). Circumcision policy statement. *Pediatrics.* 130(3), 585–586.

Borreli, L. (August 12, 2015). Watching adult films alters brain activity similar to addicts, alcoholics: The pornographic mind. *Medical Daily*, published by Newsweek Media Group. Retrieved May 20, 2018 from https://www.medicaldaily.com/watching-adult-films-alters-brain-activity-similar-drug-addicts-alcoholics-347224

Brand, M., Young, K., Laier, C., Wolfling, K., Potenza, M. N. (December 2016). Integrating psychological and neurobiological considerations regarding the development and maintenance of specific Internet-use disorders: An Interaction of Person-Affect-Cognition-Execution (I-PACE) model. *Neuroscience and Biobehavioral Reviews.* 71:252-266. Retrieved May 22, 2018 from https://doi.org/10.1016/j.neubiorev.2016.08.033

Canadian Civil Liberties Association. (May 13, 2015). Understanding Bill C-36, The Protection Of Communities And Exploited Persons Act. Retrieved May 4, 2018 from https://ccla.org/understanding-bill-c-36-the-protection-of-communities-and-exploited-persons-act/

Canadian Paediatric Society. (February 28, 2018). Position Statement on Newborn Male Circumcision. Retrieved May 4, 2018 from www.cps.ca/en/documents/position/circumcision

Clark-Flory, T. (September 30, 2014). Keeping it up. The Fix. Retrieved May 22, 2018 from https://www.thefix.com/content/keeping-it-porn-industry

CYWH. (2010). *Sports and menstrual periods: The female athlete triad.* Center for Young Women's Health. Retrieved January 15, 2013 from http://www.youngwomenshealth.org/triad.html

The Family and Christian Guide to Movie Reviews. (no date). The effects of pornography on individuals, marriage, family, and community. Retrieved May 22, 2018 from https://www.movieguide.org/news-articles/the-effects-of-pornography-on-individuals-marriage-family-and-community.html

Fight the New Drug. (2018). Retrieved May 22, 2018 from https://fightthenewdrug.org

Hess, A. (October 11, 2013). How many women are not admitting to Pew that they watch porn. *Slate.* Retrieved May 20, 2018 from http://www.slate.com/blogs/xx_factor/2013/10/11/pew_online_viewing_study_percentage_of_women_who_watch_online_porn_is_growing.html

Kinsey, A., Pomeroy, W., Martin, C. (1948). *Sexual behavior in the human male.* Philadelphia: W. B. Saunders.

Kinsey, A., Pomeroy, W., Martin, C., Gebhard, P. (1953). *Sexual behavior in the human female.* Philadelphia: W. B. Saunders.

Kravdal, H., Syse, A. (October 14, 2011). Changes over time in the effect of marital status on cancer survival. *BMC Public Health.* 11, 804.

Kuhn, S., Gallinat, J. (2014). Brain structure and functional connectively associated with pornography consumption: The brain on porn. *JAMA Psychiatry.* 71(7):827-834.

Kutchinsky, B. (Summer 1973). The effect of easy availability of pornography on the incidence of sex crimes: The Danish experience. *Journal of Social Issues.* 29(3):163-181.

Kutchinsky, B. (1991). Pornography and rape: Theory and Practice?: Evidence from crime data in four countries where pornography is easily available. *International Journal of Law and Psychiatry.* 14(1):47-64.

Ley, D. J. (July 25, 2013). Your brain on porn – it's NOT addictive. *Psychology Today*. Retrieved May 20, 2018 from https://www.psychologytoday.com/us/blog/women-who-stray/201307/your-brain-porn-its-not-addictive

Ley, D., Prause, N., Finn, P. (June 2014). The emperor has no clothes: A review of the 'pornography addiction' model. *Current Sexual Health Reports*. 6(2):94-105.

Liu, H., Reczek, C. (2012). Cohabitation and US adult mortality: An examination by gender and race. *Journal of Marriage and Family*. 74, 794–811.

Love, T., Laier, C., Brand, M., Hatch, L., Hajela, R. (2015). Neuroscience of Internet pornography addiction: A review and update. *Behavioral Science*. 5(3):388-433.

Lubben, S. (October 28, 2008). Ex-porn star tells the truth about the porn industry. Covenant Eyes. Retrieved May 22, 2018 from http://www.covenanteyes.com/2008/10/28/ex-porn-star-tells-the-truth-about-the-porn-industry/

Masters, W. H., Johnson, V. E. (1966). *Human sexual response*. Boston: Little, Brown.

Masters, W. H., Johnson, V. E. (1970). *Human sexual inadequacy*. Boston: Little, Brown.

Masters, W. H., Johnson, V. E. , Kolodny, R. C. (1988). *Human sexuality* (3rd ed.). Glenview, IL: Scott, Foresman.

Net Nanny (May 21, 2009). The "Denmark Experiment" Failed! Porn Affects Behavior. Retrieved May 22, 2018 from https://www.netnanny.com/blog/the-denmark-experiment-failed-porn-affects-behavior/

Peck, M. S. (1978). *The Road Less Traveled*. NY: Simon & Schuster.

Roelfs, D. J,. Shor, E., Kalish, R., Yogev, T. (2011). The rising relative risk of mortality for singles: Meta-analysis and meta-regression. *American Journal of Epidemiology*. 174(4), 379–389.

Sorokan, S. T., Finlay, J. C, Jefferies, A. L. (February 28, 2015). Newborn male circumcision. *Paediatrics and Child Health*. 20(6):311-315.

Stevenson, V. (September 9, 2014). Advocates: Gov't Leaves Sex Workers Out of the Discussion on Bill C-36. *The Link*. Retrieved May 4, 2018 from https://ccla.org/understanding-bill-c-36-the-protection-of-communities-and-exploited-persons-act/https://thelinknewspaper.ca/article/for-the-people-by-the-people-just-not-all-the-people

Supreme Court of Canada. (1992). *R. v. Butler*, [1992] 1 S.C.R. 452. Retrieved May 22, 2018 from https://scc-csc.lexum.com/scc-csc/scc-csc/en/item/844/index.do

Voon, V., Mole, T. B., Banca, P., Porter, L., Morris, L., Mitchell, S., Lapa, T., Karr, J. Harrison, N. A., Potenza, M. N., Irvine, M. (July 11, 2014). Neural correlates of sexual cue reactivity in individuals with and without compulsive sexual behaviours. PLOS One. Retrieved May 22, 2018 from http://journals.plos.org/plosone/article?id=10.1371/journal.pone.0102419

WHO. (2007). *Male circumcision: Global trends and determinants of prevalence, safety and acceptability*. World Health Organization and Joint United Nations Programme on HIV/AIDS. Retrieved January 18, 2013 from http://whqlibdoc.who.int/publications/2007/9789241596169_eng.pdf

Winter, K. (November 15, 2013). It's not just men who watch porn! *Daily Mail*. Retrieved May 20, 2018 from http://www.dailymail.co.uk/femail/article-2507752/Over-half-women-regularly-watch-porn-daring-40-admit-making-own.html

11 Sexually Transmitted Infections

Learning Objectives

By the time you have finished this chapter you should be able to

- Discuss HIV infection and AIDS, including transmission, disease progression, epidemiology, treatment, and prevention
- Describe hepatitis, differentiating between fecal-oral and body-fluid transmission modes
- Explain human papillomavirus infection, including prevalence, transmission, and prevention
- Summarize herpes simplex virus infection, including prevalence, transmission, treatment, and prevention
- Name the three most common STIs in the USA and differentiate these from the viral infections named above
- Discuss, in holistic terms, the root causes for global mortality from sexually transmissible infections

1 Overview

In Chapter 3: Infectious Disease you learned about infectious diseases, many of which are **communicable**; that is, they can be passed or transmitted from one person to another. In this chapter, we will look at several specific infections for which direct contact, or exchange of body fluids during sexual activities, are main modes of transmission. The *prevalence* and incidence of STIs is high: in the USA an estimated 110 million Americans have an STI, with nearly 20 million new infections occurring yearly. Young people (age 15–24) are disproportionately affected, comprising 50% of all new STIs while representing only 25% of the "sexually experienced" population (CDC, 2013).

2 HIV/AIDS

In the late 1970s and early 1980s in New York and San Francisco, young men in apparently good health began developing rare types of cancer, pneumonia, and other disorders. This disorder was subsequently named *AIDS*. The first case of AIDS in Canada was reported in 1982. Research pointed to the *human immunodeficiency virus (HIV)* as the cause.

It is now generally believed that the disease started in central Africa, where infected primates (monkeys and chimpanzees) transmitted it to humans by biting them. AIDS activists, however, typically urge us to focus less on pinpointing the origins of AIDS and more on developing effective prevention and treatment methods.

> ### *What is the difference between HIV and AIDS?*
>
> HIV is an abbreviation for "human immunodeficiency virus." It is the name of a **pathogen**. Infection with this pathogen results in HIV infection. The most common way to test whether a person is infected is to analyze his or her blood for the presence of **antibodies** to HIV. That is, rather than looking for the virus directly, the laboratory looks for the antibodies produced in response to HIV infection. A person so infected is diagnosed as "HIV positive."
>
> AIDS is an abbreviation for **acquired** (i.e., not inherited) **immune deficiency** (i.e., reduced functioning of the immune system) **syndrome** (a group of signs and symptoms that commonly occur together, usually used as diagnostic criteria). HIV infection leads to AIDS. AIDS is a later stage of the infection.
>
> The diagnostic criteria for AIDS vary in different countries. A common set of criteria is (a) being HIV positive, (b) having a T cell[1] count below 200, and (c) having one or more of some 15 specific **opportunistic infections** that are rare in people who are not HIV infected. HIV weakens the immune system, which allows these rare infections to occur. Usually an opportunistic infection is the cause of death from AIDS.

---

1   A T cell is a type of white blood cell of key importance to the immune system and at the core of adaptive immunity, the system that tailors the body's immune response to specific pathogens (MedicineNet.com, 2013).

2.1 Natural history of HIV/AIDS

Viruses enter body cells, use the cellular machinery to make copies of themselves, and destroy the host cell in the process. HIV multiplies within T cells, a type of white blood cell that is part of the immune system. This is particularly troublesome because as the HIV infection advances, it destroys an important part of the immune system. This leaves the infected person vulnerable to a range of opportunistic infections, such as rare cancers and infections that are not a health threat in people with a normal immune system.

After HIV enters someone's body, it takes a week or more to build up to concentrations that make it contagious to others (Figure 11.1). Infection is accompanied by early acute symptoms, such as fever, fatigue, and swollen lymph glands. Unless the person has reason to suspect he has been infected (e.g., an accidental needle-stick injury or an episode of high-risk sex), these symptoms are often mistaken for the flu or a cold. Viruses are difficult to detect directly in body fluids. However, their presence causes the body to produce *antibodies* against them, and these antibodies can be detected with blood tests. It takes several weeks or more after infection for the antibody levels to increase to levels that will produce a positive blood test. At this point, the person is said to be **HIV positive**. There is a window of several weeks to several months during which an HIV-infected person will test negative but will be able to infect others.

2.2 Transmission

HIV is *not* highly contagious. Casual contact with infected people is unlikely to cause transmission. Rather, transmission requires intimate contact with body fluids, especially blood, semen, vaginal fluids, and breast milk. The main routes of infection these days are through

- Unprotected intercourse
- Unsterile needles (including those used for tattooing)
- Mother to fetus or infant

A mother can infect her fetus while it is in the womb, because the virus can pass from the mother's blood to the fetal blood through the **placenta**. Infants can also be infected while breastfeeding. The WHO estimates that without intervention, mother-to-child transmission rates are between 15% and 45%. If both mother and child are supplied with antiretroviral drugs,[2] transmission is almost fully prevented (WHO, 2013b).

---

2   A brief explanation is in order to contextualize the terms **antiretroviral therapy** and **antiretroviral drugs**. Most viruses have DNA as their genetic material, which they transcribe into RNA in a host cell. Retroviruses do the reverse; their genetic material is RNA, which they transcribe into DNA after entering a cell.

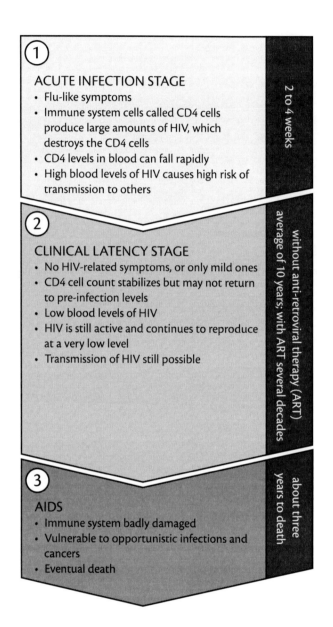

Figure 11.1. The stages in HIV infection and AIDS.

In the 1980s, thousands of Canadians were infected with HIV or the hepatitis C virus (HCV) through **transfusion** of contaminated blood. As a result of this scandal, the national blood donor system was transferred from the Canadian Red Cross to a new agency, Canadian Blood Services, in 1999. Now blood donors and blood donations are screened. The risk of infection by HIV or HCV through blood transfusion in Canada is estimated at about 1 chance in 8–12 million transfusions, and 1 chance in 5–7 million transfusions, respectively

(MacDonald, O'Brien, Delage, 2012). These risks are lower than the risk of being hit by lightning, estimated at 1 in 3 million (MacDonald, O'Brien, Delage, 2012).

Receptive anal intercourse and **vaginal intercourse** are by far the most important routes of sexual infection. Transmission of the virus is more likely to occur during anal than vaginal intercourse because

- The skin lining the rectum is thin.
- The rectum has a rich blood supply, so the virus can easily get into the blood vessels if the skin is torn.
- The rectum contains many of the white blood cells that have the receptor molecule that lets the HIV attach to it.
- The skin is often damaged during rectal penetration, which allows contact between HIV and the cells that have the receptor molecule on their membranes.
- The vagina has better natural lubrication, is thicker, and is less easily damaged.

Risk of HIV transmission by **oral-genital** contact without protection (i.e., no condom over the penis or no dental dam over the female genitals) is also considered to be low, although higher risk than kissing.

The HIV virus has also been detected in saliva, urine, sweat, and tears, but at concentrations so low that infection by these fluids is very unlikely. The WHO advises that individuals cannot become infected through ordinary day-to-day contact, such as kissing, hugging, shaking hands, or sharing personal objects, food, or water (WHO, 2013b).

2.3 Epidemiology of HIV/AIDS

Because AIDS has a well-defined and usually obvious diagnosis, it is relatively easy to accurately track its occurrence in a population, at least in industrial countries with well-established systems of recording health data. This is less true in developing countries. Also, there is concern that some countries (e.g., China) are deliberately under-reporting AIDS in the interests of maintaining a good international image.

HIV infection is more difficult to track. The HIV-positive person may be symptom-free for many years, and blood testing is done on a voluntary basis.

2.3.1 Canada

The number of new cases of *AIDS* reported annually in Canada has declined dramatically, from a peak of about 1,800 in 1993 to less than 200 (Health Canada, 2014), as shown in Figure 11.2. The number of people living with *HIV* (including AIDS) in Canada continues to rise, from an estimated 64,000 in 2008 (PHAC,

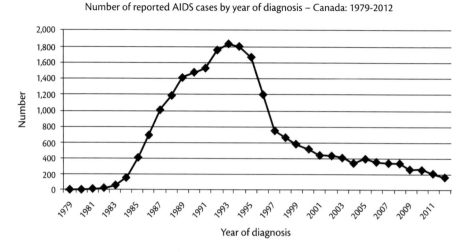

Figure 11.2. Number of reported AIDS cases in Canada by year of diagnosis.

2012c) to over 80,000 in 2014 (Health Canada, 2014). The increase in the number of people living with HIV is due to two factors:

- New treatments have improved survival of HIV-infected people.
- New infections continue to occur.

The number of new HIV infections in 2014 was reported at 2,044, down from the 2,582 reported in 2008 (Health Canada, 2014). Of those newly-infected in 2014,

- 49% were men who have sex with men (MSM).
- 13% were injection drug users (IDU).
- 10% were heterosexuals from countries where HIV infection is prevalent or **endemic**. Endemic means "regularly found among particular people or in a particular area" (The American Heritage Medical Dictionary, 2007).
- 19% were heterosexual and not from endemic countries.

Females living with HIV (including AIDS) in Canada accounted for a reported 18% of the national total (Health Canada, 2014). The two groups that were most over-represented (i.e., had more people infected with HIV than you would expect from the proportion these groups make of the total Canadian population) were

- People from HIV-endemic countries
- Indigenous people

> Do *you* know anyone with HIV infection?
>   How does your familiarity, or lack of familiarity, with HIV-infected people affect your health behaviours?

In Canada, AIDS *mortality* increased throughout the 1980s and early 1990s. It peaked in the mid-1990s and has since declined dramatically, a finding comparable to other developed countries (Norris, 2011; PHAC, 2013b).

2.3.2 United States
The epidemiology of HIV/AIDS in the United States is similar to that of Canada, with the exception that the USA has larger African American and Hispanic/Latino populations, groups in which HIV/AIDS rates are higher.

In 2016, 18,160 Americans were diagnosed with AIDS. An estimated 1,122,900 people in the USA age 13 and older are living with HIV infection, including 162,500 (15%) who are unaware of their infection. Incidence has remained stable overall in recent years, at about 50,000 new HIV infections per year (CDC, 2016).

Of those Americans newly infected with HIV (CDC, 2016),

- 67% were MSM
- 9% were IDU
- 24% were heterosexual

The two most over-represented groups in the USA were (CDC, 2016)

- Blacks (African Americans), who represent approximately 12% of the US population, accounted for an estimated 44% of new HIV diagnoses.
- Hispanics/Latinos, who represent 18% of the population, made up 25% of new HIV diagnoses.

2.3.3 Globally
HIV and AIDS are big problems globally, but in much of the world and in many ways there has been progress.

- Declines in new HIV infections are stable at about 1.9 million per year, with large regional disparities. Eastern and southern Africa saw the largest reduction in new adult HIV infection, a 4% decline. Asia, the Pacific, and western and central Africa experienced more gradual declines. Rates of new infections *increased* by 57% in eastern Europe and central Asia. Rates were relatively constant in the rest of the world (UNAIDS, 2016).

- Annual deaths from HIV/AIDS, which had increased from 300,000 in 1990 to a peak of 1.7 million in 2006, have declined since. In 2016, an estimated 1.0 million died from HIV/AIDS (WHO, 2018).
- The decrease in deaths from HIV/AIDS since 2015 has been greater in adult females than males: 33% versus 15%. This reflects higher rates of treatment among females than males: 52% versus 41% (UNAIDS, 2016).

Females age 15–24 are at particularly high risk of HIV infection. This group accounted for 20% of new HIV infections among adults globally in 2015, despite representing only 11% of the adult population. "Harmful gender norms and inequalities, insufficient access to education and sexual and reproductive health services, poverty, food insecurity and violence, are at the root of the increased HIV risk of young women and adolescent girls" (UNAIDS, 2016).

Other key populations at increased risk of HIV infection include

- Men who have sex with men
- People who inject drugs
- Sex workers
- Transgender people
- Prisoners

Again, the demographics of HIV infection vary from one region of the world to another. Injection drug users accounted for 51% of HIV infections in eastern Europe and central Asia but only 13% of new HIV infections in Asia and the Pacific. Men who have sex with men accounted for 49% of new infections in western and central Europe and North America, and for 30% in Latin America, but only 18% in Asia and the Pacific (UNAIDS, 2016).

Major goals of the UNAIDS include

- Preventing new infections
- Preventing transmission from mothers to their children *in utero* or from breastfeeding
- Treating those who are infected
- Preventing discrimination against those living with HIV or AIDS
- Caring for those orphaned because their parents died from AIDS

There is still a long way to go. Public health programs on this scale are a good investment, but they are hugely expensive. Political instability in some regions of the world, as well as global economic weakness, threatens the commitment to continue efforts against HIV and AIDS. Systemic inequalities in income and education, and social norms that disempower girls and women, pressure vulnerable groups into higher-risk lifestyles (e.g., commercial sex, unprotected intercourse). Stigmas and discrimination against key populations (e.g., same-sex relationships, drug users, sex workers) and against people living with HIV infection limit their access to HIV services.

2.4 Treatment

It currently appears that everyone (or almost everyone; see below) who gets infected with HIV will eventually die of AIDS. However, the *latent period* (time between infection with HIV and appearance of signs and symptoms of AIDS) has increased greatly in recent years due to more successful management of HIV infection by combinations of drugs. The median latent period for AIDS in industrial countries (where the drug therapy is available and affordable) is over 10 years. Overall life expectancy for HIV-infected individuals has also increased. Hogg et al. (2013) report that, in a study population of over 22,000 people in Canada and the USA, "Overall life expectancy at age 20 rose from 36.1 in 2000–2002 to 45.2 in 2003–2005, and to 51.4 in 2006–2007. The 2006–2007 estimate means a 20-year-old starting antiretroviral therapy in those years could expect to live to age 71.4."

Until recently, it seemed AIDS was incurable. It is difficult to design drugs that will kill viruses without also killing the cells they parasitize. The immune system of the infected host has trouble detecting HIV because it covers its outer proteins with rapidly mutating decoy proteins and with antibody-resistant sugar molecules called glycans (Medicalnewstoday.com, 2014).

There are, however, drugs that make it more difficult for viruses to enter cells, which slows the rate at which viruses reproduce. "Cocktails" of drugs (meaning combinations of a number of different drugs) can control the virus and keep patients healthy. Because HIV is a **retrovirus**, this treatment strategy is called **antiretroviral therapy** (ART).

In 2015 there were 17 million HIV-infected people taking antiretroviral drugs (UNAIDS, 2016). This represents huge progress compared with the 8.1 million people covered in 2011 (WHO, 2013a).

A person referred to as the "Berlin patient" may have been cured of HIV infection. He was given a bone marrow transplant to treat his cancer. It is thought that immune system cells in the bone marrow from the donor killed his own immune cells—and the HIV they contained. Six more people with HIV who got bone marrow transplants for their cancer also seem to now be free of HIV. It will be very interesting to see if these people remain HIV negative after they stop taking anti-HIV drugs (Wilson, 2017).

2.5 Prevention

There is currently *no vaccine* available to protect against HIV infection. Researchers are trying to find vaccines that either prevent infection or would control the virus so patients would be less likely to transmit it.

2.5.1 Be selective in your sexual partners

Contrary to popular myth, *it is not usually possible to tell whether someone is HIV infected by the way they look or act.* Infection occurs in all segments of society. It is safer to wait until you get to know someone well before having sex. Having a number of sexual partners increases risk. Monogamous relationships where both partners are uninfected are safe, provided both partners are faithful.

> **Do people have a chance of getting an STI even without a sex partner? What about one sex partner?**

Yes, some sexually transmitted infections can be transmitted in other ways besides sexual activity. A useful way to look at this question is from the broader perspective of transmission of infectious disease. Direct transmission can occur through exchange of body fluids, such as blood, semen, vaginal secretions, breast milk, and in some cases, saliva. It is my understanding that the concentration of pathogens in the saliva of an HIV-infected person is probably not high enough to cause transmission through kissing, even "wet kissing" or "French kissing," where the tongue of one partner enters the mouth of the other. Direct transmission can also happen with skin-to-skin contact (genitals, lips, etc.).

Hepatitis B and HIV are transmitted by exchange of body fluids. This can occur during sexual intercourse. Sharing of contaminated hypodermic needles is a common mode of transmission of these infections among injection drug users.

Sharing of personal articles such as unlaundered towels or toothbrushes can transmit yeast infections.

Young children often put toys in their mouths. A child with an oral herpes infection who sucks on a toy and then shares it with a friend can infect the friend.

Yes, you can get an STI with even one sex partner, if that person becomes infected, either through sexual contact with a third person or by non-sexual modes such as those outlined above.

> How about *you?* How well do you want to know a partner before having intercourse? The third date? Marriage?
>
>   How do you learn enough about a partner's sexual history or infection status to feel confident having sex with him or her?

2.5.2 *Practise safer sex*

Abstinence is the safest of all. Masturbation (by oneself or by a partner) is very low risk. Kissing is relatively safe. Oral sex is safer than intercourse.

2.5.3 *Use protection*

Latex condoms reduce risk during intercourse. Most condoms purchased today are latex. Condoms made from sheep intestines are available and reportedly permit greater penile sensation, but they do not provide as much protection. Disappointingly, only 58% of Canadians age 15 to 49 report using a condom the most recent time they had sex (Racco, 2018). **Dental dams** (squares of latex) can be placed over the female genitals for protection during oral sex.

The condom must be used properly to maximize protection:

- Don't store condoms for prolonged periods in the glove box of your car or in your wallet; over time, heat will cause the latex to deteriorate.
- Be careful when opening the package not to tear the condom.
- Place the condom over the erect penis, holding the tip between your fingertips to preserve a space into which the ejaculate can go. Many condoms have a receptacle tip for this purpose.
- Roll the condom down as far as it will go.
- Avoid rolling the condom down over pubic hair, as this will reduce the effectiveness with which the condom seals around the penis.
- Buy pre-lubricated condoms, or use a water-based lubricant (such as K-Y Jelly), not a petroleum-based lubricant (such as Vaseline). Petroleum-based lubricants can cause the latex to dissolve.
- Remove the penis from the vagina, anus, or mouth while the penis is still firm, and dispose of the used condom.

> Why do you think I've used the term "safer sex" above rather than "safe sex"?

2.5.4 *Communicate*

Be clear with your partner about your boundaries around sex and your expectations regarding condom use. This can be an awkward subject for new partners, but it is less difficult if discussed *before* you get in the bedroom with your clothes off.

2.5.5 Don't combine drug use and sex

Drugs change the way people think, feel, and act. People can become more adventurous and are more likely to make errors when they are high.

2.5.6 Needles

Avoid injecting drugs, but if you do, use a clean needle each time and don't share needles. Used needles can be sterilized by soaking them in a bleach solution, but this is not a foolproof procedure. If you are getting a tattoo, body piercing, or acupuncture, have the work done at a reputable establishment. Dispose of needles and surgical instruments in special containers. Don't put the needles or instruments into the regular garbage where they may cause needle-stick injuries to janitorial staff.

2.5.7 At the community level

Screen blood donations for the presence of HIV antibodies. Screen donors for risk factors and refuse donations from high-risk groups. Wear surgical gloves when you might come into contact with a person's body fluids.

2.5.8 Get a blood test

This is the only way to determine whether you are infected. Get tested regularly (e.g., yearly, or more often if you are sexually active or have multiple sex partners). The province of British Columbia offers free HIV/AIDS blood tests every five years for those age 18 to 70 and every year for people in high-risk groups (CBC, 2014). See BC Point of Care HIV Testing Program in the Additional Resources section near the end of this chapter.

> *Is it possible to get sexually transmitted diseases from sharing underwear?*

Yes. Sharing underwear probably doesn't cause enough sharing of body fluids to support infection with HIV or hepatitis B, as such fluids have probably dried by the time the second user dons the underwear. However, infection by yeast or insects such as pubic lice can happen.

3 Hepatitis

Hepatitis literally means "inflammation of the liver." Our concern here is viral hepatitis—not, for example, alcoholic hepatitis, which is not caused by a pathogen. There are five known variants of the hepatitis (hep) virus: A, B, C, D, and E.

Hep A and hep E are mainly transmitted via the **fecal-oral** route, just like cholera. Blood-borne contamination is rare. The virus is excreted in the feces of infected people and is transmitted in contaminated food and water. Prevention of hep A and hep E focuses on sanitary disposal of human wastes, provision of clean drinking water, and ensuring foods are washed or cooked before consumption

Hep B, hep C, and hep D are transmitted by the same modes as HIV—exchange of **body fluids**. The hep B antigen has been found in virtually all body fluids, but only blood, semen, vaginal fluids, and saliva have been shown to be infective. Hemophiliacs used to be at very high risk of infection. In hemophilia, a normal blood-clotting factor is lacking, and patients need regular transfusions of this factor. Since 1987, all blood products have been routinely screened in North America for the hepatitis virus. Over 80% of hemophiliacs treated with products prepared before this time contracted hepatitis. Currently, **sexual contact** and sharing of used **needles** are the main modes of transmission. Prevention of hep B, hep C, and hep D uses the same approach as prevention of HIV infection.

There is no cure for hepatitis, although antiviral drugs such as **interferons** may help. The most effective combination of current drug treatments has a cure rate of 40% to 50%. Liver transplants can be life-saving in advanced cases. Blood tests are commercially available for all types of viral hepatitis except hep E. There are vaccines effective against hep A and hep B. As hep D depends upon hep B for its replication, vaccination against hep B gives immunity against hep D as well. Researchers are working on a vaccine for hep C. Immunoglobulin (antibodies) for temporary immunity to hep A is available.

Reported cases of hepatitis C virus infection (HCV) have declined in Canada in recent years. The majority of HCV cases are among people who inject drugs (61% of new cases). Poverty and lack of social support can lead to homelessness, make people vulnerable to higher-risk behaviours, and decrease access to health services. (PHAC, 2012b).

4 Human Papillomavirus

HPV is an abbreviation for **human papillomavirus**. This is a pathogen, an infectious disease-causing agent. There are about 100 different types of HPV. More than 30 types are sexually transmitted. About 10 types are called "high risk," because they can lead to cervical and other types of cancer. Other HPV types cause skin warts.

HPV infections in the genital area are mainly transmitted by sexual activity. Hand-genital contact in a sexual way (e.g., touching yourself or touching someone else) is another, less common, route of transmission. Sharing of contaminated objects is another possible route of transmission.

HPV infection of the skin is widespread. HPV infection is the most prevalent STI, with an estimated 79 million Americans infected as of 2008 (CDC, 2013). Most sexually active men and women will probably get a genital HPV infection sometime during their lives (CDC, 2013). Estimates of the prevalence of *active* genital HPV infection vary, but may be around 10% or more of the population. A British Columbia study of almost 5,000 women age 13 to 86 participating in the provincial cervical cancer-screening program reported an overall HPV prevalence of about 17% (PHAC, 2012a). A review of over 40 studies reported a large range in prevalence of HPV infection among males, with more than half of the studies reporting prevalence of 20% or more.

There is *no treatment* for HPV infection. There are treatments for the serious diseases that HPV infection can cause (CDC, 2013). Most HPV infections clear up by themselves with no serious consequences. In 5% to 10% of infected women the infection persists beyond two years. Infections appear to clear up somewhat faster in men. Persistent infection signifies high risk of developing pre-cancerous changes to the cervix, which can lead to cervical cancer in 10 to 15 years. This large window of time provides ample opportunity to remove pre-cancerous cells if they are identified (e.g., by Pap tests).

Why is HPV so common and what are we doing to stop it?

In answer to the first part of the question, I suppose HPV infection is so common because there are many types of the pathogen. HPV infects the skin, and direct transmission from skin to skin is hard to avoid. There is a large reservoir of infected people from which others can become infected. Also, perhaps people are careless about preventing infection because they are under-informed about the prevalence, risk, or preventive strategies.

What are we doing to stop HPV infection?

Preventive strategies for HPV include sexual abstinence and condoms. Female condoms may be more effective than male condoms against HPV because the female condom covers a larger skin area. Recent research indicates that several inexpensive chemicals, including some sexual lubricants, may reduce risk of transmission.

Two different vaccines (made by two different pharmaceutical companies) have become available since 2005 to prevent infection by the types of HPV that cause most cervical cancer. The vaccine is recommended for females and males who have not yet been exposed to HPV—those who are not yet sexually active. This is somewhat controversial. Some parents are opposed to vaccinating their children against an STI on the grounds that this may unintentionally send the message that sexual activity (especially at a young age or before marriage) is acceptable or even expected.

Since 2008, all of the provinces and territories in Canada have included HPV immunization for girls and boys (some jurisdictions recommend starting at Grade 4, others not until Grade 8) in their schedule of routine immunizations. "Catch-up" programs for teens who missed vaccination when they were younger are also recommended (PHACa, 2012).

[The US Centers for Disease Control] recommends that all teen girls and women through age 26 get vaccinated, as well as all teen boys and men through age 21 (and through age 26 for gay, bisexual, and other men who have sex with men). HPV vaccines are most effective if they are provided before an individual ever has sex. (CDC, 2013)

> What do *you* think?
> Would you have your young (e.g., age 10) daughter or son vaccinated for HPV? Why or why not?

5 Herpes Simplex

A virus causes herpes. There are actually two strains of the herpes simplex virus: HSV-1 and HSV-2. Herpes appears as small lesions (like fever blisters or cold sores) on the lips, mouth, face, genitals, anus, or buttocks. Usually, facial infection is associated with type 1 and genital infection involves type 2. However, there is considerable overlap, presumably because of oral-genital transmission.

Initial infection is usually asymptomatic, although it may present with non-specific flu-like symptoms, such as fever and malaise, lasting about a week. Genital infection may have symptoms of itching, burning, soreness, and pain on urination, which are all common symptoms of many other STIs.

The World Health Organization estimates that 67% of the global population under age 50 are infected with HSV-1; another 8% have HSV-2 infection. HSV-1 rates are lower in the Americas (49% of females and 39% of males) than in the rest of the world (WHO, 2015). Blood tests of a representative sample of Canadians found that over 13% of those age 14 to 59 have HSV-2 (16% of females and 11% of males). More than 90% of those infected were unaware of their infection (Branswell, 2013).

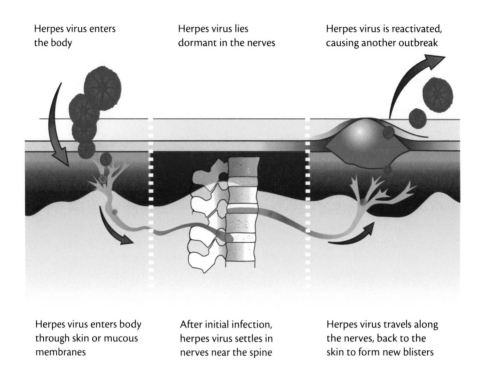

Herpes virus enters
the body

Herpes virus lies
dormant in the nerves

Herpes virus is reactivated,
causing another outbreak

Herpes virus enters body
through skin or mucous
membranes

After initial infection,
herpes virus settles in
nerves near the spine

Herpes virus travels along
the nerves, back to the
skin to form new blisters

Figure 11.3. After the initial infection, herpes viruses lie dormant in nerve cells near the spine. Recurrent lesions occur when the viruses migrate back along nerves to the surface of the skin.

Once infection has occurred, the virus remains in the body for life, living in nerve cells in the head or pelvis and migrating along the nerve fibres to erupt periodically at the skin (Figure 11.3). A number of things can trigger a recurrence: trauma, stress, menstruation, fever, overexposure of the lips to sun, or suppression of the immune system (Merck Manual, 2009).

Initially, there may be four to five attacks per year. Over the years, attacks become less frequent and less severe, and tend to clear quickly. The biggest health consequence for most people with herpes is the embarrassment associated with the lesions. The lesions can also be painful and itchy, especially in genital herpes. There are, however, more serious potential consequences. HSV infection can lead to **meningitis**, an infection of the covering of the brain. Genital herpes is a risk factor for cervical cancer, and increases risk of HIV infection by two to three times (Looker, Garnett, Schmid, 2008).

> In *your* experience, what situations are associated with cold sores—when are they more likely to occur?

HSV is highly contagious (Merck Manual, 2009). Prevention, especially of HSV-1, is difficult because the **reservoir** (number of infected people) is large, and children readily touch each other's faces, put things in their mouths, and so on. Genital herpes is easier to prevent, as transmission is almost always by sexual contact or from mother to newborn. Risk of transmission increases when active sores are present but can occur even if there are no lesions. Condoms may help. Spermicidal foams and jellies have some antiviral activity.

Infrequently, a pregnant woman can transmit HSV to her baby, usually when the mother has active lesions in her genital area. Newborns with HSV become very ill. Without treatment, two-thirds die, and even with treatment, many become brain-damaged (Merck Manual, 2009).

There is *no cure* for herpes. For decades, researchers have tried to develop a vaccine. As of May 2018, there was *no vaccine* for herpes, although reports suggest that such a vaccine might be available in the near future (Thompson, 2017). Antiviral drugs such acyclovir somewhat reduce the severity and duration of recurrent episodes. Topical anaesthetics such as benzocaine can help relieve pain (Merck Manual, 2009).

6 Other STIs

Other than HSV and HPV, which we discussed earlier in this chapter, **chlamydia**, **gonorrhea**, and **syphilis** are three of the most commonly reported STIs (CDC, 2013). These three are all caused by bacterial pathogens, and they are easy to treat (with anti-microbial agents) and cure if they are diagnosed early (CDC, 2013; Racco, 2018). Incidence of these three STIs increased steadily in Canada between 1998 and 2015, with 3-, 4-, and 9-fold increases for chlamydia, gonorrhea, and syphilis, respectively (Racco, 2018).

The US Centers for Disease Control (CDC, 2013) gives the following recommendations for screening (remember the difference between screening and testing):

- Yearly chlamydia screening for all sexually active women age 25 and under, and for older women with risk factors such as new or multiple sex partners.
- Yearly gonorrhea screening for at-risk sexually active women, such as those with new or multiple sex partners or those who live in communities with high prevalence of disease.

- Yearly screening for syphilis, chlamydia, and gonorrhea for all men who have sex with men (MSM). More frequent screening is recommended for MSM who have multiple or anonymous partners, who have sex in conjunction with illicit drug use (especially "meth"; see Chapter 13: Drugs), or whose sex partners have sex and illicit drug use.
- Syphilis, chlamydia, and gonorrhea screening for pregnant women.

6.1 Chlamydia

Blood testing of a representative sample of Canadians found that 0.7% of them were infected with chlamydia (Branswell, 2013). About 50% and 70% of infected men and women, respectively, have no symptoms (Racco, 2018). Those who do have symptoms may experience burning during urination; discharge from urethra, anus, or vagina; pain when being penetrated; or tenderness in the testicles, rectum, or in females, the abdomen (PubMed Health, 2010).

Unlike many infectious diseases, infection with chlamydia does not produce much immunity, so a person can be infected again and again.

6.2 Gonorrhea

Gonorrhea enters the body through the same portals that chlamydia does—the anus, vagina, and urethra—as well as the mouth and eyes (remember the term "portal of entry" from the chain of infection in Chapter 3: Infectious Diseases). Most symptoms resemble those of chlamydia. Sore throat is another possible symptom of gonorrhea. Symptoms can be absent, mild, or delayed (PubMed Health, 2011).

Gonorrhea can **metastasize** (remember from Chapter 5: Cancer, this means "spread through the blood stream") and cause problems in the joints, the heart, and the central nervous system.

6.3 Syphilis

Again, infection can occur through mouth, vagina, urethra, or anus. The first sign of infection is a **lesion**, or sore, at the site of infection, which appears an average of 21 days after infection. The sore lasts three to six weeks, and it disappears whether the infected person is treated or not (CDC, 2012).

If the person is not treated while the initial lesion is present, the infection can progress to a secondary stage, with more serious symptoms that include skin rash, fever, swollen lymph glands, weight loss, muscle aches, and fatigue (CDC, 2012).

If untreated, the secondary-stage symptoms will also disappear. However, about 15% of untreated people get late-stage syphilis. This manifests 10 to 30 years after initial infection as serious damage to brain, nerves, eyes, heart, blood vessels, liver, bones, and joints. It can be fatal (CDC, 2012).

> Syphilis—a disease once on the verge of elimination—began re-emerging as a public health threat in 2001. This is primarily because of a resurgence of the disease among men who have sex with men (MSM), though cases among women have also been increasing in recent years. (CDC, 2011)

The same picture presents in Canada (Racco, 2018).

Prevalence of STIs is much higher among African Americans, with rates for chlamydia 8 times, and gonorrhea 18 times, higher than among white Americans.

> A common misconception is that young African Americans simply are not as careful as whites in protecting their sexual and reproductive health. But a close examination of the extent of the HIV and STI epidemics and their underlying causes reveals a much more complex picture. (Augustine & Bridges, 2008)

Even with equal or fewer sexual risk behaviours, Black people are more affected by STIs. A holistic look at social determinants of health helps explain:

> Many African Americans are part of dense, highly-infected social networks, which means that when choosing a sexual partner, they are more likely to come into contact with an infected partner. Almost a quarter of African Americans are living in poverty, compared to 11 percent of whites. Those who live in poverty are more likely to commit crime, especially drug-related crime. They are more likely to live in unstable neighborhoods with higher rates of crime and more liquor stores. Poverty also contributes to problem alcohol use, which in turn contributes to unemployment/underemployment and unstable relationships. Unstable relationships can lead to unprotected sex if partners are afraid that insisting on condoms will endanger the relationship. Those living in poverty are also less likely to have access to medical treatment.... (Augustine & Bridges, 2008)

Also, more than 25% of African American men are incarcerated during their lifetime, and unprotected sex in prison transmits STIs. Furthermore, homosexuality is more stigmatized in the African American community, meaning that infected men who have sex with men are less likely to seek treatment, and are less likely to tell their female partners about their male sex partners (Augustine & Bridges, 2008).

6.4 Prevention

Condoms usually prevent transmission. The best form of protection in sexually active people is a monogamous relationship with an uninfected monogamous partner (PubMed Health, 2010).

6.5 Treatment

Fortunately, chlamydia, gonorrhea, and syphilis are all **bacterial** infections, and are all easily treated with **anti-microbial agents**. The problem is that the symptoms may go undetected, and thus the disease may remain untreated. Like cancer, treatment is easier when the disease is localized.

From a public health perspective, treatment includes identifying and testing all of the sexual contacts an infected person has had and treating them if they are also infected.

7 Conclusion

Each year, millions of people die from sexually transmissible infections in the world. What is the biggest reason for this? I suppose the simplest answer is "because many people are contracting diseases and are not getting treated."

> *Why are they contracting these diseases, and why aren't they getting treated?*

Let's focus on HIV/AIDS, as much of the same logic applies more or less to other STIs. People get HIV infected sexually because they practise higher-risk forms of sexual activity with at least one person who is already infected with HIV: and this includes intercourse without a condom, anal intercourse, or oral sex. Note I have used the term "higher-risk" rather than "unsafe." Instead of thinking in terms of "safe" vs. "unsafe" sex, it's more realistic to think in terms of a continuum of risk. The only guaranteed safe form of sexual activity is no sexual activity.

> *Why do people practise higher-risk sex?*

For several reasons:
- They may not understand the risks. "I don't have sex with prostitutes," "I never have sex until I get to know the person well," "I have only one sexual partner," "Only gay men get HIV"—these are several examples of misperception of risk.
- They may not feel they have control over the sexual encounter. The partner may insist on sex and refuse to use a condom. In

societies where women are more equal, they are more likely to be assertive and more likely to have their preference respected.

- In a commercial sex situation (prostitution), customers will pay more for sex with a virgin, for sex without a condom, for anal intercourse, and so on.
- Condom use may be inconsistent with religious beliefs.
- Condoms may be too hard to obtain.
- Some women consent to anal intercourse to preserve their vaginal virginity for marriage, or to reduce risk of pregnancy.
- They may not care. For example, they may be socially alienated, drug-involved street youth, who often have fled abusive homes and have nowhere else to go.
- They may make poor decisions while impaired by alcohol or other drugs.

Okay, but why aren't they getting treated?

Again, for various reasons:

- They may not know that they are infected. HIV infection has a very long latent period, during which there are no specific signs or symptoms. Shortly after infection, there may be vague symptoms (fever, headache, fatigue), but these are often mistaken for a flu-like illness.
- They may not get a blood test because they don't think they are at risk—or because they *know* they are at risk and don't want to face reality by being tested (we might say they are in denial).
- They may assume HIV infection is untreatable, so why bother?
- They may not be able to afford the treatment. The combination of medications being used to effectively fight HIV infection and prevent it from progressing to AIDS may cost tens of thousands of dollars per person per year. In industrial countries, a person's extended health-insurance plan may pay for this. In other places, health coverage is uncommon.

So, back to the main question: What *is* the main reason millions of people die annually from sexually transmissible infections? I see three main candidates:

- Lack of education about safer sex
- Low feeling of control in sexual situations
- Low disposable income

All three of these seem related to the underlying factor of socio-economic status (remember this factor from Chapter 1: Models of Health?). As the standard of living of a society increases, education and income increase, superstitions are gradually displaced by scientific knowledge, and the status of women rises.

Although dramatic progress has been made against infectious diseases such as smallpox and measles, sexually transmitted diseases remain a major global health problem. Vigorous research into better treatments and potential vaccines continues. In the meantime, community health efforts focus on raising awareness and reducing risky behaviours. There is evidence, though, that education alone has mixed effectiveness. The message seems to be that more creative and holistic approaches are indicated, targeting selected geographical areas and risk groups with interventions tailored to their specific motivations.

Study Questions

1. What does the abbreviation "AIDS" represent?
2. Outline the "natural history" of AIDS—that is, the chronological progression of the disease in an individual.
3. Identify the main routes of transmission for HIV infection.
4. What is the significance of the latent period for AIDS?
5a. What is the difference between HIV and AIDS?
5b. Why is it easier to track the epidemiology of AIDS than HIV infection?
6. How has incidence of HIV infection and prevalence of AIDS changed in Canada and elsewhere in the world?
7. Outline how risk of HIV infection can be reduced.
8. Describe how to use a condom correctly.
9a. What is hepatitis?
9b. There are different varieties of the hepatitis pathogen. State the main route of transmission of each of the two groups of hepatitis virus.
9c. Most people newly infected with hepatitis C in Canada today belong to what exposure category?
10. Why are about 10 of the 100 types of HPV called "high risk"?
11. What is the prevalence of HPV infection?
12. What is the "natural history" of HPV infection—that is, how does it normally progress?
13. What do each of the following abbreviations represent in the context of this chapter: HCV, HIV, HPV, and HSV?
14. What is the prevalence of herpes simplex virus infection?
15. Why is herpes simplex infection difficult to prevent?
16a. What *kind* of pathogen causes chlamydia, gonorrhea, and syphilis?
16b. What *kind* of pathogen causes HIV, hepatitis C, and HPV infection?

17. Some STIs are highly treatable, but infected people don't seek treatment. Why not?
18. Summarize in your own words the argument that low socio-economic status is an underlying causal factor of death from sexually transmissible infections.

Glossary

AIDS—acquired immune deficiency syndrome

HIV—human immunodeficiency virus, the pathogen that causes AIDS

antibodies—antibodies are produced by the immune system in response to an antigen; pathogens all have antigens on them, and antibodies help fight pathogens

latent period—the time from exposure to a disease-causing agent (such as a pathogen) until the onset of symptoms of the disease

prevalence—the number of people in a population with a given condition; often expressed as a rate (e.g., per 100,00 people)

syndrome—a group of symptoms that frequently occur together

Additional Resources

BC Centre for Disease Control
www.bccdc.ca
655 West 12th Avenue
Vancouver, BC, V5Z 4R4
604-707-5635

BC Point of Care HIV Testing Program
www.bccdc.ca/our-services/programs/point-of-care-rapid-hiv-testing
POCinfo@bccdc.ca
Information on HIV and other STIs is available at
www.bccdc.ca/dis-cond/a-z/_s/SexuallyTransmittedInfections/default.htm

References

Augustine, J., Bridges, E. (2008). Understanding Disparities in the HIV Epidemic. Advocates for Youth. Retrieved May 29, 2018 from http://www.advocatesforyouth.org/storage/advfy/documents/hivdisparities.pdf

Branswell, H. (April 17, 2013). The Canadian Press, reported in CTV news online. Retrieved May 23, 2018 from https://www.ctvnews.ca/health/health-headlines/one-in-7-canadians-has-genital-herpes-statscan-study-1.1241792

CBC News. (May 13, 2014). BC to offer free HIV/AIDS testing to adults every 5 years. Retrieved May 21, 2018 from http://www.cbc.ca/news/canada/british-columbia/b-c-to-offer-free-hiv-aids-testing-to-adults-every-5-years-1.2641128

CDC (Centers for Disease Control and Prevention). (September 4, 2012). *Syphilis: CDC fact sheet.* Retrieved March 6, 2013 from http://www.cdc.gov/std/syphilis/stdfact-syphilis.htm

CDC. (February 2013). Fact Sheet: Incidence, prevalence, and cost of sexually transmitted infections in the United States. Retrieved May 23, 2018 from https://www.cdc.gov/std/stats/sti-estimates-fact-sheet-feb-2013.pdf

CDC. (2016). *HIV in the United States: At a Glance.* Retrieved May 21, 2018 from https://www.cdc.gov/hiv/statistics/overview/ataglance.html

Health Canada. (2014). HIV and AIDS in Canada: Surveillance Report to December 31, 2014 – Data tables. Retrieved May 21, 2018 from https://www.canada.ca/en/public-health/services/publications/diseases-conditions/hiv-aids-canada-surveillance-report-december-31-2014/page-10-data-tables.html#t20b

Hogg, R. S., Althoff, K. N., Samji, H., et al. (2013). 7th IAS Conference on HIV Pathogenesis, Treatment and Prevention, June 30–July 3, 2013, Kuala Lumpur: Life expectancy with HIV jumps 15 years from 2000–2002 to 2006–2007 in US, Canada. Retrieved May 11, 2014 from http://www.natap.org/2013/IAS/IAS_43.htm

Looker, K. J., Garnett, G. P., Schmid, G. P. (2008). An estimate of the global prevalence and incidence of herpes simplex virus type 2 infection. *Bulletin of the World Health Organization.* 86(10), 737–816.

Lozano, R. et al. (December 15, 2012). Global and regional mortality from 235 causes of death for 20 age groups in 1990 and 2010: A systematic analysis for the Global Burden of Disease Study 2010. *The Lancet.* 380(9859), 2095–2128.

MacDonald, N. E., O'Brien, S. F., Delage, G., Canadian Paediatric Society, Infectious Disease and Immunization Committee. (December 3, 2012). Transfusion and risk of infection in Canada: Update 2012. *Paediatrics and Child Health.* 17(10), e102–e111. Retrieved April 25, 2014 from http://www.cps.ca/documents/position/transfusion-and-risk-of-infection-Canada

Medicalnewstoday.com. (May 15, 2014). *Hitting a moving target: Scripps Research Institute scientists shows AIDS vaccine could work against changeable site on HIV.* Retrieved May 31, 2014 from http://www.medicalnewstoday.com/releases/276834.php

MedicineNet.com. (August 28, 2013). *Definition of T cell.* Retrieved May 11, 2014 from http://www.medterms.com/script/main/art.asp?articlekey=11300

Merck Manual. (November 2009). *Herpes simplex virus infections.* Retrieved April 25, 2014 from http://www.merckmanuals.com/home/infections/viral_infections/herpes_simplex_virus_infections.html

Norris, S. (November 8, 2011). *HIV/AIDS–past, present and future.* Library of Parliament. Library of Parliament Research Publications. Retrieved March 6, 2013 from http://www.parl.gc.ca/Content/LOP/ResearchPublications/2011-86-e.htm

PHAC. (2012a; January 2012). *Update on human papillomavirus (HPV) vaccines.* Ottawa, ON: Public Health Agency of Canada. Canada Communicable Disease Report. Volume 38. ACS-1. Retrieved January 17, 2013 from http://www.phac-aspc.gc.ca/publicat/ccdr-rmtc/12vol38/acs-dcc-1/index-eng.php

PHAC. (2012b; May 23, 2012). *Hepatitis C in Canada: 2005–2010 surveillance report.* Ottawa, ON: Public Health Agency of Canada. Retrieved July 30, 2014 from http://www.catie.ca/sites/default/files/1109-0139-Hep%20C%20Report-EN%20FINAL.pdf

PHAC. (November 29, 2012c). *Summary: Estimates of HIV prevalence and incidence In Canada, 2011.* Ottawa, ON: Public Health Agency of Canada. Surveillance and Epidemiology Division, Centre for Communicable Diseases and Infection Control. Retrieved April 25, 2014 from http://www.phac-aspc.gc.ca/aids-sida/publication/survreport/estimat2011-eng.php

PHAC. (2013b; November 29, 2013). *At a Glance—HIV and AIDS in Canada: surveillance report to December 31, 2012.* Ottawa, ON: Public Health Agency of Canada. Retrieved April 25, 2014 from http://www.phac-aspc.gc.ca/aids-sida/publication/survreport/2012/dec/index-eng.php

PubMed Health. (June 7, 2010). Chlamydia. *PubMed Health.* A service of the National Library of Medicine, National Institutes of Health. Retrieved March 6, 2013 from http://www.ncbi.nlm.nih.gov/pubmedhealth/PMH0002321/

PubMed Health. (May 22, 2011). Gonorrhea. *PubMed Health.* A service of the National Library of Medicine, National Institutes of Health. Retrieved March 6, 2013 from http://www.ncbi.nlm.nih.gov/pubmedhealth/PMH0004526/

Racco, M. (October 16, 2017). Why STI rates are steadily going up in Canada. Global News. Retrieved May 23, 2018 from https://globalnews.ca/news/3797824/why-sti-infection-rates-are-steadily-going-up-in-canada/

Thompson, D. (January 19, 2017). Genital herpes vaccine promising in animal trials. WebMD. Retrieved May 23, 2018 from https://www.webmd.com/genital-herpes/news/20170119/genital-herpes-vaccine-shows-promise-in-animal-trials#1

UNAIDS (Joint United Nations Programme on HIV/AIDS). (2016). *Global AIDS Update 2016.* Retrieved May 23, 2018 from http://www.who.int/hiv/pub/arv/global-AIDS-update-2016_en.pdf?ua=1

WHO (World Health Organization). (2013a, June). *Consolidated guidelines on the use of antiretroviral drugs for treating and preventing HIV infection.* Geneva: World Health Organization. ISBN 978 92 4 150572 7. Retrieved July 30, 2014 from http://apps.who.int/iris/bitstream/10665/85321/1/9789241505727_eng.pdf

WHO. (2013b, October). *HIV/AIDS. Fact sheet No 360.* Geneva: World Health Organization. Retrieved April 25, 2014 from http://www.who.int/mediacentre/factsheets/fs360/en/

WHO. (2014). HIV/AIDS. Geneva: World Health Organization. Retrieved May 31, 2014 from http://www.who.int/hiv/en/

WHO. (October 28, 2015). News release: Globally, an estimated two-thirds of the population under 50 are infected with herpes simplex virus type 1. Retrieved May 23, 2018 from http://www.who.int/en/news-room/detail/28-10-2015-globally-an-estimated-two-thirds-of-the-population-under-50-are-infected-with-herpes-simplex-virus-type-1

WHO. (2018). Global health observatory data: HIV/AIDS. Retrieved May 23, 2018 from http://www.who.int/gho/hiv/en/

Wilson, C. (May 3, 2017). Immune war with donor cells after transplant may wipe out HIV. New Scientist. Retrieved May 23, 2018 from https://www.newscientist.com/article/mg23431244-400-immune-war-with-donor-cells-after-transplant-may-wipe-out-hiv/

Xu, F., Sternberg, M. R., Kottiri, B. J., McQuillan, G. M., Lee, F. K., Nahmias, A. J., Berman, S. M., Markowitz, L. E. (2006). Trends in herpes simplex virus type 1 and type 2 seroprevalence in the United States. *Journal of the American Medical Association*. 296(8), 964–973.

12 Fertility Management

Learning Objectives

By the time you have finished this chapter you should be able to

- Describe how different methods of contraception work
- Outline the advantages and disadvantages of different contraceptive methods
- List the factors people might consider in choosing how to manage (or not) their fertility
- Discuss legal, medical, and social situations regarding abortion in Canada and the United States
- Summarize trends in teenage pregnancy and abortion rates, and suggest reasons for these trends
- Summarize the processes of pregnancy and childbirth, and give advice that would help a woman have a healthy pregnancy

1 Overview

This chapter is titled "Fertility Management" rather than "Contraception" because not everyone wants to prevent pregnancy. Some people are *trying* to get pregnant. The term "management" implies one should plan—that is, make a conscious decision about if and when to get pregnant. This is a value judgment with which not everyone agrees. Some people think of children as a valued gift from God and believe that humans should let God decide when pregnancy comes and feel grateful for it when it does. As I have said elsewhere, this text does not intend to bend you to a particular point of view. However, empowerment to take control of your health is a central theme of this book.

2 Choosing a Fertility Management Plan

Some people would like to have children. Others would rather not have any children, or any more than they already have, or they would rather wait and have children later. Some couples would like children, but either the male or female is infertile. Other couples would like to practise contraception but are limited, for religious or other reasons, in the choice of methods available. There is no one course of action that is right for everybody. The following section presents factors that an individual or couple might consider when planning fertility management.

2.1 *Nature of sexual activities and relationship*

Contraception may not be an issue for gay men or lesbians, for an individual who cannot physically have intercourse, or for an individual incarcerated in solitary confinement. In other situations, a number of questions arise:

- Who decides? Female? Male? Both?
- Are children desired? Why or why not?
- When: Now? Later? Never?
- How old are the prospective parents?
- What is the financial position of the prospective parents?

2.2 *Personal, religious, and moral beliefs*

Some religions, such as the Roman Catholic Church, prohibit their followers from using any method of contraception except abstinence and the rhythm method. In some cultures (e.g., the Caribbean) having many children is seen as a symbol of male virility. In others (e.g., rural Guatemala) women don't like to touch their genitals (which certainly makes sense if it is hard to keep their hands clean), so timing ovulation by feeling the viscosity of the vaginal mucous is not practical.

2.3 *Effectiveness*

If one chooses to use contraception, it makes sense to use a highly effective method. Table 12.1 shows effectiveness of various methods, with values from two different sources.

It is important to distinguish the theoretical effectiveness from the actual effectiveness of a method. The *theoretical effectiveness* is the effectiveness of the method in a test group of people who use the method carefully, under controlled conditions. The *actual effectiveness* is the effectiveness of the method as used by the general population in regular use. The actual effectiveness is substantially lower than the theoretical effectiveness for some methods because individuals fail to use the method correctly or consistently (Table 12.2).

Table 12.1
Effectiveness of Various Contraceptive Methods

Method	Pregnancies per 100 women per year	
	(from Planned Parenthood, 2007)	(from CDC, 2011)
Vasectomy	less than 1 (< 1)	< 1
Female sterilization	< 1	< 1
IUD	< 1	< 1
Implant	< 1	< 1
Breastfeeding	2 to 9	--
Shot	2 to 9	6
Pill	2 to 9	9
Ring	2 to 9	9
Patch	2 to 9	9
Diaphragm	15 to 24	12
Male condom	15 to 24	18
Female condom	15 to 24	21
Withdrawal	15 to 24	22
Sponge	15 to 24	24 or 12*
Cervical cap	15 to 24	--
Spermicide	about 25	28
Fertility-awareness methods	about 25	24

* 24% for **parous** women (women who have given birth one or more times), 12% for **nulliparous** women (women who have never given birth).

Table 12.2
Effectiveness of Various Contraceptive Methods

Contraceptive Method	Theoretical Effectiveness	Actual Effectiveness
No method (chance)	15	15
Abstinence	100	100 (if actually abstinent)
Withdrawal	96	73
Predicting fertility	91 to 99	variable
Spermicides	82	71

Contraceptive Method	Theoretical Effectiveness	Actual Effectiveness
Male condom alone	98	85
Female condom alone	95	79
Diaphragm & spermicide	94	84

Note: Values in the table are the percentage of users who will not get pregnant in one year while using that method. Adapted from Hatcher et al. (2004). *Contraceptive technology* (18th Revised Edition). New York: Irvington.

2.4 Safety

Potential side effects are associated with many forms of contraception. Sometimes a certain method is not recommended for specific high-risk groups. For example, oral contraceptives are not recommended in older women who smoke because of the risk of circulatory problems. As another example, females who have never been pregnant are more likely to experience abdominal pain and bleeding with intrauterine devices.

2.5 Cost

Natural methods of contraception, such as the calendar method, are free. Provincial medical services plans and private extended health-insurance plans may cover some costs (e.g., tubal ligation and vasectomy, and the practitioner's time in *fitting* a diaphragm), but they sometimes don't cover other contraceptive costs, such as the diaphragm itself, oral contraceptives, or condoms. Some methods have a one-time up-front cost (e.g., surgical sterilization). Other methods, such as condoms, are inexpensive for a single act of intercourse but can become costly if one uses them often.

2.6 Accessibility

Some contraceptives are more accessible than others. Surgical methods, such as tubal ligation and vasectomy, of course require the services of a physician. A prescription is required for oral contraceptives and diaphragms, and the diaphragm needs to be fitted by a practitioner. Condoms, sponges, and foam are available without prescription in pharmacies. Condoms can also be purchased in dispensers in public washrooms.

In Canada, the teen pregnancy rate is highest in the North and in rural areas. This is reportedly because teens in these regions have less access to services such as sexual health clinics, pharmacies that sell birth control to teens, and abortion clinics. In general, "where women—and young women, in particular—have access to good health care, education and employment opportunities, teen pregnancy rates decline" (Picard, 2007).

2.7 Convenience

People are more likely to use a method consistently if it is easy. For example, it is easier to take a single pill each morning than it is to insert a diaphragm before sex.

2.8 Comfort and aesthetic considerations

Some couples find spermicidal foams and jellies messy, or feel condoms interfere with tactile sensations during intercourse. Others may prefer condoms because the semen is easier to clean up after intercourse. This is very much an individual preference.

2.9 Interference with spontaneity of sex

A method such as the condom or diaphragm, which must be applied before intercourse, may be less preferred and may be forgotten or ignored in the heat of passion. On the other hand, applying the condom can become part of the foreplay.

2.10 Active versus passive method

A passive method, such as tubal ligation, vasectomy, or intrauterine device, is done once and then may be virtually forgotten. By contrast, an active method, such as condoms or oral contraceptives, requires that one *do something* to maintain protection against conception.

2.11 Effectiveness in preventing sexually transmitted infection (STI)

Other than abstinence, barrier methods such as the condom and diaphragm are the most effective methods for disease prevention. They provide a physical barrier—a membrane of latex—between the body fluids of the two partners. Spermicidal jelly or foam (used alone or with a diaphragm) also reduces disease transmission. Some methods that are very effective in preventing *pregnancy* (e.g., sterilization, oral contraceptives) do nothing to help prevent *STIs*.

2.12 Options if contraception fails and pregnancy results

Ideally, options should be considered *before* pregnancy occurs. Options include obtaining a **morning-after pill** (a large dose of hormones to prevent conception within 24 hours after unprotected intercourse), having an abortion, offering the child for adoption, or keeping the child.

> What choices would *you* make if you found out tomorrow that you or your partner was six weeks pregnant?

2.13 Summary of factors to consider when choosing a fertility management plan

1. Nature of the sexual activities and relationship
2. Personal, religious, and moral beliefs
3. Effectiveness
4. Safety
5. Cost
6. Accessibility
7. Convenience
8. Comfort and aesthetic considerations
9. Interference with spontaneity of sex
10. Active versus passive method
11. Effectiveness in preventing sexually transmitted infection (STI)
12. Options if contraception fails and pregnancy results

3 Contraceptive Technology

3.1 Abstinence

There are two types of abstinence:

*   **Periodic abstinence:** This is a way sexually active women can prevent pregnancy. They become familiar with their fertility patterns and then they abstain from vaginal intercourse on the days they think they could become pregnant. This type of abstinence is discussed below under "Predicting fertility."
*   **Continuous abstinence:** This means not having sex play with a partner of the opposite sex at all. This is the kind of abstinence discussed here.

Practicing abstinence does not mean a person is sexless. Almost all women and men are abstinent at some time in their lives. It can be a positive way of dealing with sexuality—that is, as a well-thought-out choice regarding one's body, mind, spirit, and sexual health. Some abstinent women and men enjoy "sexy" thoughts and feelings. Others use their sexual energy for creative, physical, or intellectual activities. Sexual relationships present physical and emotional risks. Abstinence is a very good way to postpone taking those risks until you are able to handle them.

Take the time to consider fully what abstinence might mean for you. It is important to know what you are thinking and feeling, and what you need. Be straightforward about the limits you want to set. Then you can tell your partner about it. Talking with your partner about your decision to abstain from sex play is important. Partners need to be honest with each other and make sexual decisions together. These are some of the best ways to keep a relationship happy. Even so, it may not be easy to do. You may feel awkward or embarrassed.

It's best to talk about your feelings before things get sexual. For many people, it's hard to be clear about what they want when they are aroused. It is helpful to think—ahead of time—about how you can say "no" to sex play. What behaviour will be clear? What words will be best? You can practise saying the words out loud and then think about how someone could respond to you.

Abstinence can only work when both partners agree to it, so it's also helpful to keep talking to each other about why you've agreed to abstain from sex play. Your relationship may change. And your decision to be abstinent may change, too.

3.2 *Withdrawal*

Withdrawal involves the man pulling his penis out of the vagina before or when he feels he has reached the point when ejaculation can no longer be stopped or postponed. He ejaculates outside the vagina, being careful that semen does not spill onto his partner's genitals.

This method requires *skill* and *trust*. Men must be able to tell when they are reaching the peak excitement. Some men lack the experience and self-control to pull out in time. Other men say they will pull out, but they get so excited and carried away that they don't—or they never intended to. In addition, it is possible to get pregnant even if the man *does* pull out before ejaculating; almost all penises leak fluid before ejaculation, and that fluid contains sperm and can cause pregnancy.

3.3 *Predicting fertility*

Predicting a woman's fertile periods and using contraception (including abstinence) during these periods reduces the probability of pregnancy. The **ovum** (egg) lives about one or maybe two days after it is released from the ovary.

> ### How long does sperm survive in a woman?
>
> Most sperm die within the first 12 hours. Some survive for three days; if conditions are very favourable for the sperm, it might survive up to five days.

Thus, a woman has a good chance of becoming pregnant for about seven days of each monthly menstrual cycle: five days before ovulation, the day of ovulation, and possibly a day after ovulation.

Three methods can be used, separately or in combination, to predict ovulation:

- **The temperature method:** The woman takes her body temperature (in the mouth or rectum) with a sensitive thermometer every morning before rising from bed. This **basal body temperature** increases by 0.2 to 0.4 °C (0.4 to 0.8 °F) on the day of ovulation (Figure 12.1).
- **The mucous method:** This is based on changes in the appearance and texture of the woman's cervical mucous. Mucous is normally cloudy and sticky. In the few days before ovulation, it becomes clear and slippery. It will also stretch between the fingers.
- **The calendar method:** With this method, the woman charts her menstrual cycles or periods. The day when bleeding occurs is Day 1. For a woman with a 28-day cycle, ovulation usually occurs about Day 14. For women with irregular cycles, it is harder to predict fertile periods.

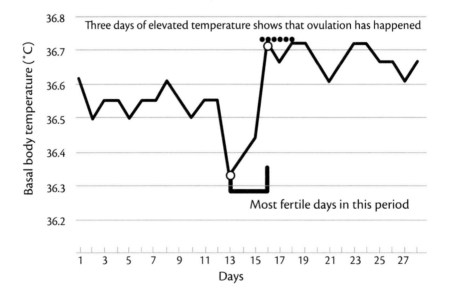

Figure 12.1. A sharp rise in basal body temperature accompanies ovulation, the most fertile time of the menstrual cycle.

Is it normal for a woman to not have a period once a month?

This is the "normal versus typical" issue again. A typical menstrual cycle is 28 days long, with the first day of menstrual bleeding counted as Day 1. With such a cycle, Day 29 would be Day 1 of the next cycle. Since there are 365 (or 366 during leap year) days in a year, the typical cycle would occur 13 times a year. So, even with a typical cycle, there would be one month that has two cycles in it.

Many women do not have a cycle that is exactly 28 days long. Here is the record for one of the women in my family (values are duration of each cycle, in days, over one year): 30, 32, 27, 35, 24, 27, 21, 51, 30, 30, 26, 26, and 19.

3.4 *Barrier methods*

Barrier methods (condom, diaphragm, and cervical cap) involve putting a physical barrier between the penis and the vagina or the cervix (Figure 12.2). These methods make it hard for sperm to join with an ovum, and also protect against STIs by providing a barrier against pathogens. Most other contraceptive methods (e.g., the Pill) do not provide this protection.

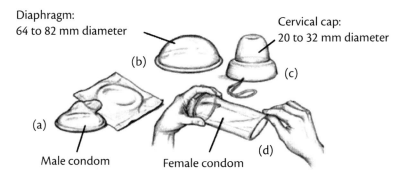

Figure 12.2. Barrier methods of contraception: (a) male condom; (b) diaphragm (c) cervical cap; (d) female condom.

3.4.1 *Condoms*

The male condom is a sheath that fits over the penis. Condoms are easy to obtain, have few side effects (though some people are allergic to latex), and are inexpensive (unless you have intercourse often, because condoms are not reusable). Condoms are convenient for people who are not sexually active at the time but may become sexually active on short notice. They are also an attractive choice for people with multiple sex partners because of the protection they provide against infectious diseases, such as HIV.

> *How can I talk with my partner about condoms?*

Don't be shy—be direct. Be honest about your feelings and needs. Talking with your partner about using condoms makes it easier for you both. It can help create a relaxed mood to make sex more enjoyable. It may be difficult to talk about using condoms. It will be easier if you are in a loving relationship that makes you feel happy and good about yourself and your partner. In any case, don't let embarrassment become a health risk. Here are some ideas for talking about condoms (Planned Parenthood, 2014):

If your boyfriend says: *I don't like using condoms.*
You can say: *Why not?*

If your boyfriend says: *It doesn't feel as good with a condom.*
You can say: *I'll feel more relaxed. If I'm more relaxed, it will be better for both of us.*

If your boyfriend says: *Condoms are gross.*
You can say: *Being pregnant when I don't want to be is worse. So is getting an STD.*

If your boyfriend says: *Don't you trust me?*
You can say: *Trust isn't the point. People can carry sexually transmitted infections without knowing it.*

If your boyfriend says: *I'll pull out in time.*
You can say: *I want to feel relaxed and enjoy this, and pulling out is just too risky. There's a chance I could get pregnant from your pre-cum, or we might get too excited to stop. And pulling out doesn't help much with sexually transmitted infections.*

If your boyfriend says: *Condoms aren't romantic.*
You can say: *Being together like this and protecting each other's health sounds really romantic to me.*

If your boyfriend says: *It just isn't as sensitive.*
You can say: *With a condom you might last even longer, and that'll make up for it. Or let's try a female condom.*

If your boyfriend says: *Putting it on interrupts everything.*
You can say: *Not if I help put it on.*

If your boyfriend says: *I'll try, but it might not work.*
You can say: *Practice makes perfect.*

If your boyfriend says: *But I love you.*
You can say: *Then you'll help me protect myself.*

If your boyfriend says: *I guess you don't really love me.*
You can say: *I'm not going to "prove my love" by risking my health. Do you really love me? Do you want me to feel safe?*

If your boyfriend says: *I'm not using a condom, no matter what.*
You can say: *I'm not having sex without a condom, no matter what. Let's not have sex.*

If you are a virgin and have decided to have sex and want to use a condom and your
boyfriend says: *Just this once without it. Just the first time.*
You can say: *It only takes once to get pregnant. It only takes once to get a sexually transmitted infection. It only takes once to get HIV.*

How does this dialogue sound to *you?*

If you wanted to be assertive about a boundary around your sexual relations, what words would you use?

When do you think would be a good time to have such a conversation with your partner?

If your partner absolutely refuses to wear a latex condom, you can use a female condom. Some men have said that the sensation is not so reduced with a female condom. Don't be afraid of being rejected. A partner who doesn't care about protecting your health and well-being is not worth your sexual involvement.

What are female condoms?

Female condoms are sheaths of latex rubber that are similar in structure to, and used for the same purposes as, male condoms. That is, they reduce probability of **conception**, which means "getting pregnant," and of STI transmission.

The difference is in the way the condom fits over the body. The male condom is a tube that comes to a rounded tip at one end. When the user takes the condom from the package, the tip is placed over the end of the penis, and then the rest of the condom is rolled down, fitting tightly over the shaft of the penis. The female condom is larger in diameter than the male condom, and the closed end goes straight across rather than coming to a point. A rubber ring is built into the condom at each end of the tube. The closed end is inserted into the vagina, and the ring of the open ends makes a loose seal over the **vulva** (the female external genitalia).

3.4.2 Diaphragms and cervical caps

These soft latex barriers cover the cervix. The **diaphragm**, which is a shallow, dome-shaped cup with a flexible rim, fits into the vagina and over the cervix (Figure 12.3). The smaller **cervical cap** fits snugly onto the cervix. Both must be used with spermicidal cream, jelly, or foam. Visit a doctor or a family planning clinic for an exam and prescription.

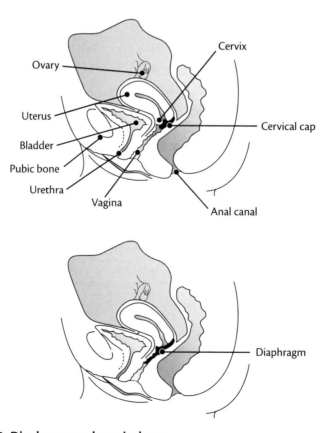

Figure 12.3. Diaphragm and cervical cap.

3.5 Hormonal methods

3.5.1 Oral contraceptives (the pill)

"The pill" contains hormones like those made by a woman's ovaries. Taking the pill daily maintains the level of hormone needed to prevent pregnancy. The pill works by preventing **ovulation** (i.e., by preventing a woman's ovaries from releasing eggs), or by thickening the cervical mucus, or by preventing fertilized eggs from implanting in the uterus.

A clinician will tell whether you can take the pill and what dosage is right for you. Have checkups at least annually. Your prescription may need to be adjusted. See your clinician right away if any problem develops. Remember to tell any other clinician you may see that you take the pill.

Taking the pill is simple, safe, and convenient. Many women who take the pill have more regular, lighter, and shorter periods. The pill does not interfere with having sex. Many women say the pill has improved their sex lives. They say they are free to be more spontaneous and do not have to worry about becoming pregnant. The pill offers many health benefits, including some protection against pelvic inflammatory disease (PID, an infection of the **Fallopian tubes**), which often leads to infertility. Other benefits included decreased risk of ovarian cancer, uterine cancer, troublesome menstrual cramps, iron deficiency anemia (which can result from heavy menstrual bleeding), acne, and premenstrual symptoms. The pill may offer some protection against osteoporosis and rheumatoid arthritis.

You should not take the pill if you are 35 or older *and* you smoke more than 20 cigarettes a day, *or* if you have high blood pressure, a history of blood clots, vein inflammation, or certain other conditions (check with your doctor). You should also not take the pill if you think you might be pregnant.

Overall, the pill is much safer than pregnancy and childbirth for healthy women, *except* smokers who are age 35 or older. This is the concept of **relative risk**, which you read about in Chapter 3: Infectious Disease, in the context of vaccination.

> *What are the risks of using birth control pills?*

A posting to the website of The Center for Young Women's Health (CYWH, 2010) addressed this:

> Most women have no side effects when taking the oral contraceptive pill. However, it is possible to have irregular periods, nausea, headaches, or weight change, especially in the first few months. Each type of oral contraceptive pill can affect a young woman differently.

Mood changes (feeling up and down emotionally) are unlikely to be caused by the pill. Very occasionally, breasts may enlarge or become tender.

> If side effects occur, they are usually mild and go away in the first three to four cycles. If you do have side effects, talk with your health care provider. If the side effects are uncomfortable or if they don't go away, your health care provider may switch you to a different kind of birth control pill.

The most serious potential side effect seems to be blood clots. Blood clots were much more of a risk with old versions of the pill that had higher doses of both estrogen and progestin than with the current versions of the pill. Current combined hormonal contraceptives are associated with a slight increased risk of blood clots.

Contraceptive hormones can also be administered through the vagina in either vaginal rings or hormonal IUDs. Vaginal delivery uses lower doses of hormones than the pill. Progestin-only pills and intrauterine devices are not associated with an increased risk of blood clots.

The Center for Young Women's Health (CYWH; 2010) also advises that if you experience any of the following symptoms, you should contact your health care provider right away. These may indicate serious side effects. Remember the acronym ACHES:

Abdominal or stomach pain (severe)
Chest pain (severe), cough, shortness of breath
Headache (severe), dizziness, weakness, or numbness
Eye problems (vision loss or blurring), speech problems
Severe leg pain (calf or thigh)

In 2011, the US Food and Drug Administration (FDA) issued a "drug safety communication" regarding possible increased risk of blood clots with birth control pills containing drospirenone. Drospirenone is a synthetic version of the female hormone **progesterone** (also known as **progestin**). The FDA then reviewed recent epidemiological studies and concluded that drospirenone-containing birth control pills may be associated with a higher risk for blood clots than other progestin-containing pills. The FDA reported that

> … Some epidemiologic studies reported as high as a three-fold increase in the risk of blood clots for drospirenone-containing products when

compared to products containing levonorgestrel or some other progestins, whereas other epidemiological studies found no additional risk of blood clots with drospirenone-containing products. (FDA, 2013)

The brand names of drospirenone-containing pills include Beyaz, Safyral, Yasmin, and Yaz.

My dental professional told me that her 22-year-old daughter was hospitalized with brain blood clots, which were believed to be due to the oral contraceptive Yasmin.

> The preceding paragraph exemplifies what type of evidence (from Chapter 2: Evaluating Health Claims)?

3.5.2 Injected contraceptives

Depo-Provera is the brand name of a prescription method of reversible birth control. It is a hormone similar to the one in implanted contraceptives. An injection of this hormone in the buttock or arm can prevent pregnancy for 12 weeks. "The shot" keeps the ovaries from releasing eggs and thickens cervical mucus to keep sperm from joining eggs. Protection is immediate if you get the shot during the first five days of your period. Otherwise, you must use an additional method of contraception for the first two weeks.

Irregular bleeding is the most common side effect for women using the shot. Periods become fewer and lighter for most women; most have no periods after five years of use. Other women have longer and heavier periods. Other, less-common side effects include increased appetite and weight gain, headache, nausea, nervousness, dizziness, and depression. Side effects may continue for up to eight months, until the hormone is cleared from your body. You may not be able to become pregnant for a full year after you stop using it.

3.5.3 Implanted contraceptives

Implanon is the brand name of a thin plastic rod that is about the length of a matchstick (Figure 12.4, next page). The rod contains a hormone. A doctor implants it under the skin on the inside of the upper arm. The hormone is slowly released into the woman's system, and continues to be effective for three years.

3.5.4 The patch

The **contraceptive patch** (brand name Evra) has been available in the USA since 2002 and in Canada since 2004. The 4 cm × 4 cm patch sticks to the skin and continuously releases small amounts of hormones (Figure 12.4). The hormones work like oral contraceptives. The patch is removed after a week and a new one is applied. However, the patch releases more hormones than

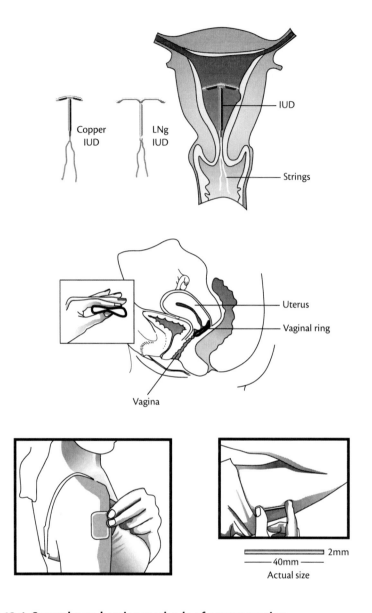

Figure 12.4. Several non-barrier methods of contraception.

was originally thought, and this increases the risk of blood clots. In 2005, the US Food and Drug Agency issued a warning about "the patch." In 2006, the manufacturer started settling lawsuits for injuries and deaths related to use of the patch. In 2015, the manufacturer stopped making Evra … but a generic alternative (Xulane) is still available. Over 3,000 women had filed suit as of 2016 (Wayne Wright Injury Lawyers, 2016).

3.5.5 *Vaginal ring*

The **contraceptive ring** (brand name *NuvaRing*) is a flexible clear plastic ring 54 mm (about two inches) in diameter. It looks like a small bracelet. The ring releases hormones that work like oral contraceptives.

The woman inserts the ring into her vagina (Figure 12.4). She does this by squeezing the ring together between thumb and forefinger, inserting the ring into the vagina, then removing her fingers. The ring opens up, and pressure against the vaginal wall keeps it in place, even during exercise or sexual intercourse. Unlike the diaphragm, it is not critical where the ring is positioned inside the vagina.

The usual approach is to leave the ring in for three weeks, remove it and have a week with no ring, insert a new ring for another three weeks, and so on.

> ### *Is it hard to get pregnant after using hormonal contraceptives?*

> No. Ovulation may start within two weeks after discontinuing use of oral contraceptives. Once you ovulate, you can become pregnant (Mayo Clinic, 2012). Most women get their menstrual period within four to six weeks of stopping oral contraceptives (American Pregnancy Association, 2003). If you get pregnant within your first cycle after stopping the pill, you may not menstruate at all (Mayo Clinic, 2012).
>
> Injected contraceptives are effective for about three months. So obviously you would have to wait longer for ovulation after an injection than after going off the pill.

3.6 *Intrauterine device (IUD)*

IUDs are small devices made of flexible plastic that contain copper or a hormone (Figure 12.4). They are placed inside the uterus (through the vagina and cervix) by a health professional, and do not normally need to be removed until a woman wishes to become pregnant. IUDs are available by prescription only. There are several types and sizes of IUD, and the health professional clinician decides the right type for each woman.

Once inserted, the IUD is immediately effective. When removed, its contraceptive effect is immediately reversed. The IUD is the most inexpensive, long-term, reversible method of contraception available in the world.

Years of negative publicity following lawsuits regarding one faulty IUD— the *Dalkon Shield*—raised many questions about the safety of all IUDs. Some manufacturers even withdrew *safe* IUDs from the North American market. But the IUD is still recognized by the World Health Organization, the American

Medical Association, and the American College of Obstetricians and Gynecologists as one of the safest and most effective reversible methods of birth control for women. The Canadian Paediatric Society notes that long-acting reversible contraceptives such as the IUD are the most effective forms of birth control available. The Society encourages doctors to recommend them to adolescent girls before any other method (Weeks, 2018). Many more Canadian women use the pill (44%) than IUDs (11%). The pill can be highly effective if it is used properly, but in real-world conditions the actual effectiveness of IUDs is up to nine times better than the pill (Weeks, 2018).

IUDs usually prevent fertilization of the egg. Scientists are not entirely sure why. IUDs seem to affect the way the sperm or egg moves. It may be that substances released by the IUD immobilize sperm. Another possibility is that the IUD prompts the egg to move through the Fallopian tube too fast to be fertilized.

The copper adds to the effectiveness of the IUD by preventing implantation. The hormone thickens cervical mucus and also affects the lining of the uterus in ways that would prevent implantation if an egg was fertilized, which is very unlikely.

IUDs have a string that is threaded through a hole in the IUD and tied in place with a knot. The string is a single strand of strong plastic. The string also allows a woman or her clinician to know if the IUD is still in the correct position, and the string allows for easier removal by a clinician when the time comes.

Many women adjust to their IUDs very quickly. Others may take several months to become entirely comfortable. Heavy bleeding and cramping in the first few months may lead women to change their minds and ask their health care providers to remove the IUD. Many clinicians prescribe medication during the first few months to lessen bleeding and cramps during menstruation.

Overall, women's level of satisfaction with the IUD is quite strong. More than 60% of women who have IUDs inserted continue to use them for more than two years.

There may be some spotting between periods during the first few months, the first few periods may last longer, and the flow may be heavier. It is not unusual for a woman to have heavier and longer periods while using an IUD. Cramping or backache may occur for several days or weeks after insertion. Simple pain medication usually clears up cramping and discomfort. If bleeding or pain is severe and does not seem to lessen, tell your clinician.

You should have a checkup after your first period. Don't wait longer than three months after your IUD has been inserted to make sure it is still in place. Women using an IUD should have checkups at least once a year to make sure everything is all right. This is usually done at the time of the annual physical and Pap test.

3.7 Emergency contraception

Emergency contraception can prevent pregnancy after unprotected vaginal intercourse. It is also called **morning-after** contraception. It is available from health care providers, Planned Parenthood health centres, and other women's health and family planning centres. It is provided either by emergency contraceptive pills (ECPs) or by insertion of an IUD. It prevents pregnancy by stopping ovulation, fertilization, or implantation. It will not affect an existing pregnancy, and it will not cause an abortion. The side effects, advantages, and disadvantages of using IUDs for emergency contraception are the same as those associated with using IUDs for ongoing contraception.

ECPs reduce the risk of pregnancy by 75% to 90%. Emergency IUD insertion reduces the risk of pregnancy by over 99%. ECPs work best if taken as soon as possible after unprotected intercourse. The closer a woman is to ovulation at the time of unprotected intercourse, the greater her chances of pregnancy.

Emergency contraception is meant for emergencies only. It is not as effective as regular use of oral contraceptives, injected contraceptives, implanted contraceptives, or IUDs. ECPs *do not* continue to prevent pregnancy during the rest of the cycle. Other methods of birth control must be used.

3.8 Permanent methods

3.8.1 Tubal sterilization

Tubal sterilization is a surgical operation that closes off the Fallopian tubes, where sperm fertilize ova (eggs). When the tubes are closed, sperm cannot reach the egg, and pregnancy cannot happen (Figure 12.5). The procedure can be reversed in some cases, but your decision not to have a child in the future must be firm.

Tubal sterilization is often the answer for women who have completed their families and for women who do not want children. Sterilization does not decrease a woman's sexual pleasure. It is very unlikely sterilization will affect the sexual organs, or your sexuality. No glands or organs will be removed or changed. All of the hormones will still be produced. The ovaries will release an egg every month. The menstrual cycles will most likely follow their regular pattern. Sterilization will not cause symptoms of menopause or make menopause happen earlier.

Tubal sterilization is low-risk surgery. Complications can occur with any kind of surgery. The complications that can occur during or after sterilization include bleeding, infection, or reaction to the anesthetic. Very rarely, the bowel or blood vessels are injured. Major surgery may be required to repair this. Deaths resulting from tubal sterilization are extremely rare.

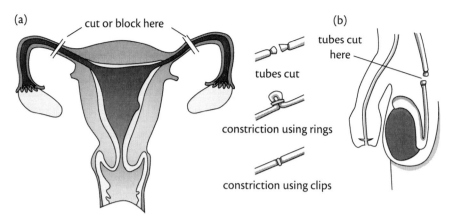

Figure 12.5. Surgical methods of contraception.

3.8.2 Hysterectomy

This means removal of the uterus (womb), and it is major surgery, usually used to correct significant medical conditions and not for sterilization per se. Hysterectomy ends menstruation as well the possibility of pregnancy. It does not necessarily affect the Fallopian tubes. However, some medical conditions also call for the removal of a tube or ovary, on one side or both. Women need to spend several days in the hospital. They usually spend several weeks at home recuperating.

3.8.3 Vasectomy

Vasectomy is a surgical operation that causes sterility by blocking the **vas deferens**, thus keeping sperm out of the ejaculate (Figure 12.5). It can sometimes be reversed, but it is meant to be permanent; that is, it is intended for men who do not want any (or any more) children. Vasectomy is nearly 100% effective and is the most effective birth control for men (Planned Parenthood, 2014).

Usually a local anesthetic is first injected into the area. Alternatively, the patient may be "put under" with a general anesthetic. Then the doctor makes a cut or puncture on each side of the scrotum, or sometimes a single cut is made in the centre. In most procedures, a small section of each tube is removed. Tubes may be tied off, sealed with heat, or blocked with surgical clips.

Vasectomy does not affect masculinity, the ability to get hard and stay hard, or sexual pleasure. The hormones and sperm continue being produced. The ejaculate looks like it always has, and there will be about as much of it as before. The semen is only about 2% to 5% sperm. The rest is seminal fluid from the prostate and other glands. The change in the amount of fluid is too little to notice. After a vasectomy, sperm continue to be produced by the testes. The sperm dissolve and are absorbed into the body.

Vasectomy is not immediately effective. Sperm remain beyond the blocked tubes. You must use other birth control until the sperm disappear, which usually takes about three months. A simple semen analysis shows when there are no more sperm in the ejaculate. Very rarely, tubes grow back together again and pregnancy may occur.

Vasectomy is low-risk surgery, but complications can occur with any kind of surgery. The most serious risk is that of infection. Other complications include swelling, bruising, and formation of lumps. These usually clear up by themselves.

As with any surgery, there's some discomfort after the operation. It will be different for each man. However, most men say the pain is "slight" or "moderate," as opposed to "excessive." An athletic supporter, ice bag, and medication may help ease the pain. Avoid strenuous physical labour or exercise for three to five days.

3.9 *Breastfeeding as a contraceptive*

Breastfeeding can prevent pregnancy quite reliably. Using breastfeeding as birth control can be effective for six months after delivery under the following conditions (Planned Parenthood, 2014):

- The woman does not substitute *any* other foods for a breast milk meal. That is, the baby should not eat anything other than breast milk.
- The woman feeds her baby at least every four hours during the day and every six hours at night.
- The woman has not had a period since she delivered her baby.

Less than 1 out of 100 women who practise continuous breastfeeding perfectly will become pregnant.

It should also be noted that giving the baby a pacifier may reduce the **efficacy** (effectiveness) of breastfeeding as a reliable contraceptive (Smith, 2012).

> Considering your circumstances, what form of fertility management is most suitable for *you* at this time in your life?

4 Abortion

Abortion means termination of pregnancy. A significant minority (perhaps 30%) of all pregnancies result in **miscarriage**, also known as *spontaneous abortion*. This can cause the woman (and her partner) profound loss, grief, and guilt. Most fetuses that are miscarried are defective in some way and would never have survived even if they had been carried for the full term. Abortions that are medically induced are called **therapeutic abortions**. Usually when the word "abortion" is used, it means therapeutic abortion, and that is the way we will use it in this chapter.

4.1 Demographics of abortion

In Canada in 2013, 12.6 abortions were performed for every 1,000 women age 15 to 44 (CIHI, 2013). This represents a decrease from the rate of 15.4 in 2002 (Statistics Canada, 2005). Note that the denominator commonly used to present **abortion rates** is not the *whole* population, or even the *whole female* population. Instead, the 15-to-44 age range is used, because it is the section of the population most likely to become pregnant, so-called women of childbearing age. This way, the abortion rate isn't skewed by changing population demographics (e.g., an increasing portion of the population is over age 65). The Western European rate is also 12 (Guttmacher & WHO, 2012). The picture is similar in the United States, where the 2014 abortion rate was 12.1 (CDC, 2017), down from 19.4 in 2005 and 23.3 in 1990, the latter being the year that the US abortion rate peaked (Associated Press, 2008). In both Canada and the USA, most abortions were for women in their 20s (Statistics Canada, 2005; CIHI, 2013; CDC, 2017). Globally, the abortion rate declined from 35 per 1,000 women of childbearing age in 1995, to 29 in 2003, and a bit more to 28 in 2008 (Guttmacher & WHO, 2012).

The Guttmacher Institute and the World Health Organization (2012) have expressed concern about **unsafe abortions**, which they define as abortions performed by individuals who lack the necessary skills and/or in an environment that does not meet minimal medical standards. Almost half (49%) of all abortions worldwide in 2012 were unsafe. *Almost all* abortions in Africa and Latin America were unsafe (97% and 95%, respectively). Globally, an estimated 47,000 women died from unsafe abortion in 2008. A therapeutic abortion performed by a qualified physician in a proper medical setting is safer for the mother than an illegal abortion. In the USA, *legal* abortion results in only 0.6 maternal deaths per 100,000 procedures. Worldwide, *unsafe* abortions account for 220 deaths per 100,000.

In developing countries, poor women have the lowest access to fertility management services, the fewest resources to pay for safe abortions, and the highest risk of complications related to unsafe abortions. Laws that strictly limit abortions are *not* associated with lower abortion rates. For example, in Africa and Latin America, where abortion is illegal under most circumstances in most countries, abortion rates are 29 and 32 per 1,000—more than twice the rate in Western Europe, where abortion laws are more liberal (Guttmacher & WHO, 2012).

The abortion rate in Eastern Europe is 43, more than three times the rate in Western Europe. "The discrepancy in rates between the two regions reflects relatively low contraceptive use in Eastern Europe, as well as a high degree of reliance on methods with relatively high user failure rates, such as the condom, withdrawal and the rhythm method" (Guttmacher & WHO, 2012). Given that (a) legal abortion is much safer for the woman, (b) abortion is more common when less effective contraception is used, and (c) strict abortion laws do not reduce demand for abortion, then a logical response may be to address the unmet need for effective contraception.

4.2 Legal and social issues in abortion

United States abortion law is based on the landmark Supreme Court decision *Roe v. Wade*. It's a fascinating story. Norma McCorvey, an unmarried woman who wanted to end her pregnancy, filed a class-action suit challenging a Texas statute that made abortion a crime unless a woman's life was at stake. To protect her identity, she used the name "Jane Roe." She had a tough life: she was a ninth-grade dropout, had suffered abuse, rape, and substance abuse, had spent some time in reform school, was married at age 16, had two children (one raised by her mother, the other by its father), and was pregnant for the third time at age 21 when the suit was filed in 1970. Henry Wade was then the district attorney of Dallas, Texas. Roe's challenge was denied at the state level, and eventually she appealed to the Supreme Court. While waiting for the appeal, she gave birth to a girl, who was given up for adoption. In 1973, the Supreme Court ruled in her favour, striking down the Texas statute (and similar laws in many other states) on the grounds that the state could not interfere in a person's right to privacy around contraceptive and reproductive matters. Subsequently, Norma McCorvey publicly revealed her identity and supported abortion rights. Then, in 1995, she was baptized as a born-again Christian, and is now a vigorous *opponent* of abortion.

The Supreme Court decision stated the right to privacy was not absolute, and that the state has valid interests in safeguarding maternal health, maintaining medical standards, and protecting potential life. The Court said this last point could not be considered "compelling" until fetal viability, which means the point at which the fetus could live on its own if delivered. The Supreme Court divided pregnancy into three equal periods, or trimesters:

- In the **first trimester**, the abortion decision was left to the woman and her physician.
- In the **second trimester**, the state could impose some limits, such as the type of facility where the abortion could be performed.
- In the **third trimester**, states were allowed to ban all abortions except those necessary for the mother's life or health.

Medical advances have undermined the logic upon which the *Roe v. Wade* decision was based. In 1973, a fetus was not viable at less than 28 weeks. A fetus delivered at the beginning of the third trimester (29th week) could live *if* provided with special medical care. It is now possible to save a fetus born in the 24th week, which has blurred the neat legal division of pregnancy into three trimesters.

In Canada, from 1969 to 1988 federal law specified that abortion was illegal unless

- It was performed by a licensed physician.
- It was performed in an accredited hospital.
- The hospital had an abortion committee (consisting of three to eighteen people, of which at least three had to be physicians).
- It was performed for the "life or health" of the mother.

In January 1988, the Supreme Court of Canada ruled that Canada's abortion law was unconstitutional because it violated a woman's right to privacy. The British Columbia Social Credit government immediately announced that the Medical Services Plan (MSP) would not pay for any abortions performed in the province. The BC Human Rights Coalition challenged this policy, and the policy was ruled unconstitutional. The BC Medical Services Plan now covers the cost for physician services and anesthetics for all abortions, regardless of whether the abortion is performed in hospital or in a **free-standing abortion clinic** (which means it's not part of a hospital). In Canada in 2013 somewhat more than half of all reported abortions were performed in clinics (CIHI, 2013). To locate abortion clinics in British Columbia, see Options for Sexual Health in the Additional Resources section near the end of this chapter.

Currently no Canadian law covers abortion. Rather, abortion is governed by the limitations and policies of medical practice. In general, abortion is less risky to the woman than delivery, unless abortion is performed quite late in pregnancy. Almost 98% of abortions reported by Canadian hospitals in 2013 had no maternal complications (CIHI, 2013). Abortion is not normally performed after the 20th week of pregnancy because of the increased risk of complications. In 2012, more than 85% of abortions performed in Canadian hospitals were for pregnancies of 12 weeks or less (CIHI, 2013). US figures are similar, with 92% of abortions performed at 13 weeks or earlier (CDC, 2017).

There is considerable support for **abortion on demand**. Proponents of this view (i.e., those who refer to themselves as **pro-choice**) believe a female has the right to determine what is done to her body and should not be prevented by law from having an abortion if she wants one. The male partner seems to have fewer rights concerning his offspring. Whichever way you think, the whole question underscores the value of a couple's discussing their options before conception.

Opponents of abortion (i.e., those who refer to themselves as **pro-life**) argue that abortion is murder, and that nobody has the right to choose murder. This argument turns on the question "Is the fetus a person?" Some people believe that the embryo[1] is a human being from the moment of conception, and it is immoral to deliberately take the life of a human being. Others do not consider the fetus to be a human being until after birth, or at least until it would be capable of surviving if delivered prematurely. Before then, they consider the fetus to be part of the woman's body, and believe it is a woman's right to decide what she will do with her body.

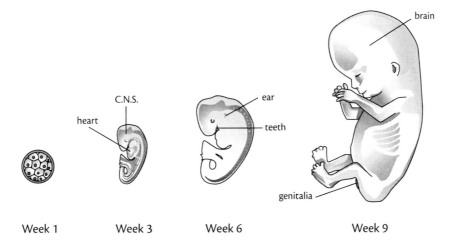

Week 1   Week 3   Week 6   Week 9

Figure 12.6. Selected stages in the development of the human embryo and fetus.

What is *your* opinion?

Should there be legal limits on abortion in Canada, or should the situation continue to be a matter for a woman and her doctor? If you think there should be limits, what limits would you propose?

a) No abortion under any circumstances?

b) Abortion only if the fetus has a serious genetic abnormality?

c) Abortion if a woman becomes pregnant as a result of rape?

d) Or ...?

---

1   An **embryo** is the earliest stage of development, from the time of first cell division. The human embryonic stage is considered to last for the first eight weeks or pregnancy. After eight weeks, the embryo becomes a **fetus**. The developing embryo/fetus becomes increasingly recognizable as a human infant over time (Figure 12.6).

5 Pregnancy and Childbirth

5.1 Pregnancy

Pregnancy is the 38-week period during which the fertilized ovum grows and develops in the uterus, nourished by its mother via an ***umbilical cord*** and ***placenta***, which in turn is attached to the uterine wall.

Pregnancy is usually divided into three equal trimesters:

- In the **first trimester** most women experience **morning sickness**, a nausea that can actually occur any time during the day. The risk of miscarriage—losing the embryo or fetus—is highest in the first trimester. For this reason, many people wait until the second trimester before announcing they are pregnant. The embryo is tiny at first. By the end of the first trimester, the fetus is still only about 8 cm (about 3 in.) long and weighs about 30 g (about 1 oz.).
- The pregnant woman's abdomen starts to swell noticeably in the **second trimester**. During this period, the mother usually starts to feel the baby move inside her. Some sources say the woman may feel the baby move between 14 and 18 weeks. Other sources say around 20 weeks.
- The fetus grows most rapidly during the **third trimester**. Weight gain by the mother is natural and desirable; a woman of normal weight before pregnancy should gain about 11 to 16 kg (25 to 35 lb.) during a healthy pregnancy.

> ***Can a woman tell if she is having twins?***

You might suspect you are carrying more than one baby if
- You seem bigger than you should be for your dates.
- Twins run in your family.
- You have had a fertility treatment.

It is usually possible to find out if you're having twins (or other multiples) through your dating ultrasound scan (the scan used to estimate delivery date), which occurs when you are 8 to 14 weeks pregnant.

5.2 Childbirth

At the end of the 38 or 40 weeks of a normal pregnancy, the fetal head is positioned at the bottom of the uterus, against the cervix. Birthing begins with maternal abdominal contractions, which become increasingly frequent and strong. Simultaneously, the cervix dilates. The mother may experience considerable pain. Eventually, the fetus is pushed down the **birth canal** (the

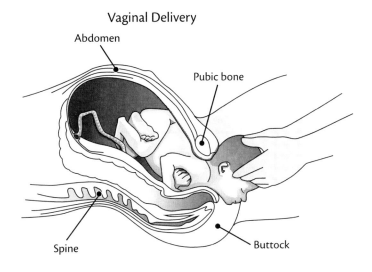

Vaginal Delivery

Abdomen

Pubic bone

Spine

Buttock

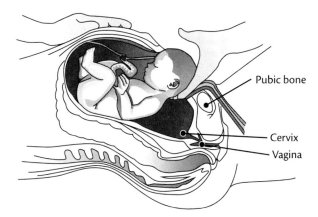

Caesarian Delivery

Pubic bone

Cervix

Vagina

Figure 12.7. In a vaginal birth (a) the newborn is delivered through the birth canal (cervix and vagina). With a Caesarian section (b) the newborn is delivered through an incision in the abdomen and uterus.

dilated cervix and vagina) and enters the world, still connected to the mother via the abdominal cord. **Labour** lasts an average of 13 hours, which can be quite exhausting. Other tissues, such as the **perineum** (i.e., the membrane between the vagina and the anus) may stretch or tear, and are repaired surgically.

The newborn soon begins to breathe air, and shortly thereafter (as quickly as one minute in hospitals, usually longer in birthing centres), the umbilical cord is clamped. The cord is subsequently cut (this is painless because the cord has no nerves), and then tied. The place where it is tied becomes the infant's **navel** (belly button).

Usually within 15 to 30 minutes of birth, the placenta is expelled. This is called the **afterbirth.** The human placenta is about 22 cm × 2 cm (9 in. long and 1 in. thick) and weighs about 500 g (about 1 lb.). Many cultures have rituals around the disposal of the placenta (burying it, eating it, etc.). In Western culture, the placenta is usually incinerated (burned), like other biological hospital waste.

Increasingly, women in Canada are delivering by *Caesarian section*, or *C-section.* This involves cutting through the woman's abdomen and uterus and removing the newborn surgically (Figure 12.7, previous page). This is sometimes done for medical reasons (e.g., the baby is not coming through the birth canal correctly) and sometimes for the convenience of the mother (who skips the hours of labour) and the obstetrician (who can time the delivery rather than being called in the middle of the night when labour reaches the critical stage). Complications are more common for C-sections than for vaginal deliveries.

> *Is it necessary for women to stay in bed for a month after giving birth?*

No. I have heard this may be common in China, but it would be very unusual in Canada or the United States.

A normal vaginal delivery is both physically and psychologically stressful for the mother. It is typical for the mother to have a period following delivery during which she is relieved of some of her duties. From a medical perspective, one or two days of rest and monitoring in hospital following delivery may be indicated. On the other hand, before the 20th century, hospital deliveries were uncommon, with most babies born at home, often under the supervision of a midwife rather than a physician. The point is that modern society has, to some extent, **medicalized** delivery, turning it from a dramatic but normal part of life into a medical problem that needs medical treatment. Currently about 30% of births in Canada are done via Caesarian section, which involves more cutting and sewing than normal deliveries, so a somewhat longer stay in hospital seems warranted.

A review of over four million childbirths in US community hospitals in 2008 revealed that 33% of childbirths were by C-section, up from 21% in 1997 (Podulka, Stranges, & Steiner, 2011). C-sections were, overall, the most commonly performed operating-room procedure in US hospitals. This study reported the mean (average) length of hospital stay for various types of childbirths as follows:

All deliveries combined	2.6 days
Vaginal delivery without complication	2.1
Vaginal delivery with complication	2.7
C-section without complication	3.1
C-section with complication	4.5

5.3 *Having a healthy pregnancy*

According to Government of Canada guidelines (2008; revised 2012), you can increase your chances of having a healthy pregnancy by doing the following:

- **Eat sensibly**. In the second and third trimesters, you need to eat a bit more to support the growing fetus.
- **Keep in mind** that pregnant women are at increased risk of infection; accordingly, avoid raw fish (e.g., sushi), unpasteurized cheeses and juices, and foods made with raw or undercooked eggs (e.g., homemade Caesar salad dressing).
- **Avoid sodium nitrite and nitrate**, which are food preservatives found in hot dogs and deli meats.
- **Ensure adequate intake of folic acid** (one of the B-vitamins, also known as **folate**) to minimize risk of **neural tube defects** in the fetus. The neural tube develops into the spinal cord and brain. Folic acid levels should be checked—and if necessary, increased—*prior to* a planned pregnancy, because neural tube formation is complete by the time a woman knows she is pregnant. Good food sources of folic acid include dark green leafy vegetables, corn, beans, peas, oranges, and orange juice. Grain products fortified with folic acid are another good source. Consider supplements.
- **Avoid alcohol**. There is no safe dose. Even one drink per day can damage the fetus, causing **fetal alcohol syndrome** (FAS) or a less serious variation of this condition called fetal alcohol effects (FAE); collectively, this range of disorders is now referred to as fetal alcohol spectrum disorder (FASD).
- **Get a balance** between moderate physical activity and rest.
- **Avoid smoking**, including cannabis. Smoking tobacco or cannabis is associated with lower birth weight babies.
- **Enjoy normal sexual intercourse**. This is safe for both mother and fetus during pregnancy, although sexual desire may be lower than it was before pregnancy.
- **Avoid drugs, toxins, and heavy metals**, such as mercury (e.g., in large-sized fish, such as tuna) and lead (house paint used to contain lead; new paints don't have lead, but sanding existing painted surfaces can release lead dust from old paint into the air). Heavy metals adversely

affect neural development. The fetus and newborn are more susceptible to heavy metal toxicity than adults are.

- **Try to breathe clean air and drink clean water**. Air and drinking water contaminants are also associated with birth defects and with problems for the child later in life. Pollution is discussed in Chapter 15: Environment.

5.4 Teenage pregnancy

The United Nations Population Fund regards teenage pregnancy as a huge problem.

- "Most of the world's births to adolescents—95 per cent—occur in developing countries, and nine in 10 of these births occur within marriage or a union" (UNFPA, 2013, p. iv).
- "Every year in developing countries, 7.3 million girls under the age of 18 give birth" (UNFPA, 2013, p. 1).
- Two million of these births happen to girls under 15 (UNFPA, 2013, p. 4).
- "The risk of maternal death for mothers under 15 in low- and middle-income countries is double that of older females" (UNFPA, 2013, p. iv).

Young pregnant girls are at increased medical risk of complications from their pregnancy and delivery.

- "Annually, 70,000 adolescent deaths occur globally from complications of pregnancy and childbirth" (UNFPA, 2013, p. v). Teen mothers are also at risk from unsafe abortions if they seek to end their pregnancy.
- Each year, adolescents experience 3.2 million **unsafe abortions** (UNFPA, 2013, p. v).
- "Compared to adults who have unsafe abortions, adolescents are more likely to experience complications such as haemorrhage [bleeding], septicaemia [blood infection], internal organ damage, tetanus, sterility and even death" (UNFPA, 2013, p. 21).

In addition to these physical risks, young mothers have reduced educational and employment opportunities, and other psychosocial issues around the abrupt transition from childhood to motherhood. Globally, the roots to the adolescent pregnancy issue are complex, involving the status of women in society, power imbalance in relationships, sexual violence and coercion, and access to education, contraceptives, health services, and prenatal care.

The babies of teen mothers are also more likely to have health problems, including low birth weight and premature birth, which are associated with increased risk of respiratory, digestive, vision, cognitive, and other problems (*WebMD*, 2012).

American **teen pregnancy rates** have declined steadily over the last 25 years (HHS 2016; CDC, May 2017). This decline seems due to a combination of more adolescents waiting to have sexual intercourse and increased contraception use by those teens who are sexually active. The **birth rate** in 2008 among Americans age 15 to 19 has also declined almost continuously over the same period, and is at its lowest recorded level. Teen birth rates in the USA vary greatly from state to state, and even by county within states. In the USA, teen birth rates are lowest among Asians and Pacific Islanders and highest among Hispanics and Blacks (CDC, May 2017). Overall, the American teen birth rate remains above that of other developed countries, including Canada and the United Kingdom (HHS, 2016).

The **teen pregnancy rate** in Canada fell by 40% from 1974 to 2003. The teen birth rate declined by more than 60% over the same period, due to higher teen abortion rates (Picard, 2007). Over the ensuing decade, the decline in teen pregnancy rate leveled off, and it *went up* substantially in four provinces: New Brunswick, Nova Scotia, Newfoundland, and Manitoba. Researchers explain this latest change in socio-economic terms. These regions of Canada have seen economic hard times, with outmigration of many young people. Those who remain may feel pessimistic about the future, making them less likely to delay childbearing to pursue education or employment opportunities (Bielski, 2018). In the USA, low education and low income levels of a teen's family contribute to high teen birth rates. For example, teens living in foster care have a higher rate of pregnancy than their counterparts not in foster care (CDC, May 2017). We explore the issue of fertility rate as a function of socio-economic development in the Population section of Chapter 15: Environment. Not surprisingly, teen pregnancy rates drop when young, economically challenged women have better access to long-term, reversible contraception (Bielski, 2018).

6 Conclusion

Scientific and medical advances such as oral contraceptives, intrauterine devices, female condoms, and implanted hormones have increased the range of contraceptive options available. There is still no *best* or *ideal* contraceptive, and there probably never will be. What is suitable for one individual or couple won't be for others. This individual variability is also reflected in regional and global differences in attitudes toward contraception and in the type and extent of contraceptive use. Contemporary health educators largely agree that health is promoted by

- Providing choices.
- Providing education so people can make informed choices.
- Empowering people so they can feel inspired and competent to take charge of their lives.

Globally, family planning is most effective when it is consistent with prevailing local social customs, religious beliefs, and political and economic realities. Global population growth is covered in Chapter 15: Environment.

Study Questions

1. Explain, with the aid of diagrams, how each of the following methods of contraception works:
    - Intrauterine device (IUD)
    - Condom
    - Diaphragm
    - Vasectomy
    - Tubal ligation
2. Discuss the relative advantages and disadvantages of each of the following contraceptive methods:
    - Abstinence
    - Hormonal methods
    - Intrauterine device
    - Predicting fertility
    - Barrier methods
    - Withdrawal
    - Surgical methods
3. What is the difference between "theoretical" and "actual" effectiveness of contraception?
4. What four criteria need to be met in order for breastfeeding to be effective at preventing conception?
5. What is the difference between a spontaneous abortion and a therapeutic abortion?
6a List the questions that prospective parents should consider.
6b. Ideally, at what stage of the pregnancy should these questions be considered?
7. Describe the current situation around therapeutic abortion in Canada and the United States.

8. Outline the arguments for and against therapeutic abortion.
9. Summarize the events in a normal pregnancy.
10. Summarize the advice for having a healthy pregnancy.
11a. What is the difference between a vaginal delivery and a Caesarian section?
11b. Which one is safer for the mother?
11c. What would account for the increasing prevalence of Caesarian section as a delivery method in Canada and the United States?
12a. Are teenage pregnancy rates in Canada increasing or decreasing?
12b. What about teenage abortion rates?
12c. Suggest explanations.

Glossary

actual effectiveness—effectiveness rate is the opposite of failure rate. Thus, if a method is 90% effective at preventing pregnancy, then 10% of the couples who use this method will become pregnant. The *actual effectiveness* is effectiveness "in the field," which includes not only using the method correctly but remembering to use it consistently (examples of *in*consistent use are forgetting to take an oral contraceptive one day, and not using a condom sometimes).

Caesarian section (C-section)—a surgical method of delivering a baby; a cut is made through the abdomen into the uterus (womb) and the baby is lifted out, rather than being pushed through the cervix and vagina (birth canal) in a normal delivery

hysterectomy—surgical removal of the uterus (womb); this renders a woman unable to have further children, but the procedure is usually done for medical reasons, such as cancer, rather than for contraceptive purposes

placenta—an organ that connects the developing fetus to the uterine wall to allow nutrient uptake, waste elimination, and gas exchange via the mother's blood supply

spontaneous abortion—an accidental terminator of pregnancy; also known as a miscarriage

theoretical effectiveness—the best-case effectiveness of a contraceptive method in preventing pregnancy (see *actual effectiveness*)

therapeutic abortion—a deliberate termination of pregnancy

tubal sterilization—a procedure in which the oviducts (Fallopian tubes) are cut or tied closed or otherwise sealed

umbilical cord—a tough tube, about 60 cm (24 in.) long, that contains arteries and veins that connect the fetus with the mother's placenta

vasectomy—a procedure in which the vas deferens is cut and tied off

Additional Resources

Options for Sexual Health (formerly Planned Parenthood BC)
    3550 Hastings Street, East Vancouver, BC v5к 2A7
    604-731-4252
    1-800-739-7367 (BC only)
    info@optbc.org
    https://optionsforsexualhealth.org
The Sensible Guide for a Healthy Pregnancy
    Public Health Agency of Canada, Government of Canada
    www.HealthyCanadians.gc.ca/pregnancy
United for Life
    Box 12045 Murrayville RPO, Langley, BC v3A 9J5
    604-534-4828
    info@unitedforlifebc.ca
    http://unitedforlifebc.ca/

References

Associated Press. (January 18, 2008). US Abortion rate at lowest level since 1974. *CTV. ca.* Retrieved April 11, 2008 from http://www.ctv.ca/servlet/ArticleNews/story/ CTVNews/20080118/abortion_080118?s_name=&no_ads=

Bielski, Z. (May 11, 2018). Why teen pregnancy is on the rise again in Canada. Retrieved May 26, 2018 from https://www.theglobeandmail.com/life/health-and-fitness/ health/why-teen-pregnancy-is-on-the-rise-again-in-canada-and-spiking-in-these-provinces/article7927983/

CDC (Centers for Disease Control and Prevention). (2011). *Effectiveness of contraceptive methods.* US Department of Health and Human Services. Centers for Disease Control and Prevention. Retrieved April 25, 2014 from http://www.cdc.gov/repro-ductivehealth/UnintendedPregnancy/Contraception.htm

CDC; National Center for HIV/AIDS, Viral Hepatitis, STD, and TB Prevention. (February 2013). Incidence, prevalence, and cost of sexually transmitted infections in the United States. CDC Fact Sheet.

CDC. (May 9, 2017). About teen pregnancy. Retrieved May 26, 2018 from https://www. cdc.gov/teenpregnancy/about/index.htm

CDC. (November 16, 2017). CDCs Abortion Surveillance System FAQs. Retrieved May 26, 2018 from https://www.cdc.gov/reproductivehealth/data_stats/abortion.htm

CIHI (Canadian Institute for Health Information). (2013). Abortions in Canada. Retrieved May 26, 2018 from https://www.cihi.ca/en/ta_11_alldatatables20140221_ en.pdf

CYWH Staff. (2011). *Birth control pills: Side effects.* Center for Young Women's Health. Boston Children's Hospital. Retrieved January 21, 2013 from http://www.youngwom-enshealth.org/birth_control_pill_side_effects.html

FDA. (February 15, 2013). FDA Drug Safety Communication: Updated information about the risk of blood clots in women taking birth control pills containing drospirenone. US Food and Drug Administration. Retrieved April 25, 2014 from http://www.fda.gov/Drugs/DrugSafety/ucm299305.htm

Government of Canada. (2011). The Sensible Guide to a Healthy Pregnancy. Retrieved May 26, 2018 from https://www.canada.ca/content/dam/phac-aspc/documents/services/health-promotion/healthy-pregnancy/healthy-pregnancy-guide-eng.pdf

Guttmacher Institute & WHO (World Health Organization). (January 2012). Facts on induced abortion worldwide. Retrieved May 26, 2018 from http://www.who.int/reproductivehealth/publications/unsafe_abortion/induced_abortion_2012.pdf

Hatcher et al. (2004). *Contraceptive technology* (18th Revised Edition). New York: Irvington. As cited by Chard, D. (2007). *Effectiveness of contraceptive methods. Options for sexual health.* Retrieved April 8, 2008 from http://www.optionsforsexualhealth.org/birth-control-pregnancy/birth-control-options/effectiveness

Mayo Clinic. (2012). *Birth control pill FAQ: Benefits, risks and choices.* Retrieved January 17, 2013 from http://www.mayoclinic.com/health/birth-control-pill/WO00098

Options for Sexual Health. (January 2018). Where can I get an abortion in BC? Retrieved May 26, 2018 from https://www.optionsforsexualhealth.org/birth-control-pregnancy/abortion-resources/abortion-providers

Picard, A. (May 17, 2007). Teen pregnancies drop to a new low, abortions continue decline. *Globeandmail.com.* Retrieved April 11, 2008 from http://www.theglobeandmail.com/servlet/story/RTGAM.20070517.wxlpregnancy17/BNStory/special-ScienceandHealth/home

Planned Parenthood Federation of America. (2007). *Comparing effectiveness of birth control methods.* Retrieved April 25, 2014 from http://www.plannedparenthood.org/health-topics/birth-control/birth-control-effectiveness-chart-22710.htm

Planned Parenthood Federation of America. (2014). *Birth control.* Retrieved April 25, 2014 from http://www.plannedparenthood.org/health-topics/birth-control-4211.htm

Podulka, J., Stranges, E., Steiner, C. (April, 2011). *Hospitalizations related to childbirth, 2008.* Statistical Brief #110. Retrieved January 18, 2013 from http://www.hcup-us.ahrq.gov/reports/statbriefs/sb110.jsp

Racco, M. (October 16, 2017). Why STI rates are steadily going up in Canada. Global News. Retrieved May 23, 2018 from https://globalnews.ca/news/3797824/why-sti-infection-rates-are-steadily-going-up-in-canada/

Smith, A. (2012). *Breastfeeding and birth control.* Retrieved May 10, 2014 from http://www.pregnancy.org/article/breastfeeding-and-birth-control

UNFPA. (2013). *Motherhood in childhood: Facing the challenge of adolescent pregnancy.* United Nations Population Fund. Information and External Relations Division. The State of World Population 2013. Retrieved July 31, 2014 from http://www.unfpa.org/webdav/site/global/shared/swp2013/EN-SWOP2013-final.pdf

HHS (US Department of Health & Human Services; Office of Adolescent Health). (June 2, 2016). Trends in teen pregnancy and childbearing. Retrieved May 26, 2018 from https://www.hhs.gov/ash/oah/adolescent-development/reproduc-

tive-health-and-teen-pregnancy/teen-pregnancy-and-childbearing/trends/index.
html

Wayne Wright Injury Lawyers. (December 27, 2016). Ortho Evra birth control: A dangerous history lesson for women. Retrieved May 26, 2018 from https://www.waynewright.com/blog/ortho-evra-birth-control-patch-lawsuit-timeline.cfm

WebMD. (July 7, 2012). *Teen pregnancy: Medical risks and realities.* Retrieved April 25, 2014 from http://www.webmd.com/baby/guide/teen-pregnancy-medical-risks-and-realities

Weeks, C. (May 31, 2018). Canadian Paediatric Society says doctors should offer IUDs as first-line birth control option for young girls. *The Globe and Mail.* Retrieved May 31, 2018 from https://www.theglobeandmail.com/canada/article-canadian-paediatric-society-says-doctors-should-offer-iuds-as-first/

13 Drugs

Learning Objectives

By the time you have finished this chapter you should be able to

- Define "drug" and "psychoactive drug"
- Explain the implications of the routes of administration of drugs
- Describe the acute and chronic effects of commonly used psychoactive drugs
- Explain different models of addiction
- Offer explanations for why people take psychoactive drugs
- Discuss the issues around drug use and misuse, including prevention, enforcement, and legalization

1 Overview

A **drug** is "any substance other than food or water that is taken in order to change the structure or function of the body." This is a very broad definition. Some drugs are **prescription drugs**, which means they are only available with a prescription from a medical doctor. Other drugs are available **over the counter** (OTC) without a prescription. When people think of drugs, especially in the context of drug misuse, they are usually referring to *psychoactive drugs*. Psychoactive drugs act on the psyche; that is, they exert their effect on the brain, causing a change in perception, mood, thinking, or behaviour.

In this chapter, we won't try to cover all the major psychoactive drugs. Instead, we will look at seven examples:

- Caffeine
- Nicotine

- Cocaine
- Amphetamines
- Cannabis
- Alcohol
- Opiate narcotics, such as heroin and fentanyl

In addition, we will deal with some general concepts, including

- Routes of administration (the various ways drugs are taken)
- Why people take psychoactive drugs
- Models of drug abuse
- Strategies to address substance misuse, including an exploration of the enforcement-versus-decriminalization controversy.
- A more complete study of psychoactive drugs would also include
- Club drugs, such as MDMA (ecstasy), GHB, ketamine, and Rohypnol
- Hallucinogens, such as peyote, "magic mushrooms," and LSD
- Tranquilizers (central nervous system depressants), such Valium, Ativan, and Xanax

Regardless of the way in which psychoactive drugs are taken, the drug molecules must get to the brain to have their effect. People don't inject drugs into their brain. So, how do the drugs get to the brain? The drug molecules are carried in the bloodstream, and as the blood moves into the brain, they cross the **blood/brain barrier**. The blood/brain barrier is a network of blood vessels and tissue made of closely spaced cells. It is a protective physical barrier that keeps many substances out of the brain. After the drug molecules reach the brain, they bind (attach) to specific sites on the surface of nerve cells. This leads to changes in the nerve cell activity, such as making certain nerve cells more or less active, which causes the drug effects.

2 Routes of Administration

Drugs that are injected **intravenously (IV)**—that is, directly into the bloodstream—reach the brain quickly (Figure 13.1). So do drugs that are smoked. Swallowed substances appear in the blood more slowly. Drugs can also be absorbed across the mucous membranes of the mouth (chewing tobacco or coca leaves, or placing Ativan tablets under the tongue), nose (snorting cocaine), or rectum (suppositories containing medicines which a vomiting patient would not be able to hold down if ingested).

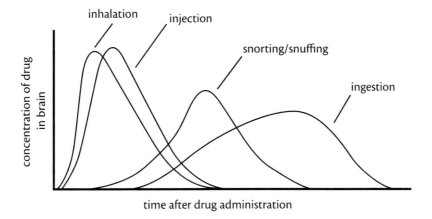

Figure 13.1. The time it takes drugs to reach and accumulate in the brain depends on the method used to administer the drug.

These ***routes of administration*** (various ways of getting drugs into the body) influence the health effects of a specific drug in three main ways:

- Injecting or smoking drugs is more likely to cause **dependence**. This is because a strong stimulus-response pairing occurs. The drug effects occur soon after taking the drug, which creates a more powerful association or memory.
- Drugs that are injected or smoked **wear off quickly**, so the user needs to take another hit in order to maintain the high. This causes more frequent stimulus-response pairs, which again fixes the behaviour more deeply in memory, making it harder to unlearn. Smoking crack (the smokable form of cocaine) is a perfect example. So is smoking tobacco.
- The **method** of taking drugs can cause health problems independent of the effects of the drug itself. For example, needles that are contaminated with pathogens can transmit infections such as hepatitis and HIV. Smoking (tobacco or cannabis) damages airways.

> Cannabis can be ingested (eaten)—baked in cookies, for example. This would eliminate all of the health consequences of smoking it.
> Why do *you* think eating cannabis is so much less popular than smoking it?

3 Common Psychoactive Drugs

3.1 Caffeine

The most widely used psychoactive drug in North America (and probably the world) is caffeine. The most common sources of caffeine—coffee, tea, energy drinks, cola beverages, and chocolate—are readily available and relatively inexpensive, and consumption is widely acceptable. Caffeine can also be taken in pill form, such as the OTC preparations Wakeups and No-Doz.

The effects of caffeine use are relatively harmless. Caffeine is a mild stimulant. It causes a general activation of the sympathetic nervous system (remember the alarm stage of the general adaptation syndrome from Chapter 9: Mental Health). This includes increased heart rate and blood pressure, increased metabolic rate, and increased alertness. Excess consumption can cause shaking, difficulty concentrating, insomnia, and in some people, irregular heartbeat. The regular user who stops taking caffeine often experiences irritability, drowsiness, and headache.

> *Does drinking coffee negatively or positively affect our heart rate or life expectancy?*

Coffee is a complex beverage. It contains caffeine, but also many other compounds. Some of these are known carcinogens in rodents, but probably the amount one would get from normal coffee drinking is too low to cause any meaningful risk of cancer in humans. On the other hand, coffee also contains antioxidants, which reduce risk of heart disease, cancer, and Alzheimer's disease.

The method used to prepare coffee also matters. For example, one method of decaffeinating coffee uses solvents, and residues of these solvents remain in the beverage. In addition, drip coffee can carry residues from the filter paper into the beverage.

The main negative effects of coffee drinking appear to be gastro-intestinal problems (e.g., stomach ulcers), adverse effects on the fetus, anemia (coffee interferes with absorption of iron from food), and effects related to the stimulant effect of caffeine if consumed in excess (e.g., increased blood pressure, nervousness, shaky hands, and insomnia).

On the other hand, there are a number of positive health effects of coffee drinking, including reduced rates of some types of cancer, decreased constipation, and protective effects on the heart and brain.

Overall, regular moderate coffee consumption seems to confer a net benefit at the population level and is associated with a moderate increase in life expectancy.

To what extent do *you* use caffeine as a stimulant?

How do you feel about this?

Suggest at least three strategies that could give you the "lift" or "energy" you get from caffeine in other ways.

3.2 *Tobacco*

The leaves of the tobacco plant are dried, cured, and shredded. The tobacco is then rolled into cigarettes or cigars, or is chewed. Tobacco contains many compounds, including the psychoactive drug nicotine. **Nicotine** is a mild stimulant, and the acute (short-term) effects of tobacco smoking reflect this. Like cocaine, heroin, and marijuana, nicotine increases levels of the neurotransmitter **dopamine**, which affects the brain pathways that control reward and pleasure (NIDA, 2012c).

Tobacco use is the leading preventable cause of disease, disability, and death in the United States (NIDA, 2012c) and Canada (Desjardins, 2013).

The tars in tobacco are carcinogenic; they cause cancers of the lip, mouth, and throat in all users, and of the lung in smokers. Also, "poisons in cigarette smoke weaken the tumour fighters." In addition, "… tobacco smoke helps tumours grow. It can undo the benefits of chemotherapy" (Benjamin, 2010, p. 6). Tobacco smoke causes your lungs to make more mucus and damages the **cilia**. Cilia are tiny hairs that line the airways; they are covered with a layer of mucus onto which foreign particles stick (Figure 13.2). In the healthy lung, the cilia move in a coordinated fashion, like a team of rowers pulling on their oars in unison. This ciliary action sweeps out mucus and the material it has trapped. Smoking damages cilia (Richardson, 2003). Surprisingly, stopping smoking allows the cilia to repair and regenerate in as few as three days.

Chronic (long-term) smoking causes other lung diseases, including **bronchitis** (inflammation of the airways) and **emphysema** (destruction of lung tissue, causing shortness of breath). Chemicals in cigarette smoke irritate cells that line the lungs. The USA Surgeon General's Report (Benjamin, 2010) compares this to spilling drain cleaner on your skin. "If you did this many times a day, your skin would not have a chance to heal. It would stay red, irritated, and inflamed" (p. 2).

"Tobacco smoke scars your lungs … Years of smoking can damage your lungs so much that they no longer stretch and exchange air" (Benjamin, 2010, p. 10).

Non-smokers exposed to second-hand smoke at home or work increase their risk of developing heart disease by 25% to 30% and lung cancer by 20% to 30% (NIDA, 2012c).

Smoking is strongly associated with cardiovascular disease (CVD), which kills more smokers than lung cancer. Smoking also makes it harder to control diabetes (Benjamin, 2010, pp. 12–13 and p. 14).

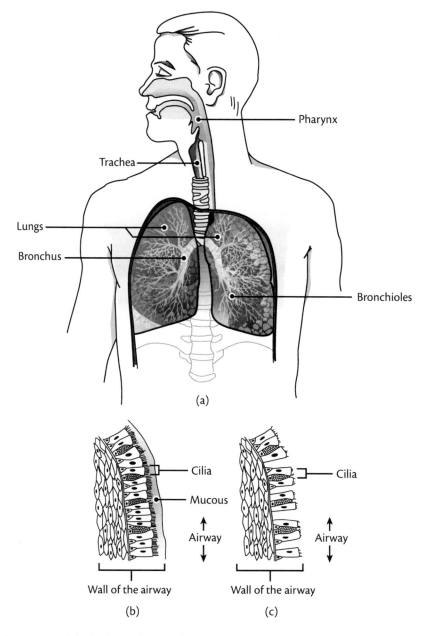

Figure 13.2. (a) The bronchus and bronchioles are tubes that allow gas to enter and leave the lungs. (b) The airways are lined with tiny hairs called cilia, covered with a layer of mucus. (c) Smoking damages the cilia, allowing mucus to accumulate in the lung, and causing the classic "smoker's cough."

Smoking by pregnant females increases risk of miscarriage and of low-birth-weight infants. Maternal smoking may also be associated with learning and behavioural problems in children. Smoking more than one pack of cigarettes per day during pregnancy nearly doubles the risk that the affected child will become addicted to tobacco if that child starts smoking (NIDA, 2012c).

> ### Can you cancel out smoking by exercising?

No. It doesn't work this way.

Smoking certainly adversely affects exercise performance. And exercise does help improve heart and lung function. However, smoking damages the body in many ways, and no amount of exercise will offset these effects. The only way to cancel out the effects of smoking is to stop smoking.

3.2.1 Smoking in Canada

In 2015, 13% of Canadian adults smoked (Statista, 2016), down from 25% in 1999 (Health Canada, 2013). The percentage of Canadians age 15 to 19 smoking is also down: 28% in 1999, 11% in 2012 (Health Canada, 2013), and 10% in 2015 (University of Waterloo, 2016).

3.2.2 Reasons why people smoke

Knowledge among young people of the health effects of smoking is high. However, knowledge alone is not enough to change behaviour. Young people may not be highly motivated by fear of lung cancer, as the effects seem so remote. Also, there is a theme of invincibility among the young, a sense that "it won't happen to me."

Smokers typically start as adolescents or young adults, initially smoking in social situations. They "just wanted to try it," or they thought it was "cool" to smoke (American Cancer Society, 2014b). Young smokers believe they can easily quit, and few believe they will be long-term smokers. But tobacco use is strongly addictive—both the nicotine in the tobacco and the smoking behaviour. (Christensen, 2014). The younger people are when they begin to smoke, the more likely they are to become addicted to nicotine. Nearly 9 out of 10 adult smokers started by age 18, and 99% started by age 26 (American Cancer Society, 2014b).

Despite regulations limiting advertising of tobacco products, tobacco companies continue to market their products aggressively (e.g., on the largely unregulated Internet and by showing smoking in movies).

There is also some evidence that other chemicals in cigarette smoke may act with nicotine to make it harder to quit smoking (American Cancer Society, 2014b).

3.2.3 Quitting smoking

Many people find it hard to quit smoking, but it can be done. Quit-smoking programs, like treatments of other addictions, often have fairly low success rates. But that doesn't mean they're not worthwhile or that the smoker should be discouraged (American Cancer Society, 2014a).

From 70% to 90% of smokers say nicotine withdrawal symptoms—such as anxiety, irritability, sleep disturbances, trouble concentrating, restlessness or boredom, and headaches—are their only reasons for continuing to smoke. That is, smoking is no longer pleasurable; it just fends off the unpleasant withdrawal symptoms.

The American Cancer Society (2014a) lists the following aids to quitting smoking:

- Counselling, including counselling over the telephone
- Support groups
- Support of family and friends
- Quit-smoking programs (e.g., through employers, hospitals, and wellness centres)
- Prescription drugs

There is little scientific evidence to support other methods, such as hypnosis, acupuncture, magnets, lasers, or herbs. The most effective method seems to include the following steps:

1. Decide on a "quit day."
2. Make a plan.
   Successful quitting is a matter of planning and commitment, not luck. Decide now on your own plan. Some options include using nicotine replacement or other medicines, joining a stop-smoking class, going to Nicotine Anonymous meetings, using self-help materials such as books and pamphlets, or some combination of these methods. For the best chance at success, your plan should include at least 2 of these options. (American Cancer Society, 2014a)
3. Deal with withdrawal symptoms.
4. Manage your stress levels—not just the stress from quitting smoking, but in other areas of your life—because "smokers often mention stress as one of the reasons for going back to smoking" (American Cancer Society, 2014a).

Nicotine replacement therapy (NRT) allows the user to overcome the *psychological* aspects of addiction by providing maintenance doses of nicotine in chewing gum, patches, sprays, or inhalers to prevent *physical* withdrawal. Combining nicotine replacement therapy with behavioural counselling increases the success rate compared with nicotine therapy alone. The nicotine in NRT has some adverse health effects per se, which is a concern for people with cardio-vascular disease and pregnant women. In addition, there is the possibility of nicotine overdose, although this is rare. However, quitting smoking, with or without NRT, greatly reduces your risk of future health problems.

3.2.4 *Electronic cigarettes*

Also known as **e-cigarettes**, these electronic nicotine-delivery systems (ENDS) typically consist of a mouthpiece, battery, heating element, and container of liquid. The heating element turns the liquid into a vapour, which is then inhaled (Figure 13.3).

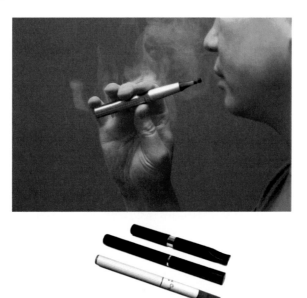

Figure 13.3. Examples of e-cigarette devices.

This is a relatively new field. Little is actually known yet about the effectiveness or safety of e-cigarettes (Bam et al., 2014). Use seems to be increasing rapidly, and represents a multi-billion-dollar industry, with multinational tobacco companies as major players (Bam et al., 2014).

Because they deliver **nicotine** without burning tobacco, e-cigarettes *appear* to be a safer, less toxic alternative to conventional cigarettes. However, the vapour inhaled still contains nicotine and other potentially harmful chemicals. Nicotine is a highly addictive drug. Recent research suggests nicotine exposure may also prime the brain to become addicted to other substances (NIDA, 2013c). Fetal and adolescent nicotine exposure has potential detrimental consequences for brain development. In high doses, nicotine can cause death by poisoning (WHO, 2014).

E-cigarette vapour (which should more properly be called "aerosol," meaning a gaseous suspension of fine solid or liquid particles) contains some of the same carcinogenic compounds and other toxicants found in tobacco smoke—at average levels of only 1% to 10% of the levels found in tobacco smoke, but still higher than in nicotine inhalers (WHO, 2014). Also like tobacco smoke, e-cigarette vapour contains tiny particles, though at levels lower than in tobacco smoke. Bystanders are exposed to the aerosol, creating the same health issues as second-hand tobacco smoke (Bam et al., 2014; WHO, 2014). "The fact that ENDS exhaled aerosol contains on average lower levels of toxicants than the emissions from combusted tobacco does not mean that these levels are acceptable to involuntarily exposed bystanders" (WHO, 2014).

Nicotine levels in each puff can vary a great deal. Another worry is the refillable cartridges used by some e-cigarettes. Users may expose themselves to potentially toxic levels of nicotine when refilling them. Also, cartridges could be filled with substances other than nicotine, thus possibly serving as a new and potentially dangerous way to deliver other drugs (NIDA, 2013c). Furthermore, the ingredients in e-cigarettes are not labelled. The manufacturers say the ingredients are safe, but it's not clear if they are safe to inhale; many substances that are safe to *eat* can harm delicate tissues inside the lungs.

The rise of e-cigarette use has created a deep division among tobacco control advocates. "Whereas some experts welcome ENDS as a pathway to the reduction of tobacco smoking, others characterize them as products that could undermine efforts to denormalize tobacco use" (WHO, 2014). On the one hand, e-cigarettes may cause non-smokers (especially children) to become addicted to nicotine and subsequently transfer this addiction to tobacco smoking. This is the so-called **gateway effect**. On the other hand, e-cigarettes are a way for smokers to maintain their nicotine addiction while getting rid of many of the harmful effects of smoking tobacco (Branswell, 2015). So far, however, there is limited evidence for the effectiveness of e-cigarettes as a method for quitting tobacco smoking (WHO, 2014). "Because the American Cancer Society doesn't yet know whether e-cigarettes are safe and effective, we cannot recommend them to help people quit smoking" (American Cancer Society, 2014a).

Concern has also been raised that the popularity of e-cigarettes will undermine the de-normalization of tobacco use that has underpinned the success of tobacco control in developed countries over the last half-century. "Everything that makes ENDS attractive to smokers may enhance the attractiveness of smoking itself and perpetuate the smoking epidemic. ENDS mimic the personal experience and public performance of smoking" (WHO, 2014). Finally, since many e-cigarettes closely resemble tobacco cigarettes in appearance and public performance, "it is likely that their use where smoking is banned will make enforcing smoke-free policies more difficult" (WHO, 2014).

The World Health Organization (WHO, 2013) has concluded that "until such time as a given ENDS is deemed safe and effective and of acceptable quality by a competent national regulatory body, consumers should be *strongly advised not to use any of these products, including electronic cigarettes*" [emphasis added] (WHO, 2013).

Health Canada had been slow to regulate e-cigarettes. In the absence of action by the federal government, a number of provinces and municipalities have enacted their own laws limiting e-cigarettes (Branswell, 2015). In April 2018, the Canadian federal government passed legislation (Bill S-5) that prohibits the sale of vaping products to minors, bans the promotion of vaping products containing flavours that appeal to youth, and restricts advertising of vaping products (Norris & Tiedemann M, 2017).

3.3 *Cocaine*

Cocaine is a stimulant derived from the leaves of the **coca plant**, grown in the mountains of South America. For centuries, people in this region have chewed the leaves to reduce hunger and fatigue. Elsewhere in the world, cocaine is usually taken as a white powder, which is snorted into the nose or mixed with water and injected. Cocaine smoked in a pipe is called "crack" because of the crackling sound the small "rock" of cocaine makes as it is heated (NIDA, 2013a).

Cocaine is a strong stimulant. It causes a rapid heart rate and breathing rate, dilated pupils, sweating, paleness, and decreased appetite. In addition, users experience an exaggerated perception of alertness, competency, and power. Large doses can cause nausea, twitching, tremors, and chest pain. Overdose can cause death from heart irregularities. There appears to be no safe dose—that is, no dose low enough to avoid such health risk. The high is rather short and may be followed by a deep low and the desire to use again. Repeated use can lead to insomnia, weight loss, impotence, and exhaustion. Impurities in street cocaine may produce a fatal allergic reaction.

Cocaine is powerfully addictive (NIDA, 2013a). Habitual use can be expensive ($500+ per day for those who inject it). So cocaine users are more likely to do criminal activities to support their habit than are users of drugs such as cannabis or ethanol. Over time, snorting causes holes in nose tissue and nose bleeds. Injecting causes collapsed veins, scarring, and infections. Chronic use can cause personality changes, including aggression and paranoia (NIDA, 2013a). For example, a user may believe the mail carrier is an undercover police agent, or shoot at her through the letter slot. Babies born to mothers who used cocaine regularly during their pregnancy also become addicted.

3.4 Amphetamines

Amphetamines are powerful stimulants with effects similar to cocaine. Amphetamines are used medically, but most amphetamines these days are manufactured by illegal labs for non-medical use. **Methamphetamine** (also known as meth, speed, or crank) is a commonly abused amphetamine. It can be snorted, swallowed, smoked, or injected intravenously. **Ice** is a high-purity, crystalline form of methamphetamine that is mainly smoked or injected (NADRC 2012).

Estimates from Health Canada (2014) for prevalence of use of speed or methamphetamine in the past year are not available because of high sampling variability in the data they obtained.

Chronic amphetamine use produces tolerance. Over three-quarters of dependent meth users report some mental health problems. Regular use at high doses produces **amphetamine psychosis** (similar to schizophrenia) or very powerful psychological dependence and extremely compulsive patterns of use. Withdrawal symptoms include feeling depressed, irritable, restless, fatigued, and having physical complaints such as stomach cramps, aches, nausea, and rapid heartbeat (NADRC, 2006). In addition, about half of dependent meth users suffer poor physical health, including disturbed sleep, weight loss, and chest pain. Other facets of health are also compromised. Dependent meth users are more likely to engage in unsafe sexual behaviours compared with their peers.

> Other problems experienced by some methamphetamine users include social isolation, relationship breakdowns, and financial difficulties. Some methamphetamine users also become involved in crime, such as drug dealing or theft, to support their drug use. Over half of regular users have been arrested and one-third have been to prison. (NADRC, 2006)

Methamphetamine use has become quite a problem in parts of the USA. Meth can be concocted relatively easily from readily available ingredients, such as crushed antihistamine pills, lighter fluid, and drain cleaner. This makes it a cheap and available drug. As a stimulant, it wards off sleep and increases stamina for work. These characteristics may seem especially attractive at a time when the economy is depressed.

3.5 Cannabis

Cannabis seems to be the most difficult psychoactive drug for the non-expert to investigate. I have read focused reports by what I consider credible, non-biased government- or university-affiliated health organizations (not law enforcement) and found that pro-cannabis and anti-cannabis feelings are strong, and positions at either end of this spectrum are quite polarized.

Marijuana, hashish (hash), and hash oil are all products of the cannabis plant. This plant grows well both outdoors and indoors. Cannabis is usually smoked in a pipe or rolled into cigarettes called "joints." Tetrahydrocannabinol (**THC**) and other similar cannabinoids are the psychoactive drugs in cannabis. THC acts on specific molecular targets on brain cells. THC activates the reward system in the same way that nearly all drugs of abuse do—by stimulating brain cells to release the chemical **dopamine** (NIDA, 2012a).

3.5.1 Prevalence

Cannabis is the most widely used illicit drug (NIDA, 2010, p. 23). Over 12% of Canadians 15 years and older report using cannabis, up from 5.6% in 1985 (CBC, 2018). This compares with 1.1% reported past-year cocaine or crack use and 0.6% ecstasy use (Health Canada, 2014). Between 2004 and 2015, cannabis usage rates remained stable for males age 15 to 17 but went *down* among females of the same age, and went down among members of both sexes in the 18-to-24 age range (CBC, 2018). Statistics Canada estimated that in 2017, almost 5 million Canadians consumed cannabis, 90% of them for illegal non-medical use. The estimated $5.7 billion Canadians spent on cannabis compares with the $20 and $16 billion dollars Canadians spent on alcohol and tobacco, respectively, the same year (Evans, 2018).

3.5.2 Acute effects

Cannabis use is not "safe." Instead, acute and chronic use both increase risk for a number of health conditions. Acute effects of cannabis use include mild euphoria and heightened perception. Effects start within a few minutes of smoking and persist for several hours. Red eyes, increased appetite, euphoria, and drowsiness are common. Distortion of time and space, plus decreases in concentration and attention span, make it hazardous to participate in any activity requiring motor coordination, such as driving, using power tools, or playing sports. Subjects who smoked marijuana under experimental conditions made significantly more errors on a driving course (e.g., failing to stop at stop signs) than their placebo-controlled counterparts. In contrast with other drugs (e.g., alcohol, cocaine, amphetamines), cannabis use is rarely associated with violence.

3.5.3 Chronic physical effects

The main probable long-term physical effects concern the lungs. Marijuana smoke is an irritant to the lungs, so it is not surprising that cannabis smokers experience many of the same respiratory problems as tobacco smokers (NIDA, 2014). Cannabis smokers are probably at increased risk of respiratory diseases associated with smoking, including cancer (NPIC, 2011a).

> *Are the health effects of smoking cigarettes the same as smoking other substances such as cigars and marijuana?*

Burning anything produces, among other things, carbon monoxide and carbon dioxide. These substances are inhaled with the tobacco smoke and interfere with the blood's ability to carry oxygen to cells.

The paper rolled around tobacco or marijuana and the matches used to light the material contribute additional compounds.

Cigars and cigarettes are both made from tobacco. Tobacco contains many compounds, some of which are carcinogenic. Cigar smokers typically take fewer puffs of tobacco smoke in a day than cigarette smokers do, and cigar smokers don't usually inhale the smoke into their lungs. Instead, they take it into just their mouth and nose. Thus, risk of lung cancer is probably a lot lower in cigar smokers than in cigarette smokers. However, risk of cancers of the lip and mouth may be similar between the two types of smokers.

Marijuana (cannabis) has not been studied as well as tobacco has. Cannabis also contains lots of compounds, some of which are carcinogens. The mode of smoking cannabis differs from that of tobacco smoking. Cannabis smokers typically inhale deeply and then hold the smoke in their lungs to maximize the time for the psychoactive chemicals to move from the lungs into the blood. This would logically increase risk of cancer. On the other hand, cigarette smokers typically smoke a pack of 20 or more cigarettes in a day, while typical cannabis consumption is at a much lower daily level. This would reduce risk of cancer due to cannabis compared with tobacco.

Another consideration is that cannabis, not being a legally controlled substance, is much more variable in quality and composition.

Poorer grades of cannabis may be contaminated with agricultural chemicals, cow dung, and so on. Hydroponically grown cannabis is probably purer in general.

I don't believe the evidence on cannabis and lung cancer is definitive. However, I think an association has been demonstrated between cannabis smoking and other lung diseases, such as bronchitis (inflammation of the upper airways) and asthma (periodic constriction of the airways, leading to shortness of breath).

In conclusion, smoking anything probably causes some health harm. The safest way to smoke cannabis is probably in a vaporizer, a device that heats the dried cannabis leaves to the point that the THC vaporizes and collects in a glass chamber or a plastic balloon. The smoker then inhales the vapour through a tube.

3.5.4 Intellectual and emotional health

A number of studies have linked chronic marijuana use and mental illness ... [with] depression, anxiety, suicidal thoughts among adolescents, and personality disturbances, including a lack of motivation to engage in typically rewarding activities. More research is still needed to confirm and better understand these linkages. (NIDA, 2014)

Cannabis use may trigger schizophrenia in those who are already at risk of developing the disorder, and cannabis use has been clearly shown to make psychotic symptoms worse in people who already have a psychotic disorder such as schizophrenia (NPIC, 2012). "Although some people say the use of cannabis alleviates their symptoms of depression, there is evidence that smoking cannabis may make depression worse" (NPIC, 2012). Cannabis use is also associated with decreased memory and learning abilities, and decreased motivation in areas such as study, work, or concentration (NPIC, 2011a). Children of women who used cannabis when they were pregnant are more likely to have problems with attention, memory, and problem-solving (NIDA, 2014). However, the strong *associations* that are often found between cannabis use and mental health symptoms do not necessarily imply a *causal* link (NPIC, 2012).

3.5.5 Socio-economic health

Cannabis impairs judgment and motor coordination, which increases risk of car crashes (NIDA, 2014). Because it is illegal, cannabis possession can lead to criminal prosecution and a criminal record (ADAI, 2013). Cannabis use is associated with relationship problems, less academic and career success, and increased absences, tardiness, and accidents at work (NIDA, 2014). Long-term cannabis use has also been associated with **amotivational syndrome** (NIDA, 2012a), although it may be that people with low motivation to study or work are attracted to using cannabis, rather than that cannabis use *causes* the decreased motivation.

3.5.6 Young users

Concern about the broad range of health effects associated with cannabis use seems especially focused on young users. "Generally speaking, people who start smoking cannabis at a younger age (early adolescence) and smoke heavily are more likely to experience negative consequences" (NPIC, 2012). This seems to be due to the importance of social development in adolescence. "Adolescence is a period when many developmental changes are occurring. It is a time when a young person's intellectual capacities expand and their friends and peers become increasingly influential" (ADAI, 2013).

Using cannabis at an early age is associated with higher levels of (ADAI, 2013)

- Leaving the family home
- Immature sexual activity, which can result in unplanned pregnancy
- Driving while under the influence of marijuana
- Being in an accident (risk more than doubled)
- Criminal behaviour, such as motor vehicle theft and break-and-enter offences, to pay for drug use
- Poor school performance
- Absences from school
- Dropping out without graduating
- Impaired emotional development
- Dissatisfaction with life
- Depression, anxiety, psychosis, or other mental illness

The pronounced effect of cannabis on young users is partly due to brain development.

> A recent study of marijuana users who began using in adolescence revealed substantially reduced connectivity among brain areas responsible for learning and memory. And a large long-term study in New Zealand showed that people who began smoking marijuana heavily in their teens lost an average of 8 points in IQ between age 13 and age 38. Importantly, the lost cognitive abilities were not fully restored

in those who quit smoking marijuana as adults. Those who started smoking marijuana in adulthood did not show significant IQ declines. (NIDA, 2014)

3.5.7 Dependence

"Historically, cannabis was not seen as a drug of dependence like heroin or alcohol, but cannabis dependence is now well recognised in the scientific community" (NCPIC, 2011b). The NIDA (2012a) says that an estimated 9% of people who use marijuana will become dependent on it. Australia's NCPIC (2011b) concurs, estimating that about 10% of those who have tried cannabis at least once in their lifetime will become dependent. The more often a person uses cannabis, the more likely he is to become dependent. If someone uses cannabis every day, he has a 50/50 chance of becoming dependent. Young people develop cannabis dependence more quickly than adults (NCPIC, 2011b).

> Think about the acute effects of cannabis as described above.
> In what ways would smoking cannabis likely affect a person's academic performance in university?

3.6 Ethanol

Ethanol is the proper name for alcohol that we drink. Other alcohols (e.g., methanol) are poisonous. Ethanol is absorbed from the stomach and the small intestine, and takes only a few minutes to reach the brain (NADRC, 2010).

Ethanol is a central nervous system (CNS) depressant. Yet the acute effects of moderate consumption make it *seem* like a stimulant. After a couple of drinks at a party, people typically become more talkative and animated, because the ethanol is suppressing inhibition at the higher levels of the brain (NADRC, 2010). Even if you normally feel shy, after a few drinks you may feel more uninhibited and talkative—and may find yourself saying things you later wish you had kept to yourself!

Acute effects of low doses of ethanol include mild euphoria and relaxation. Moderate intake alters judgment and causes decreased balance, coordination, and reaction time. These effects explain why ethanol (and other drugs) is strongly associated with accidents such as car crashes. Stimulants, such as caffeine and amphetamines, counteract the CNS-depressant effects of alcohol, but they do not counteract the loss of coordination. Some ethanol users become aggressive.

Alcohol use in Canada is common. Health Canada (2014) reports that over 78% of Canadians age 15 and over say they used alcohol in the last year. This figure is comparable to the 80% of Australians age 14 and over who reported in a 2010 survey that they used alcohol in the past year (NADRC, 2010).

Back to Canada: a higher percentage of males than females reported past-year alcohol use (84% vs. 74%). Among drinkers, 19% reported exceeding low-risk guidelines for chronic drinking, and 13% reported exceeding guidelines for acute drinking (Health Canada, 2014).

Alcohol affects every organ in the drinker's body (NIDA, 2012b). Chronic effects of ethanol consumption include

- **Gastritis**, which is inflammation of the stomach.
- **Pancreatitis**, which is inflammation of the pancreas, another digestive organ.
- **Cardiovascular disease**. A J-shaped dose-response *association* exists between alcohol consumption and cardiovascular disease (Figure 13.4). This does not prove that drinking *reduces* risk of heart disease; it may be that those with the lowest current levels of alcohol consumption used to be heavy drinkers until they got sick, and then they reduced their intake. Heavier consumption, including periodic binge drinking, is clearly associated with most types of CVD, but not heart attack (Wood, Wood, Kaptoge, Butterworth et al., 2018).

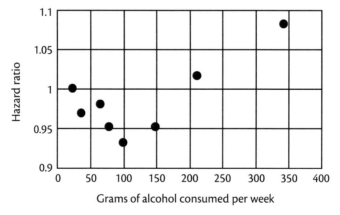

Figure 13.4. The dose-response relationship between alcohol consumption and cardiovascular disease of all types. By convention, the relative risk or hazard ratio is set to 1.0 for the group with the lowest exposure level. Note that relative risk rises beyond consumption of 100 g of ethanol (about 6 glasses of wine) per week.

- **Liver disease**, which includes cirrhosis (in which healthy liver cells are replaced by scar tissue) and liver cancer.
- **Cancers of the mouth and throat**. Ethanol is not a carcinogen itself, but it is a solvent in which carcinogens such as the "tar" in tobacco can dissolve and be carried more efficiently to target tissues.

- **Malnutrition**. Ethanol increases the rate at which B-vitamins are metabolized and thus need to be replenished. Also, in heavy drinkers, ethanol may make up 50% or more of the daily caloric intake, and ethanol contains no vitamins, minerals, or other nutrients.
- **Mental illness**, including depression (NADRC, 2010) and psychosis.
- **Brain damage**, including inability to remember recent events or learn new information. Yes, alcohol kills brain cells. Long-term consumption of too much alcohol can damage almost every major system in the body. The brain is one of the organs most sensitive to alcohol consumption. Chronic heavy drinking impairs memory and increases risk of dementia.
- **Reproductive effects**, including impotence (in men), infertility (in men and women), miscarriage, premature delivery, low-birth-weight infants, and **fetal alcohol syndrome** (FAS). Alcohol and other drugs in the mother's blood pass to her fetus. Babies with fetal alcohol syndrome can have mental retardation, defects of the heart and joints, small head and body, and behaviour abnormalities. Although FAS is associated with chronic heavy drinking, **fetal alcohol effects** (FAE) occur at much lower doses. Attention deficits and learning disorders have been related to FAE. Most health experts advise women to not drink or use drugs at all while they are pregnant.
- **Absenteeism** from school or work, as well as making more errors, being less productive, and having more accidents.
- **Accidents**. Regular drinkers are more likely to suffer from falls, fires, poisoning, drowning, and motor vehicle accidents.
- **Violence**. Regular drinkers are more likely to commit suicide, assault, and homicide.
- **Effects on the family** can include spousal abuse, child abuse, and divorce.

In the USA, binge drinking (i.e., more than five drinks for males or four for females) has increased since the early 2000s among females, older people, and minorities. "Epidemiologists say that excessive and binge drinking begins in college, and that for many it continues through early adulthood with after-work happy hours" (Glaser, 2017). Another worrisome phenomenon that seems most common among young adult women is to deliberately eat very little before going out for a night of drinking, a strategy apparently employed to save money and calories.

A 2010 survey in Australia rated alcohol as the drug of *most concern* to society, but also the drug *most approved of* for general use (NADRC, 2010).

These outcomes suggest tobacco and alcohol are more dangerous and costly to Canadian society than illegal drugs. If so, why are tobacco and alcohol legal, controlled substances (e.g., you have to be a certain age to purchase them), rather than completely banned?

3.7 Opiate narcotics

Opium, **heroin**, **methadone**, **morphine**, **codeine**, **Demerol**, and **Oxycodone** are all either derived from the opium poppy or are synthetic analogues (compounds with a molecular structure closely similar to another). Opium is usually smoked, heroin is usually injected, and medical narcotics are usually taken orally. Narcotics are used medically to suppress pain or cough. Narcotics produce euphoria, which is described by users as a great sense of well-being. Other effects are similar to the other CNS depressants such as ethanol: slowed breathing, slurred speech, and impaired balance and coordination. Pupils constrict. Nausea is common.

The National Institute for Drug Abuse estimates that in 2011, about 1.6% of Americans age 12 and older had used heroin at least once in their life, and about one out of four of those who use heroin become dependent on it (NIDA, 2013b). Health Canada (2014) does not report estimates for prevalence of past-year use of heroin because of high sampling variability in their data.

Fischer et al. (2013) report that non-medical use of prescription opioids, and associated health problems, are much higher in North America than in other parts of the world. The authors attribute these findings to several factors, including "generally high levels of psychotrophic drug use, dynamics of medical-professional culture (including patient expectations for 'effective treatment'), as well as the more pronounced 'for-profit' orientation of key elements of health care (including pharmaceutical advertising)." Canada is the second-largest per capita consumer of prescription opioids in the world, behind only the United States. A 2015 Health Canada survey found that more than one in eight Canadians age 15 and older had taken an opioid in the previous year (CIHI, 2017). Non-medical use of prescription opioids strongly parallels prescriptions for these drugs; that is, a portion of prescribed opioids apparently get diverted from their intended medical use (Fischer et al., 2013).

At higher doses, narcotics cause stupor and unconsciousness, and can be fatal (e.g., accidental overdose) due to suppression of the brain's respiratory centre and subsequent stoppage of breathing (NIDA, 2013b). Some users die when they vomit and choke on their vomitus (this is true with ethanol and barbiturate use also). As with cocaine use, one of the main health problems (using the term holistically) is that regular use can be expensive and force users into a criminal lifestyle (e.g., theft, dealing drugs, prostitution). Other major health problems associated with heroin use are infection (e.g., hepatitis, HIV) from sharing needles or from sexual activity, as well as malnutrition and exposure from living on the street.

An opioid overdose crisis is underway in North America. Overdose rates in the USA increased by 30% in one year and now account for 140 deaths per day (BBC, 2018). "Over the past two decades, more than 200,000 people have died in the United States from overdoses involving prescription opioids" (Meier, 2018). From 1999 through 2015, drug-overdose deaths approximately tripled in the United States, and the majority of such deaths now involve an opioid. In 2016 alone, there were 64,000 drug-overdose deaths in the United States (Wood, 2018). In Canada in 2016, there were 2,946 apparent opioid-related deaths, and at least 2,923 from January to September 2017. Almost all (92%) of these deaths were unintentional (Health Canada, 2018).

The crisis seems rooted in over-prescription of opioids by medical doctors (Wood, 2018). Since synthetic opioids were introduced to the prescription market in the 1950s, the USA and Canada have become the highest and second-highest, respectively, per-capita consumers of opioids in the world (Ubelacker, 2017). It seems unlikely that North Americans experience pain more acutely than the rest of the world. Rather, aggressive (and sometimes dishonest) marketing by drug manufacturers to doctors appears to have triggered opioid use. For example, for years after officials of the company that manufactured **OxyContin** knew their product was being abused, they continued to promote it as less prone to lead to addiction and abuse—a claim not based on any research (Meier, 2018). Finally, in 2007, the company and three executives pleaded guilty to various charges and paid a total of over $600 million in fines (Meier, 2018).

By then, much damage had already been done. OxyContin's maker reformulated it so the pills couldn't be crushed and snorted. But with so many people now addicted to opioids, this didn't solve the problem. Instead, addicts found another source. "When the demand is so high and there's so much money to be made, when you try to restrain the supply side [by reformulating OxyContin pills] people will need something. And to avoid withdrawal, they'll turn to whatever they can get their hands on" (Ubelacker, 2017). This "whatever" has become **fentanyl** pills, manufactured overseas and sold illegally on the streets of North America (Ubelacker, 2017). From January to September 2017, 72% of accidental apparent opioid-related deaths involved fentanyl or fentanyl analogues, compared to 55% in 2016 (Health Canada, 2018). Fentanyl is 100 times more potent than morphine and up to 50 times stronger than heroin (Ubelacker, 2017). The potency of fentanyl makes it easy to accidentally overdose, especially when potency varies from one batch to another, as is common with black market drugs.

Canada has responded to the crisis (Wood, 2018). In 2016, the Canadian government made the overdose-reversal drug naloxone available without a prescription. British Columbia has produced enforceable standards aimed at reducing unsafe prescribing of narcotic pain relievers. A service has been developed that would allow anonymous drug users to test the contents of drugs before using them. Vancouver's Insite facility allows users to inject drugs with medical personnel on site to respond to overdoses. The federal government is making it easier for doctors to prescribe methadone or heroin to opioid addicts.

More can be done. Health professionals need to be educated about evidence-based addiction treatment. There is inadequate community-based care available for those recently released from jail (Wood, 2018). And while we are dealing with those who are currently addicted, we need to more holistically address why people take drugs, with the hope of curtailing the number of new opiate addicts.

4 Why People Take Drugs
4.1 Why do people start taking drugs?
According to the National Institute for Drug Abuse (NIDA, 2010, p. 6) people generally *begin* taking drugs for one or more of the following reasons:

- **To feel good:** Most abused drugs initially produce strong feelings of pleasure, power, self-confidence, energy, or relaxation.
- **To feel better:** Some people deal with distressing feelings of anxiety, pressure, social awkwardness, depression, and so on by taking drugs.
- **To do better:** That is, to improve physical or cognitive performance.
- **Because they're curious:** Experimentation is a normal part of growing up. The sign on the park bench says Wet Paint. Is it really? Touch it and find out! Will a pencil eraser fit in your nose? What happens if you touch your tongue to a flagpole in the middle of winter? Can you really get high by smoking dried banana skins? Unfortunately, some people who experiment with drugs, especially adolescents, get hooked and become chronic users.
- **Because others are doing it:** Drug use may also have an aura of maturity, danger, excitement, non-conformity, sophistication, or belonging to a certain social subgroup. Drug-abusing peers can sway others to try drugs for the first time.

4.2 Why do people continue taking drugs?

A combination of biological and psychosocial factors account for why people *continue* to use drugs to the point of harm—that is, to the point of drug abuse or addiction (see the following section, Models of Drug Abuse).

- **Pleasure centres** in the brain are next to regions associated with hunger, thirst, and sexual desire. The biological urge to take drugs may be as powerful as these other basic drives. Experimental animals (e.g., rats, monkeys) can be instrumented so that pressing a lever causes an electrical stimulus to the drug centres in their brains. In such experiments, animals will press the lever repeatedly for hours, foregoing food, water, and sleep until they collapse, exhausted.

- **Genetic factors** are estimated to account for between 40% and 60% of a person's vulnerability to addiction (NIDA, 2010, p. 8). The classic test for genetic versus environmental influences involves sets of identical twins reared separately. The extent to which the twins' drug use as adults is similar despite their growing up in different environments gives an indication of how much of the drug use is genetically influenced.

- **Home environment**, especially during childhood, can make an individual more likely to abuse drugs.

    In a cohort of over 1,000 people who were dependent on alcohol and over 4,000 who were dependent on nicotine, Elliott et al. (2014) found that childhood physical, sexual, and emotional abuse, as well as physical neglect, predicted subsequent dependence on alcohol and nicotine, even when the investigators controlled for other childhood adversities such as poverty and parental divorce.

    Darke and Torok (2013) report a similar finding for a different cohort. Analysis of responses to structured interviews of 300 injection drug users in Sydney, Australia, showed both that severe childhood physical abuse was associated with earlier onset of drug use and that any level of childhood physical abuse was associated with more extensive and recent drug abuse.

    Child abuse can cause feelings of shame and self-blame ("I was punished because I was bad"), which can lead to low self-confidence and poor self-image. The abuse also constitutes a violation of trust, which causes the victim to doubt her ability to trust her judgment or feelings. Drugs can be a way to feel better, or at least to feel nothing. She may find acceptance and companionship among drug-using peers.

This cycle can repeat into the next generation. The drug user may be a poor parent himself, perhaps abusing his own children or providing inconsistent parenting. Consistent parenting is crucial for healthy child development. But the child of a drug user may come home from school one day and find his father high. Dad may give the child some money to go out for a pizza or to the video store. The next day, the child may again find Dad high, but this time Dad may criticize or demean the child. So, the child doesn't know what to expect, and learns not to trust.

- **Academic failure or poor social skills** increase risk for drug abuse.
- **Route of administration** makes addiction more likely when it produces a rapid high, such as smoking or injecting it into a vein.
- **Early age of onset**. The earlier a person begins to use drugs, the more likely she is to progress to more serious abuse, maybe partly because the drug use interferes with the brain development that would normally happen during youth and young adulthood.

In one positive note, perception of risk seems to be a positive factor. The National Institute for Drug Abuse notes that drug use goes *down* when perceived risk goes *up* (NIDA, 2010, p. 14).

4.3 Is some drug-taking inevitable?

When science began to study addictive behavior in the 1930s, people addicted to drugs were thought to be morally flawed and lacking in willpower ... As a result of scientific research, we know that addiction is a disease that affects both brain and behavior. We have identified many of the biological and environmental factors and are beginning to search for the genetic variations that contribute to the development and progression of the disease. (NIDA, 2010, p. 1)

The initial decision to take drugs is mostly voluntary. However, when drug abuse takes over, a person's ability to exert self-control can become seriously impaired. Brain imaging studies from drug-addicted individuals show physical changes in areas of the brain that are critical to judgment, decision making, learning and memory, and behavior control. Scientists believe that these changes alter the way the brain works, and may help explain the compulsive and destructive behaviors of addiction. (NIDA, 2010, p. 7)

It has been argued that drug-taking is a natural and unpreventable human activity. Indeed, most societies throughout history have used some kind of intoxicant.

Perhaps instead of investing so much in trying to stop people from taking drugs, we should focus on trying to develop safe, affordable psychoactive drugs.

> What do *you* think about the argument in this last paragraph? How would society be different if safe, affordable drugs were widely available and condoned?

5 Models of Drug Abuse

The **classical model of drug abuse** defines addiction in physical terms. There are three stages in this process:

1. As one takes a drug regularly, ***tolerance*** develops. It takes more of the drug to get the same effect. This occurs because of increased ability of the liver to process and remove the drug and because of desensitization of brain cells to the drug when the drug is often present in the blood.

2. The second stage in the classical model is ***dependence***. Here, the user needs the drug to function normally. It's not that he *thinks* he needs it; he really *does* physically need it. For example, the chronic alcohol drinker may wake with a headache and shaky hands, which go away after he has a couple of drinks. The drinks return him to a normal state.

3. Physical addiction is confirmed by the third stage of this model, ***withdrawal***. When the user stops taking the drug, unpleasant and potentially fatal symptoms occur for a number of days. Generally, withdrawal symptoms are the reverse of the drug effects. So withdrawal from regular caffeine use induces lethargy, fatigue, and sleepiness. Conversely, withdrawal from central nervous system depressants, such as alcohol or barbiturates, causes agitation, restlessness, insomnia, and possible convulsion or coma.

There are a couple of problems with this model:

*   It does not fit well with cannabis or hallucinogens, which do not appear to cause physical dependence.
*   The term "addiction" was a barrier to treatment for many individuals, people who may have acknowledged that they were drinking or using drugs too much but didn't see themselves as "alcoholics" or "addicts."

The **substance dependence model** doesn't focus just on physical dependence. According to this model, a person is dependent if she experiences three or more of the following during a 12-month period:

- Tolerance
- Withdrawal
- Loss of control (i.e., taking the substance in larger amounts or over longer periods than was intended)
- A persistent desire to reduce substance use
- Compulsive use (i.e., spending a great deal of time thinking about the substance, obtaining it, using it, and recovering from its effects)
- Reducing important school, work, or recreational activities because of substance use
- Continued use despite perceived consequences

> What kind of "perceived consequences" have *you* experienced or witnessed in others in relation to drug use?

According to the **social deviance model**, drug misuse is defined as drug use that goes beyond the bounds of social norms and conventions. For example, the person who gets drunk to the point that he staggers and falls down at a party, passes out, or ends up vomiting in the bushes could be viewed as an alcohol misuser. Another example is a person who drives while intoxicated.

The **compulsive behaviour model** views any behaviour that is so compelling or time-consuming that it detracts from a balanced life as unhealthy; that is, it's a **negative addiction**. Thus, compulsive drug use compares with compulsive gambling, Internet use, video gaming, shopping, sex, exercise, or work; the main problem is the compulsivity of the behaviour. For example, you may tell yourself you will play an hour of video games before doing your homework, but you continue playing all day. In a *Global News* (2014) report, a Vancouver psychiatrist who specializes in addictions claims that some children spend up to 20 hours a week gaming on popular applications such as Candy Crush and Angry Birds. These games are not just fun; they are very compelling, reportedly because "gaming and gambling stimulate the same part of [the] brain that cocaine would stimulate" (Global News, 2014).

With all such behaviours, *most* people can participate at a recreational level without major consequences, but *some* people are vulnerable to loss of control.

> Which model of drug abuse do *you* think makes the most sense? Why?

6 Strategies to Address Substance Misuse

In 2000, the City of Vancouver launched its **Four Pillars** drug strategy. A pillar is like a large post that supports a building (Figure 13.5).

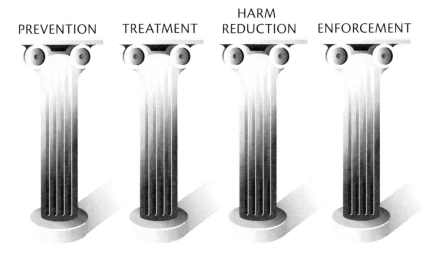

The Four Pillars drug strategy

Figure 13.5. The Four Pillars concept is a holistic way to respond to the problem of psychoactive drug abuse.

6.1 Prevention

This part of the plan aims to delay onset of first substance use and reduce incidence and prevalence of substance use through initiatives such as

> public education, employment training and jobs, supportive and transitional housing and easily accessible healthcare. They also call for prevention efforts tailored to Vancouver's youth and its diverse ethno-cultural and Aboriginal communities. The recommendations address marijuana grow operations and methamphetamine labs, as well as the need for a syringe recovery system. (see City of Vancouver, Four Pillars drug strategy https://vancouver.ca/people-programs/four-pillars-drug-strategy.aspx)

6.2 Treatment

The first step in treatment is the decision by the user that she wants to make a change. Change is difficult enough when one *wants* to change. Change imposed from without (e.g., court-ordered treatment) rarely succeeds. Efforts to keep the user from using by throwing out drugs or by policing behaviour are similarly futile; users can be very motivated and creative in obtaining and hiding their drugs and drug use.

It is common for drug and alcohol misusers to **deny** their drug use is a problem. "I can stop any time I want," "I only have a couple of drinks a day," "I'm just a recreational user," or "Leave me alone and mind your own business" are typical rebuffs to suggestions that a drug user seek help. The friends and family of drug users often unwittingly play a role in protecting and covering up for the drug user. For example, a wife may make up a story to explain her husband's absence from work, and parents may hire a lawyer to have impaired driving charges dropped against their child. This **enabling** behaviour allows the drug user to continue using, and the problem worsens because it reinforces the denial.

Successful treatment is multifaceted. The user

- Works on improving self-image
- Finds ways to manage drug urges and to manage stress without drugs
- Learns to recognize situations that may lead to drug use
- Rebuilds relationships with family and other people

Stopping drug use may involve a complete change in lifestyle, which could include

- Changing jobs
- Moving residence
- Leaving a dysfunctional or enabling relationship
- Developing substitute interests and activities
- Finding new, non-using friends

Some people succeed in quitting on their own. Others find helpful the support and guidance available in individual or group **counselling**, either through publicly funded programs (see the Additional Resources section near the end of this chapter) or private programs paid for by the individual or her employer. This counselling can be done on an **outpatient** basis (i.e., come for a one-hour appointment once a week and then go home) or as **residential** treatment (usually four weeks).

People with strong physical dependencies (e.g., on alcohol, barbiturates, or narcotics) are at risk of dying during withdrawal. In these cases, medically supervised **detox** may be appropriate.

Self-help groups are very effective for some substance abusers. **Alcoholics Anonymous** (AA) and other **12-step programs** view substance use as a disease over which the victim has no control. The alcoholic is encouraged to accept that he is powerless and to appeal to a "higher power." He vows to stop drinking or using drugs "one day at a time." Frequent meetings are encouraged. At meetings, participants share the effect alcohol has had on their lives and their struggle to overcome it. Groups are non-profit and anonymous; only first names are used at group meetings. The success of the AA concept has spawned a number of similar **support groups**, including Narcotics Anonymous, Alateen (for teenagers with drinking parents), Al-Anon (for families of those with alcohol problems), Cocaine Anonymous, Marijuana Anonymous, and Gamblers Anonymous.

> ### Does relapse to drug abuse mean treatment has failed?

The National Institute on Drug Abuse answers this:

> No. The chronic nature of the disease means that relapsing to drug abuse is not only possible, but likely. Relapse rates (i.e., how often symptoms recur) for drug addiction are similar to those for other well-characterized chronic medical illnesses such as diabetes, hypertension, and asthma, which also have both physiological and behavioral components. Treatment of chronic diseases involves changing deeply imbedded behaviors, and relapse does not mean treatment failure. For the addicted patient, lapses back to drug abuse indicate that treatment needs to be reinstated or adjusted, or that alternate treatment is needed. (NIDA, 2010, p. 26)

6.3 Harm reduction

This may involve substituting a less harmful drug for the misused drug. In methadone-maintenance programs, heroin users are medically prescribed **methadone**, a drug that is intended to satisfy their craving for heroin without making them "high." This supposedly frees the user from the criminal activities and associations she might otherwise have in order to support her heroin habit. To prevent users from selling their methadone, they may be required to come in daily and take their methadone under supervision.

Needle exchange programs (NEPs), in which injection drug users are given clean needles for free in exchange for used needles, reduce the harm associated with reusing or sharing needles. NEPs have been shown to decrease needle sharing and increase use of bleach to sterilize needles.

6.4 Enforcement

One enforcement approach is **zero tolerance**, which views *no* amount of a controlled substance as acceptable. Most of those arrested in this approach are individual users in possession of small amounts of the substance for their own use, or perhaps to sell to others on a small scale. The mindset behind this enforcement approach is presumably to reduce *demand* for the product. An alternate enforcement strategy targets large producers, importers, or distributors. This is a *supply-side* philosophy: make it harder for people to get illegal drugs so fewer people will use them.

6.4.1 The Insite experiment

The most conspicuous and perhaps most controversial manifestation of Vancouver's Four Pillars strategy is the Insite facility. Insite is North America's first legal supervised injection site. Insite uses a harm-reduction rather than an abstinence model. It provides a place where people can inject illicit drugs (acquired elsewhere) in a medically safer setting than if they injected on the street. Clean needles are provided. Users inject under supervision of nurses. Emergency medical care is available to respond to accidental overdose. Insite also connects users with other health services, such as primary illness care, addiction treatment, and housing support.

The evidence is compelling. More than 3.6 million clients have injected illicit drugs under supervision by nurses at Insite since it opened in 2003. There have been 48,798 clinical treatment visits and 6,440 overdose interventions without any deaths (Vancouver Coastal Health, 2018). Since 2007, new HIV infections among Vancouver injection drug users have fallen 50% per year. Detox program use increased by more than 30% among Insite users. Open drug use in the Downtown Eastside has decreased. Drug-related crime has not increased (British Columbia Centre for Excellence in HIV/ADIS, 2011). Fatal overdoses within 500 m of Insite decreased by 35% after the facility opened, much greater than the 9% decrease in the rest of Vancouver (Marshall et al., 2011).

> The research is unambiguous: Needle exchanges reduce the spread of bloodborne diseases like hepatitis C and H.I.V. and do not increase drug use. They've been shown to reduce overdose deaths, decrease the number of needles discarded in public places and make it more likely that drug users enter treatment. They also save money: One recent study estimated that $10 million spent on needle exchanges might save more than $70 million in averted H.I.V. treatment costs alone. (Katz, 2018)

Insite was consistently attacked by the Harper Conservative federal government, which argued that the model encouraged drug use. The federal government tried to close Insite by refusing to renew its exemption from existing drug laws. The Supreme Court of Canada's unanimous 2011 decision ordered the federal government to allow Insite to continue operating, noting that "Insite has been proven to save lives with no discernible negative impact on the public safety and health objectives of Canada" (MacQueen, 2015).

6.4.2 The case for prohibition

The production, sale, and consumption of alcohol was illegal in the United States from 1920 to 1933, in most of Canada from 1900 to the 1920s, and up to 1948 in PEI. The "failure" of national prohibition is widely cited as a rationale for the decriminalization or legalization of cannabis, but analyzing the success or failure of national prohibition (NP) is complex (Hall, 2010). For example,

- The laws prohibited production and sale of alcohol but not possession or consumption.
- Much of the evidence is incomplete and often circumstantial; for example, there are insufficient data connecting estimates of per capita alcohol consumption with measures of hospital admissions for liver disease and measures of violent crime.
- Prohibition laws were poorly enforced.
- Other major social events, such as World War I, the Great Depression, and increases in the number of single males, complicate the picture.

It's certainly true that NP did not completely stop alcohol consumption. NP also seems to have been associated with increased crime and corruption of public officials around the illegal sale of alcohol, decreased respect for the law by otherwise law-abiding citizens, and loss by government of huge tax revenue (Hall, 2010). But it may be a mistake to judge NP as a failure because

> Despite their limitations, all indicators suggested that alcohol use had declined substantially during the early years of national prohibition. There were steep and sustained declines starting in the late teens [i.e., the period around 1918] in liver cirrhosis deaths, hospitalizations for alcoholic psychosis and arrests for drunkenness. (Hall, 2010, p. 1167)

Outcomes of changes in the minimum legal drinking age (MLDA) in the USA provide useful insight for a different approach—*limiting* rather than prohibiting alcohol. In the 1970s, many US states lowered the MLDA to 18 or 19 years. Then, in the 1980s, many states raised the MLDA to 21 years. The increased MLDA led to an estimated 19% reduction in odds of traffic deaths, after factoring in other effects, such as laws requiring use of seat belts and defining maximum blood-alcohol concentration for drivers. Hall (2010, p. 1171) concludes, "Experience with the raising the MLDA in the United States shows that *partial* prohibitions can produce substantial public health benefits at an acceptable social cost, in the absence of substantial additional expenditure on enforcement" [emphasis in original].

More recently, governments and law enforcement agencies have tried to slow the use of cocaine and cannabis by locating and arresting suppliers. Despite the expense of these efforts and the large seizures that have been made, drug use continues. There is continued demand, and decreasing supply only has the effect of raising price, which makes the venture more profitable for suppliers.

6.4.3 Changing drug laws

Social acceptance of cannabis use seems to be growing. In 2012, voters approved legalization of cannabis in the US states of Colorado and Washington. At the time of this writing, eight US states and the District of Columbia have legalized cannabis for recreational use. Medical cannabis is legal in another 22 states, while the remaining 20 states have no broad laws legalizing cannabis (e.Republic, 2018).

In 2013, the small South American country of Uruguay enacted new legislation and policy around cannabis use. The Uruguay system appears very organized and regulated. Individuals who wish to legally consume cannabis must register for one of three methods of access:

- Home growing: up to six female plants allowed, with production of up to 480 g per year
- Cannabis clubs: cannabis is grown collectively, with limits on number of plants and total annual production
- Commercial: up to 10 g per week may be purchased at pharmacies that choose to sell cannabis

In addition, the law licenses commercial growers, prohibits advertising of cannabis, and bans cannabis use in indoor public spaces where tobacco smoking is banned (Hudak, Ramsey & Walsh, 2018).

The Canadian government intends to legalize and regulate cannabis with the proposed Cannabis Act. The broad goals are to protect youth, permit adults access to limited amounts of quality-controlled cannabis, protect public health, reduce the burden on the criminal justice system, and deter organized crime. More specifically, the Act would

- Prohibit selling (or giving) cannabis to anyone under age 18
- Allow possession of 30 g or less of dried cannabis or the equivalent
- Penalize people who illegally grow, possess, sell, or transport cannabis

There would also be penalties for cannabis-impaired driving in drug-impaired driving legislation. The federal government would set industry-wide standards, while the provinces and territories would license and oversee distribution and sale of cannabis. The provinces and territories could also set stricter laws in their jurisdictions, for example, by raising the minimum age or lowering the personal possession amount (Government of Canada, 2018).

Persuasive arguments support these changes.

- The health effects of cannabis use are relatively benign compared with the effects of tobacco or alcohol.
- Cannabis use has increased despite legal prohibition.
- Cannabis is easy to grow, but because most users cannot obtain it legally, it is much more expensive than it would be if it were legal.
- The big profits in large-scale **trafficking** (growing and selling) of cannabis have attracted organized crime.
- Thousands of cases of simple possession (vs. possession for the purpose of trafficking) have created long delays in the court system.
- Enforcement and prosecution cost the government huge sums, money that could be used for health care, education, and so on.
- A conviction for simple possession can restrict an individual's ability to travel, hold political office, or work in certain occupations.

On the other hand, if possession of small amounts of cannabis was permitted, if cannabis was sold in government-controlled stores with restrictions on purchasing age (like alcohol is), and if cannabis was sold at current prices, this would undermine the incentives of organized crime and generate huge tax revenues for the government.

The stated objections to legalizing or decriminalizing cannabis seem to centre on two things:

- Drug use is bad (morally wrong).
- Decriminalizing cannabis would send the message that cannabis use is acceptable, and this **endorsement** would cause more people to use it.

Another approach to prevention involves understanding why people use drugs, and trying to *satisfy these needs with alternatives.* For example, the needs for affiliation, belonging to a peer group, excitement, and stimulation may be found in a group of drug-using friends—or these needs can be met by playing basketball. Programs intended to keep preteens (age 10–12) from starting to use drugs can teach self-acceptance, positive self-image, assertiveness, and refusal skills (i.e., how to say no to peers who encourage them to try drugs). If people take drugs to relieve stress, they can be taught other stress-management techniques.

7 Conclusion

A wide variety of psychoactive drugs are more or less available in Canada today. Many drugs have adverse acute and chronic health effects, influenced to a large degree by the amount, frequency, time, and method in which they are used, and in the motivation for using them. Taking a holistic perspective, the health effects of drug misuse and abuse extend beyond the physical effects on the users and currently impose large costs on Canadian society. Most drugs also have some benefit, again depending on how and why they are used. Therefore, a "Say No to Drugs" approach seems over-simplistic.

The common term "alcohol and drugs" belies the fact that alcohol is also a drug, and points to the moral judgments that often colour social views of drug use. Most human societies have sought mind-altering substances. Many people take drugs despite knowledge of the associated risks. Substantial evidence argues against the wisdom of simple prohibition. A more effective public health approach would probably be multi-faceted, addressing the root causes of drug misuse and abuse, providing treatment and harm-reduction options, and combining economic and social incentives and disincentives with law enforcement to reduce the involvement of organized crime in supplying drugs.

> The preceding paragraph says that drug misuse and abuse imposes substantial costs on Canadian society. To what costs do you think this refers?
>
> Hint: you will find bits of the answer in this chapter. For a complete answer, you will need to think—holistically, of course.

Study Questions

1. What is a drug? What is special about a psychoactive drug? Why has concern regarding drug misuse focused on psychoactive drugs?
2. What characteristics do all psychoactive drugs share?
3. What are the three main ways in which the route of administration of a drug influences the health effects of the drug, aside from the properties of the drug itself?
4. What is the most widely used psychoactive drug in North America?
5. What is the psychoactive drug in tobacco?

6.   Name four stimulant drugs.

7a. Why do many people start smoking, even though its serious effects are well known?

7b. Other than education regarding the risks of smoking, what strategies might reduce the percentage of teenagers who begin smoking?

8.   Outline the adverse effects of tobacco. In your answer, take a holistic view of health.

9a. Describe strategies that help smokers quit.

9b. For those who wish to quit smoking, combining nicotine replacement therapy with what doubles the success rate compared with nicotine therapy alone?

10. What are the adverse acute and chronic health effects of cocaine use?

11. Which psychoactive drug is the most highly abused psychoactive substance in our society? Explain.

12. Explain in a few sentences the roots of the current opioid crisis in North American.

13. If ethanol is a central nervous system (CNS) depressant, why do small doses seem to act like a stimulant?

14. What are the adverse acute and chronic health effects of ethanol (alcohol) use?

15a. What are the adverse health effects of cannabis use?

15b. For what age group does cannabis use seem to have the greatest adverse effects?

16. Summarize the arguments for and against decriminalization of cannabis in Canada, relating this to the North American experience with alcohol prohibition in the early 20th century.

17. In addition to their potential for dependency, what adverse health effects do cocaine use and heroin use have in common?

18a. According to this text, why do people use psychoactive drugs?

18b. What strategies might help reduce drug use?

19a. Explain briefly the three stages in the classical model of addiction.

19b. According to this model, what is the proof that a person is or was addicted?

19c. What are the two main problems or limitations of this model?

20. How does the social deviance model define drug misuse?

21. What are the "four pillars" in Vancouver's drug strategy?

22. What is the first step in the treatment of substance misuse?

23. Describe the options for treatment of people who misuse substances.

24. Explain the concept of "harm reduction," giving two different examples.

Glossary

dependence—needing a specific drug to function normally

psychoactive drug—a drug that exerts an effect on the brain, causing a change in perception, mood, thinking, or behaviour

route of administration—the way in which the drug is taken into the body

tolerance—more of the drug is needed to obtain the same effect

withdrawal—when a regular user stops taking the drug, uncomfortable (and sometimes fatal) symptoms occur; this is proof that the person was physiologically addicted to the drug

Additional Resources

The British Columbia Lung Association hosts a program called QuitNow
1-877-455-2233
Text QUITNOW to 654321
www.quitnow.ca/

The Alcohol and Drug Information & Referral Service
Lower Mainland: 604-660-9382
BC: 1-800-663-1441
Yukon: 1-866-980-9099
Funded by the BC Emergency Health Services Commission and the Yukon Ministry of Health, the Alcohol and Drug Information & Referral Service is available for people across the province and territory who need help locating alcohol and drug rehab programs, needle exchanges, detox, medical marijuana, impaired driving counselling, and so on.

Centre for Addiction and Mental Health, Toronto
www.camh.ca/en/hospital/Pages/home.aspx

References

ADAI. (June 2013). *Adolescents and marijuana.* Alcohol and Drug Abuse Institute, University of Washington. Retrieved April 28, 2014 from http://learnaboutmarijuanawa.org/factsheets/adolescents.htm

American Cancer Society. (February 6, 2014a). *Guide to quitting smoking.* Retrieved April 28, 2014 from http://www.cancer.org/healthy/stayawayfromtobacco/guidetoquittingsmoking/index

American Cancer Society. (February 13, 2014b). *Why do people start smoking?* Retrieved April 28, 2014 from http://www.cancer.org/cancer/cancercauses/tobaccocancer/questionsabo...alth/questions-about-smoking-tobacco-and-health-why-do-people-start

Bam, T. S. et al. (EC/ENDS Working Group). (October 7, 2014). Summary position statement on e-cigarettes (ECs) and electronic nicotine delivery systems (ENDS)

2014. International Union Against Tuberculosis and Lung Disease. Retrieved May 26, 2018 from https://www.theunion.org/what-we-do/publications/technical/english/The-Union-Summary-Position-Statement-ECs-ENDS-Update-2014-dec-2015.pdf

BBC. (March 6, 2018). Opioid crisis: Overdose rates jump 30% in one year. Retrieved May 26, 2018 from http://www.bbc.com/news/world-us-Canada-43305340

Benjamin, R. M. (2010). *A report of the surgeon general: How tobacco smoke causes disease*. Department of Health and Human Services. Centers for Disease Control and Prevention. Retrieved January 21, 2013 from http://www.cdc.gov/tobacco/data_statistics/sgr/2010/consumer_booklet/pdfs/consumer.pdf

Branswell, H. (May 13, 2015). Health Canada slow to regulate e-cigarettes. The Canadian Press. Retrieved May 26, 2018 from https://globalnews.ca/news/1994306/health-canada-slow-to-regulate-e-cigarettes/

British Columbia Centre for Excellence in HIV/AIDS. (September 7, 2011). *Supreme Court rules Insite can stay open*. Retrieved May 3, 2014 from http://www.cfenet.ubc.ca/news/our-news/supreme-court-rules-insite-can-stay-open

CBC. (February 21, 2018). More Canadians overall smoking pot than in 1985, says StatsCan. Retrieved May 26, 2018 from http://www.cbc.ca/news/politics/statis-tics-canada-cannabis-use-1.4544838

Christensen, J. (January 13, 2014). We know it can kill us: Why people still smoke. *CNN News*. Retrieved April 28, 2014 from http://www.cnn.com/2014/01/11/health/still-smoking/

CIHI (Canadian Institute for Health Information). (2017). *Pan-Canadian Trends in the Prescribing of Opioids, 2012 to 2016*. Ottawa: CIHI. ISBN 978-1-77109-651-5 (PDF).

Collin, C. (2006a). *Substance abuse issues and public policy in Canada: IV. Prevalence of use and its consequences*. Library of Parliament; Parliamentary Information and Research Service. Retrieved April 7, 2008 from http://www.parl.gc.ca/information/library/PRBpubs/prb0619-e.htm

Collin, C. (2006b). *Substance abuse issues and public policy in Canada V. Alcohol and related harms*. Library of Parliament; Parliamentary Information and Research Service. Retrieved April 7, 2008 from http://www.parl.gc.ca/information/library/PRBpubs/prb0620-e.htm

Darke, S., Torok, M. (2013). The association of childhood physical abuse with the onset and extent of drug use among regular injecting drug users. *Addiction*. 109, 610–616.

Desjardins, L. (May 31, 2013). Smoking tobacco still a leading cause of death in Canada. *Radio Canada International*. Retrieved May 4, 2014 from http://www.rcinet.ca/en/2013/05/31/smoking-tobacco-still-a-leading-cause-of-death-in-canada/

Elliott, J. C., Stohl, M., Wall, M. W., Keyes, K. M., Goodwin, R. D., Skodol, A. E., Krueger, R. F., Grant, B. F., Hasin, D. S. (2014). The risk for persistent adult alcohol and nicotine dependence: The role of childhood maltreatment *Addiction*, 109, 842–850.

e.Republic. (March 30, 2018). State Marijuana Laws in 2018 Map. Retrieved May 31, 2018 from http://www.governing.com/gov-data/state-marijuana-laws-map-medical-recreational.html

Evans P. (January 25, 2018). Canadians spent $5.7B on marijuana last year, StatsCan estimates. CBC News. Retrieved May 26, 2018 from http://www.cbc.ca/news/business/marijuana-industry-1.4503152

Fischer, B., Keates, A., Buhringer, G., Reimer, J., Rehm, J. (2014). Non-medical use of prescription opioids and prescription opioid-related harms: Why so markedly higher in North America compared to the rest of the world? *Addiction.* 109, 177–181.

Glaser, G. (December 29, 2017). America, can we talk about your drinking? *The New York Times.* Retrieved December 29, 2017 from https://www.nytimes.com/2017/12/29/opinion/sunday/alcohol-binge-drinking.html

Global News. (January 14, 2014). *Watch: Unfiltered—Feeding the online gaming addiction.* Retrieved May 3, 2014 from http://globalnews.ca/news/1083273/watch-unfiltered-feeding-the-online-gaming-addiction/

Government of Canada. (March 13, 2018). Legalizing and strictly regulating cannabis: the facts. Retrieved May 26, 2018 from https://www.canada.ca/en/services/health/campaigns/legalizing-strictly-regulating-cannabis-facts.html

Haberkorn, L. (May 3, 2014). Uruguay leader calls Colorado pot law 'a fiction.' *Associated Press. ABC News.* Retrieved May 3, 2014 from http://abcnews.go.com/International/wireStory/uruguay-leader-calls-colorado-pot-law-fiction-23574662

Hall, W. (2010). What are the policy lessons of National Alcohol Prohibition in the United States, 1920–1933? *Addiction.* 105, 1164–1173.

Health Canada. (October 1, 2013). Canadian tobacco use monitoring survey (CTUMS) 2012. Retrieved April 27, 2014 from http://www.hc-sc.gc.ca/hc-ps/tobac-tabac/research-recherche/stat/ctums-esutc_2012-eng.php

Health Canada. (April 8, 2014). Alcohol and drug use monitoring survey. Summary of results for 2012. Retrieved April 27, 2014 from http://hc-sc.gc.ca/hc-ps/drugs-drogues/stat/_2012/summary-sommaire-eng.php

Health Canada. (March 27, 2018). Apparent opioid-related deaths. Retrieved May 30, 2018 from https://www.canada.ca/en/health-canada/services/substance-abuse/prescription-drug-abuse/opioids/apparent-opioid-related-deaths.html

Hudak, J., Ramsey, G., Walsh, J. (March 2018). Uruguay's cannabis law: Pioneering a new paradigm. Center for Effective Public Management at the Brookings Institute. Retrieved May 31, 2018 from https://www.brookings.edu/wp-content/uploads/2018/03/gs_032118_uruguaye28099s-cannabis-law_final.pdf

Katz, J. (April 27, 2018). Why a city at the center of the opioid crisis gave up a tool to fight it. *New York Times.* Retrieved May 8, 2018 from https://www.nytimes.com/interactive/2018/04/27/upshot/charleston-opioid-crisis-needle-exchange.html

MacQueen, K. (July 20, 2015). The science is in. And Insite works. *Macleans.* Retrieved May 26, 2018 from https://www.macleans.ca/news/canada/the-scientists-are-in-insite-works/

Marshall, B. D. L., Milloy, M. J., Wood, E., Montaner, J. S. G., Kerr, T. (2011). Reduction in overdose mortality after the opening of North America's first medically supervised safer injecting facility: A retrospective population-based study. *Lancet.* 377(9775), 1429–1437.

Meier, B. (May 29, 2019). Origins of an epidemic: Purdue Pharma knew its opioids were widely abused. *New York Times.* Retrieved May 29, 2018 from https://www.nytimes.com/2018/05/29/health/purdue-opioids-oxycontin.html

NADRC. (2010). *Alcohol facts.* National Alcohol and Drug Research Centre, University of New South Wales, Australia. Retrieved April 28, 2014 from http://ndarc.med.unsw.edu.au/resource/alcohol

NADRC. (2012). *"Ice" facts.* National Alcohol and Drug Research Centre, University of New South Wales, Australia. Retrieved April 28, 2014 from http://ndarc.med.unsw.edu.au/sites/default/files/ndarc/resources/ICE%20FACT%20SHEET%202.pdf

NADRC. (2006). Methamphetamine use and health. National Alcohol and Drug Research Centre, University of New South Wales, Australia. Retrieved April 28, 2014 from http://ndarc.med.unsw.edu.au/sites/default/files/ndarc/resources/ICE%20USE%20AND%20HEALTH.pdf

NCPIC. (October 1, 2011a). *What is cannabis? Factsheet 1.* National Cannabis Prevention and Information Centre, Australia. Retrieved April 28, 2014 from http://ndarc.med.unsw.edu.au/sites/default/files/ndarc/resources/NCPIC%20Cannabis%20fact%20sheet.pdf

NCPIC. (October 1, 2011b). Cannabis and dependence. National Cannabis Prevention and Information Centre, Australia. Retrieved April 28, 2014 from http://ncpic.org.au/workforce/alcohol-and-other-drug-workers/cannabis-information/factsheets/article/cannabis-and-dependence

NCPIC. (June 1, 2012). Cannabis and mental health. National Cannabis Prevention and Information Centre, Australia. Retrieved April 28, 2014 from http://ncpic.org.au/workforce/alcohol-and-other-drug-workers/cannabis-information/factsheets/article/cannabis-and-mental-health

NIDA. (August 2010). *Drugs, brains, and behavior: The science of addiction.* National Institute on Drug Abuse, National Institutes of Health, USA NIH Pub No. 10-5605.

NIDA. (July 2012a). *Marijuana.* Research Report Series. National Institute on Drug Abuse, National Institutes of Health, USA NIH Publication Number 12-3859.

NIDA. (December 2012b). *Alcohol.* National Institute on Drug Abuse, National Institutes of Health, USA Retrieved April 28, 2014 from http://www.drugabuse.gov/drugs-abuse/alcohol

NIDA. (December 2012c). *DrugFacts: Cigarettes and other tobacco products.* National Institute on Drug Abuse, National Institutes of Health, USA Retrieved April 28, 2014 from http://www.drugabuse.gov/publications/drugfacts/cigarettes-other-tobacco-products

NIDA. (April 2013a). *DrugFacts: Cocaine.* National Institute on Drug Abuse, National Institutes of Health, USA Retrieved April 28, 2014 from http://www.drugabuse.gov/publications/drugfacts/cocaine

NIDA. (April 2013b). *DrugFacts: Heroin.* National Institute on Drug Abuse, National Institutes of Health, USA Retrieved April 28, 2014 http://www.drugabuse.gov/publications/drugfacts/heroin

NIDA. (November 2013c). *DrugFacts: Electronic cigarettes (e-Cigarettes)*. National Institute on Drug Abuse, National Institutes of Health, USA Retrieved April 28, 2014 from http://www.drugabuse.gov/publications/drugfacts/electronic-cigarettes-e-cigarettes

NIDA. (January 2014). *DrugFacts: Marijuana*. National Institute on Drug Abuse, National Institutes of Health, USA Retrieved April 28, 2014 from http://www.drugabuse.gov/publications/drugfacts/marijuana.

Norris, S., Tiedemann, M. (September 20, 2017). Legislative Summary of Bill S-5: An Act to amend the Tobacco Act and the Non-smokers' Health Act and to make consequential amendments to other Acts. Ottawa: Library of Parliament. Retrieved May 30, 2018 from https://lop.parl.ca/About/Parliament/LegislativeSummaries/bills_ls.asp?Language=E&ls=s5&Parl=42&Ses=1&source=library_prb

Richardson, M. (2003). The physiology of mucus and sputum production in the respiratory system. *Nursing Times*. 99(23):63-64.

Statista. (2016). Share of adults who smoke in Canada from 1999 to 2015. Retrieved May 26, 2018 from https://www.statista.com/statistics/448420/share-of-adults-who-smoke-in-canada/

Ubelacker, S. (April 25, 2017). The inside history of Canada's opioid crisis. Macleans & The Canadian Press. Retrieved May 26, 2018 from https://www.macleans.ca/society/inside-the-history-of-canadas-opioid-crisis/

University of Waterloo. (2016). Tobacco use in Canada. Retrieved May 26, 2018 from https://uwaterloo.ca/tobacco-use-canada/youth-tobacco-use

Vancouver Coastal Health. (2018). Insite user statistics. Retrieved May 26, 2018 from http://www.vch.ca/public-health/harm-reduction/needle-exchange

WHO. (July 9, 2013). *Questions and answers on electronic cigarettes or electronic nicotine delivery systems (ENDS)*. Retrieved April 28, 2014 from http://www.who.int/tobacco/communications/statements/eletronic_cigarettes/en/index.html

WHO. (September 1, 2014). Electronic nicotine delivery systems. Report to the Sixth Session of the Conference of the Parties to the WHO Framework Convention on Tobacco Control. Retrieved May 26, 2018 from http://apps.who.int/gb/fctc/PDF/cop6/FCTC_COP6_10Rev1-en.pdf?ua=1

Wikipedia. (April 28, 2014). *Insite*. Retrieved May 3, 2014 from https://en.wikipedia.org/wiki/Insite

Wood, A. M., Kaptoge, S., Butterworth, A. S. et al. (2018). Alcohol consumption affects different CVD events in different ways. *The Lancet*. 391(10129):1513-1523.

Wood, E. (April 26, 2018). Strategies for reducing opioid-overdose deaths – lessons from Canada. *The New England Journal of Medicine*. 378:1565-1567.

14 Health Care Delivery Systems

Learning Objectives

By the time you have finished this chapter you should be able to

- List and explain in your own words the values and guiding principles on which the Canadian health care system is based
- Discuss current challenges to these principles
- Explain how the Canadian health care delivery system operates, outlining the roles of the federal government, provincial government, BCMA, and BCMSC
- Contrast the Canadian model of health delivery with the models of several other countries
- Identify the strengths and weaknesses of the Canadian system
- Discuss the issue of physician and nurse supply in Canada
- Describe trends in expenditures on the major categories of health care in Canada
- Explain the concept of "extra-billing"

According to the holistic model of health presented in Chapter 1: The Concept of Health, one factor that influences an individual's health is health care. That's what this chapter is about.

> How many of the other elements of the holistic model do you remember from Chapter 1?

1 Overview

In this chapter, we turn our attention to the way in which health care is delivered in Canada. We will see that a central feature of the Canadian model is the notion of a **welfare state**, in which the federal and provincial governments are in charge of health care in order to assure all Canadians have access to quality care, regardless of where they live or how much they earn. We will look behind the scenes at the mechanics of this system, and see the central role physicians play as gatekeepers, directing the flow of patients and health care resources. We will examine growing cracks in the Canadian system as governments struggle to decrease their deficits in the face of a growing and aging population. Finally, we will compare the Canadian model with the health care delivery systems of the USA, Cuba, and France.

2. Health Care in Canada

2.1. Values on which the Canadian health care system is based

In March 1994, a health care conference was held in Edmonton, Alberta, at which the values of participants toward health care were systematically recorded and analyzed. This exploration is significant because the *values* that underpin the structure of the current publicly funded and administered Canadian health care system rarely enter current discussions regarding health-care-system reform. Rather, *economic* and other *sociopolitical* forces now seem to be having a major impact on plans and actual changes within the health care system.

The conference participants identified three dominant values:

- The dignity of the human person as an individual and social being
- Respect for pluralism and difference
- Accountability

These values were found to be strong, in that they sustain a focus on the common good. The common good is the core of the Canadian health care system and is enshrined in the 1984 Canada Health Act (Wilson & Kieser, 1996).

2.2 Guiding principles

A royal commission headed by Justice Emmett Hall outlined the guiding principles for the Canadian health care system in 1963. The Hall Commission stated that any health care delivery scheme with which the federal government was involved should have the following five features:

- Universality
- Portability

- Comprehensiveness
- Accessibility
- Administration by government

Universality means the system should apply to all residents. New immigrants may have to wait (e.g., for three months) before they are eligible.

Portability means health care coverage should be transferrable between provinces. For example, an Ontario resident who needs medical care on a visit to British Columbia is entitled to this care in BC, with the costs of this care covered by her Ontario health plan.

The plan should be **comprehensive**, which means all medically necessary services provided by hospitals, physicians, and dentists (when the service is provided in a hospital) must be insured.

Accessibility means all Canadians should have equal access to health care, without any barriers due to age, financial status, health condition, where the person lives, and so on. For example, an individual living in a small community in northern Canada has the same right as one living in a major urban centre to have access to a highly specialized piece of diagnostic equipment or a complex surgical procedure. If the small community clinic does not have the equipment or personnel to perform a procedure, the health care plan should cover the costs of transporting the individual to the nearest location where such equipment or personnel are available.

The **government administration** of health care by agencies of the various provincial governments distinguishes the Canadian system from a system in which health care is administered by private parties, such as insurance companies, hospitals, or practitioners.

2.3 *Funding*

Health care in Canada is a *provincial* responsibility. The federal government sets the general standards for health care (e.g., the Canada Health Act mentioned above) and gives the provinces billions of dollars each year to help pay for health care, but each province has the power to administer its own health care delivery system. We will focus our discussion on the British Columbia system, although most of this applies to other provincial health care delivery systems.

Most of the health care costs are at the extremes of the lifespan. In 2015, Canada spent an average of over $17,000 per person for those age 80 to 84 and over $11,000 for those less than one year old, but less than $4,000 for those between age 1 and 64 (CIHI, 2017a).

A large fraction of government budgets in Canada pay for health care. British Columbia's health budget was $16 billion in 2012/2013, consuming about half the government's total budget (de Jong, 2012). By 2015, BC's 2015 health budget had increased to $18 billion (Mason, 2015). Nationwide, health spending accounted for about 37% of total provincial and territorial government program expenditures (e.g., on health, education, transportation and communication, and social services) in 2015 (CIHI, 2017a).

The public sector pays for about 70% of the costs of health care in Canada: 65% from provincial and territorial governments and 5% from the federal and municipal level. Public sector health spending is largely funded by federal and provincial income taxes. British Columbia is one of only three provinces (the others are Ontario and Quebec) that require individuals to pay **health insurance premiums,** and is the only one of these three not collecting premiums through income tax. BC plans to replace health insurance premiums with an employer health tax, starting in 2019. Four other provinces (Ontario, Quebec, Manitoba, and Newfoundland and Labrador) have similar employer health taxes.

2.4 Administration
2.4.1 Physicians
A physician must be licensed to practise in the province. A physician must complete four steps to obtain a licence:

1. Graduate from an accredited medical school, which normally takes four years. Most individuals begin medical school after at least four years of university training. Thus, a physician has usually had at least eight years of schooling after graduation from high school.
2. Pass an examination. This examination is administered by the Medical Council of Canada and by each province's medical council.
3. Finish an internship. The internship is similar to an apprenticeship. The requirements for the internship differ from province to province. A provincial professional association called the *College of Physicians and Surgeons* sets the requirements for the internship in each province. The College also sets other standards and monitors the performance of its members.
4. Pay a licence fee to the provincial College of Physicians and Surgeons.

Figure 14.1 shows how the health care delivery system in British Columbia works.

The average age of Canadian physicians is about 50. The proportion of Canadian physicians who are female is increasing. In 2014, 39% of Canada's physicians were female. Of those under age 40, 53% are female. Across all provinces, females represent a larger proportion of *general practitioners* (44% female) than of *specialists* (34% female; CIHI, 2015). Approximately one-quarter (25.5%)

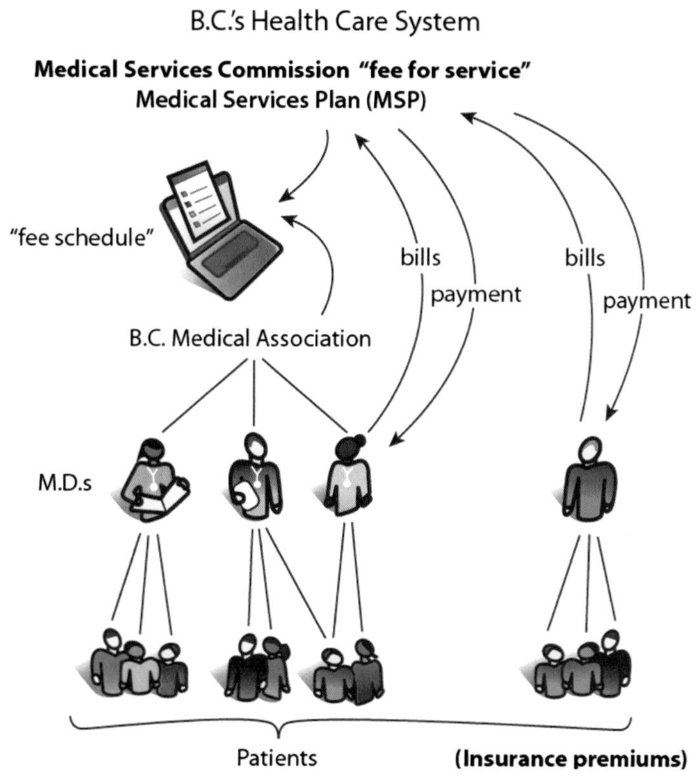

B.C.'s Health Care System

Medical Services Commission "fee for service"
Medical Services Plan (MSP)

"fee schedule"

bills

bills

payment

payment

B.C. Medical Association

M.D.s

Patients   **(Insurance premiums)**

Figure 14.1. How various players in British Columbia's health care delivery system interact with each other.

of Canada's physicians received their MD degree outside of Canada. Canada is gaining more physicians from international migration than it is losing (CIHI, 2015).

Those practising in rural Canada compose 8.6% of the overall physician pool and 14.6% of family physicians. As 18% of Canada's population lives in rural areas, the ratio of physicians per population, especially specialists, is lower in rural than in urban Canada (CMAJ, 2013).

Do *you* have a family physician? If not, why not?
  a) Perhaps you had a family physician when you lived with your parents, but now you are away at school.
  b) Perhaps you have not been able to find a doctor with whom you feel rapport.
  c) Perhaps when you need medical care you go to a walk-in clinic and see whichever physician is available.
  What are the advantages of having a family physician whom you see all the time?

2.4.2 British Columbia Medical Association (BCMA)

The *BCMA* is a voluntary organization, founded in 1990, to which physicians may belong and to which they pay dues. Most physicians belong. The BCMA acts as a bargaining agent and a lobby group for physicians. The BCMA has been successful in lobbying for increases in the *fee schedule* and in establishing a government-funded pension plan for BC physicians.

2.4.3 Physician supply

In the 1960s, Canada fell short of the World Health Organization recommended ratio of physicians to population. Canada increased physician supply by increasing the number of spaces in Canadian medical schools. This strategy succeeded, with a peak of new medical graduates in 1985. Then a report in 1984 and another in 1991 recommended *reducing* medical school spaces to avoid a surplus of physicians. This recommendation was implemented. In 1999, there was a recommendation to increase medical school intake to 2,000 per year.

In 2016 Canada had over 98,000 physicians, or 270 physicians for every 100,000 people, up from 210 per 100,000 in 2000. About half (47%) were family physicians (also known as general practitioners or primary care physicians), down slightly from 48% in 2000 (OECD, 2018). The remaining 52% or 53% of the physicians were specialists, such as cardiologists, orthopedic surgeons, gynecologists, and so on. For the 10th year in a row, the number of physicians increased at a faster rate than the number of people in the population, resulting in more physicians per person than ever before (CIHI, 2017a).

2.4.4 Nurses

In Canada in 2016, there were over 420,000 nurses. Registered nurses (RNs), including nurse practitioners, made up 71%, while 28% were licensed practical nurses (LPNs) and the remainder were registered psychiatric nurses (CIHI, June 2017). In 2010, about 93% of RNs and LPNs and 77% of RPNs in Canada were female. The average Canadian nurse was about age 45, with the average increasing, except for the LPN category (CIHI, 2010).

Nurses face many challenges. Illness and absenteeism are high. Long work shifts and overtime are common. Low job satisfaction leads to high turnover; each year, about one in five Canadian nurses quits. The highest turnover occurs in intensive care units, where the annual turnover rate is 26.7%. Each nurse turnover costs an average of $25,000, mostly due to the cost of hiring temporary replacements and the lower productivity of new hires (O'Brien-Pallas, Tomblin, Murphy & Shamian, 2008).

Nurses' skills may be under-utilized in the current system. They could arguably make a larger contribution if they were better integrated with other members of the health care team.

2.4.5 Medical Services Plan of BC

All BC residents are eligible—and *required*—to enrol in the **Medical Services Plan (MSP)**. The MSP operates much like an automobile insurance plan, with each user paying a "premium." When you visit your physician, you usually do not pay the physician directly for the services she performs. Almost all Canadians are covered by a health insurance plan. The MSP covers virtually all British Columbia residents.

The **Medical Services Commission (MSC)** administers the MSP on behalf of the Government of British Columbia. Remember, one of the guiding principles of the Canadian health care system is that it should be government administered. The MSC is a nine-member body with three representatives each from the BC Government, the British Columbia Medical Association (BCMA), and the public, jointly nominated by the BCMA and the Government to represent MSP beneficiaries.

2.4.6 Extra billing

In 1979, Justice Emmett Hall was asked to chair another royal commission, this time to investigate **extra-billing**. Extra-billing is when a health care practitioner requires the patient to pay a fee in addition to the fee the practitioner receives from the provincial health insurance plan—thus, it is an "extra bill."

Under the 1984 Canada Health Act, extra-billing is defined as "the billing for an insured health service rendered to an insured person by a medical practitioner or a dentist [i.e., a dentist providing insured surgical-dental services in a hospital setting] in an amount in addition to any amount paid, or to be paid, for that service by the health care insurance plan of a province or territory." For example, if a physician was to charge a patient any amount for an office visit that is insured by the provincial or territorial health insurance plan, the amount charged would constitute extra-billing. Extra-billing is seen as a barrier or impediment for people seeking medical care, and is therefore contrary to the accessibility criterion.

The Hall Commission strongly recommended a prohibition on extra-billing. In 1984, the federal government responded to this recommendation with the Canada Health Act. This act empowered the federal government to withdraw funds from provinces that permitted extra-billing or that charged any user fees (e.g., charges for visiting hospital emergency departments, daily charges to stay in hospital, fees for visiting a physiotherapist). For each dollar of extra billing in a particular province, the federal government withholds one dollar of transfer payments. For example, if $90 million worth of extra-billings are made in Ontario, the federal government gives Ontario $90 million less.

2.4.7 Services covered

The provincial medical services plans cover many, but not all, health care items and services. This varies from province to province; remember, the provinces are the ones that decide, not the federal government. Some items *not* covered by British Columbia's MSP include

- Services that are deemed not medically required, such as **cosmetic surgery**
- **Dental** services, except as outlined under benefits
- Routine **eye examinations** for people age 19 to 64
- **Eyeglasses**, **hearing aids**, and other equipment or appliances
- Prescription **drugs**
- Chiropractic, massage therapy, naturopathy, physical therapy, and non-surgical podiatry services (except for MSP beneficiaries with premium-assistance status)

> What kind of health insurance do *you* have?
> a) Do you have a British Columbia Services Card?
> b) Who pays the premiums? Do you? Do your parents? Does your employer?
> c) Do you have "extended" health insurance? If so, what does it cover?

A provincial program called PharmaCare provides financial assistance to British Columbia residents for eligible prescription drugs and designated medical supplies. When a person buys prescription drugs, part of the cost is for the drug itself and part of the cost is a dispensing fee.

2.4.8 Fees for services

Most Canadian physicians work on a *fee-for-service* basis. That is, when they do something for the patient (provide a service) they are entitled to a fee. The specific services covered and the fee the physician is paid for each service is determined by negotiations between the MSC and the *BC Medical Association (BCMA)*. Over time, there has been a growing shift toward alternative payment plans in place of fee-for-service payments. In 1999–2000, alternative payments (i.e., not fee-for-service) made up 10.6% of total gross clinical payments. Since 2008, this trend has stabilized, with fee-for-service payments accounting for about 71% of total clinical payments; alternative payments accounted for the balance (CIHI, 2015).

It is important to note that most Canadian physicians are *self-employed*. Although they are mainly reimbursed by government-administered health insurance plans, they are *not* government employees. The government, through the MSC, sets the fees practitioners will be paid for various services. However, the Supreme Court has ruled that the government cannot regulate what geographical area physicians can practise in.

Table 14.1 shows some sample services and the corresponding fees.

Table 14.1

Fees Paid to Health Care Practitioners in British Columbia

Code	Description	Fee
12100	Visit in office (age 0 to 1)	$32.75
00100	Visit in office (age 2 to 49)[1]	$29.79
16100	Visit in office (age 60 to 69)	$34.23
17100	Visit in office (age 70 to 79)	$38.70
18100	Visit in office (age 80+)	$44.67
00101	Complete physical examination and history (age 2 to 49)[2]	$66.20
00120	Individual counseling in office (age 2 to 49)[3]	$51.84
01730	Graded exercise test: technical fee	$30.97
01731	Graded exercise test: professional fee	$45.18
02015	Eye exam by ophthalmologist	$48.90
08534	X-ray ankle	$33.62

Source: British Columbia Ministry of Health, May 1, 2018

1. If a practitioner sees more than 50 patients in a day, she is only paid 50% of the normal rate for patients #51 to #65, and nothing for more than 65 patients in a day.
2. Routine or periodic physical examination (checkup) is not a benefit under MSP. This includes any associated diagnostic of laboratory procedures unless significant pathology is found. Patient is responsible for payment.
3. Minimum 20 minutes per visit. Maximum four such services per patient per year.

Do the preceding figures surprise you?

Did you know, for example, that your doctor is paid over $30 each time you see him?

Does this seem like a reasonable fee? Why or why not?

3 Strengths of the Canadian Medical Care System

Canada provides a *high quality* of care to *almost everyone* at a *reasonable cost.* The Canadian system is a ***welfare state*** model; that is, the government is considered to be responsible for the welfare of its citizens. In Canada, health care is treated like education or roads—the government provides it to all citizens. A majority of Canadians who use the system are highly satisfied with the quality and standard of care and strongly endorse the concept of government-administered health care rather than an American-type system.

3.1 *Comparison with the American system*

The American health care system is fundamentally a ***free-enterprise*** system, in which health care is treated like any other service, such as that of an accountant or an automobile mechanic. The cost and distribution of these services are determined by supply and demand. Those who can afford to pay more theoretically get more or better or faster health care. Health care facilities are largely owned and operated by private-sector businesses. Health practitioners are mainly paid on a fee-for-service basis, as in Canada. Unlike a pure free-enterprise model, the federal and state governments also participate to a significant extent.

The USA is the only industrialized nation in the world that *does not have universal health care.*

> In most countries, health spending is largely financed out of taxes or social security contributions, with private insurance or "out-of-pocket" payments playing a significant but secondary role. The United States together with Mexico and Chile are the only OECD countries where less than 50% of health spending is publicly financed. (OECD, 2013c)

The Organization of Economic Cooperation and Development (OECD) is a group of 35 developed countries, mostly in Europe and North America but also including Japan, Chile, Turkey, and Israel.

The American system is complicated, which is one reason it is expensive. Instead of having to deal with a single-payer system (e.g., a provincial medical services plan), American health care practitioners have to deal with state and federal government programs, with a number of different insurance companies, and with **co-payments** billed directly to patients (e.g., the service costs $100, but the insurance company will only pay $60 and the patient is billed for the other $40).

The **high administrative costs** are wasteful. Employer-funded health insurance coverage is a drag on the US economy. High health care costs figure large in personal bankruptcies. The USA pays twice as much for health care, as a portion of GDP, than other members of the OECD, yet lags behind other wealthy nations in such measures as infant mortality and life expectancy. Most OECD countries have enjoyed large gains in life expectancy over the past decades. In the United States, life expectancy at birth increased by almost nine years between 1960 and 2011, but this is less than the average increase across the OECD. As a result, while life expectancy in the United States used to be 1.5 years above the OECD average in 1960, it is now almost 1.5 years *below* the average (OECD, 2013c). In 2016 and 2017, life expectancy in the US actually *decreased*.

Despite the relatively high level of health expenditure in the United States, there are fewer physicians per capita (2.5 per 1,000 population) than the OECD average of 3.2. On the other hand, there were 11.1 nurses per 1,000 people in the United States in 2011, compared with the OECD average of 8.7 (OECD, 2013c).

The number of hospital beds in the United States in 2014 (the latest year available) was also lower than the OECD average (OECD, 2018). As in most OECD countries, the number of hospital beds per capita has fallen over the past 25 years in the United States. This decline has coincided with a reduction in average length of stay in hospitals and an increase in day surgeries (OECD, 2013c). Unlike the Canadian system, in which an individual can choose any physician she wants, in the USA people with private or government insurance are limited to medical facilities that accept the particular type of medical insurance they carry. Insurance companies negotiate with doctors and get a discounted rate. In return for this discount, the insurance company includes the doctor as part of its network. If a patient gets treatment from someone outside of the network, the patient will be billed for that service, often at rates much higher than the group rate the insurance company negotiated.

The USA system has been called a "patchwork quilt," which means it is stitched together from a number of different pieces. For example,

- The Veterans Health Administration operates hospitals for former members of the armed forces, but if the individual's medical problem isn't related to his military service, then he is charged for the treatment.
- The Indian Health Service operates facilities, but these are open only to Native Americans from recognized tribes.
- A federal program called **Medicare** covers those over age 65.
- A joint state-federal program called **Medicaid** covers those with low income or with disabilities.
- Government programs directly cover some 28% of the population (83 million), including people who are older, disabled, children, or veterans, and some people with low incomes.

- Most hospitals are operated as non-profit societies, and county and city governments own some hospitals, while other hospitals are privately owned for profit.
- Most of the population under 65 is insured by their or a family member's employer. Health insurance benefits are not taxable under US law, which makes them an attractive way for employers to increase the salary of employees. It has been argued that these benefits increase demand: "Hey, I'm entitled to $250 every two years for prescription eyeglasses; I haven't had new glasses for a while. I better use this benefit." However, employer-funded insurance is decreasing as companies try to cut costs. The government for the most part pays for health insurance for public-sector employees.
- A portion of Americans purchase health insurance on their own, through private providers such as Metropolitan Life Insurance Company or Blue Cross/Blue Shield.
- An estimated 27 million Americans have *no* health insurance. Lack of insurance is associated with increased mortality; one study found that uninsured working-age Americans had 40% greater mortality than their insured counterparts (Cecere, 2009).

Attempts to change the US health care system have encountered resistance. The powerful insurance-company and health-care-industry **lobbyists** oppose change. Wealthy people as a group don't want to subsidize the insurance costs of poor people. This seems partly the result of ideology. Access to health care is not a guaranteed right in the USA. Free-enterprise advocates have branded the Canadian system "socialist." This is inaccurate. In a socialist system, the government owns health care facilities, and health care workers are employees of the government. Cuba works this way. So did the former USSR. Not Canada.

3.1.1 Obamacare

The Patient Protection and Affordable Health Care Act (AHCA), which Democratic president Barack Obama signed into law March 23, 2010, aimed to reduce the number of uninsured Americans. This act, widely referred to as Obamacare, contains several key features (*The Economist*, 2014):

- It prevented insurers from charging sick people higher rates than healthy ones.
- It required all Americans to have insurance or pay a fine.
- It set up online health "exchanges" where people can shop for coverage.
- It expanded Medicaid (public health care for people with low incomes).
- It offered subsidies to low-income people.

One way the AHCA tried to insure all Americans for a reasonable cost was to *require* everyone to have health insurance. The way insurance programs work is by **pooling risk**. Let's consider the hypothetical example of a disease that costs $500,000 to treat, and assume that the lifetime prevalence of this disease is 1%. If 100 people each put $5,000 into a joint account, then when one of them gets the disease, the account can pay the full costs. You'd need to scale this plan up for it to actually work, because probabilities become more reliable when applied to larger numbers. So, let's say 10,000 people each contribute $5,000, for a total of $50 million—which will cover the cost of treatment for the predicted 100 people who get sick. Fine. But what if not everyone wants to pay the $5,000 lifetime insurance cost? Maybe I consider myself really healthy, with much less than a 1% chance of getting the disease. So, I don't buy into the plan, leaving it $5,000 short. The plan has to charge everyone else a bit more to cover this. If others follow my lead, the cost for those remaining goes up further. Then the higher cost causes others to reconsider, and they drop out, too—leaving us with a high-cost plan and a portion of uninsured people.

Obamacare was strongly opposed by many Republicans and passed by narrow margins in both houses of the US Congress. Along the way, compromises weakened the plan. For example, expanded "hardship" exemptions allowed more people to opt out of buying health insurance (*The Economist*, 2014). Obamacare was deeply unpopular among many voters, for various reasons (*BBC News*, 2014):

- It was seen as an "inappropriate government intrusion into the massive healthcare industry and an affront to personal liberty."
- Insurance costs increased for some people.
- Some people object to having to purchase insurance at all. "I don't need health insurance myself. Why should I have to join and help pay for the cost of other people's illness?"

Others (notably conservative Republicans) opposed the AHCA because its reforms did not go far enough.

Since taking office in 2017, the Republican president Donald Trump has tried to repeal and replace the AHCA. On December 22, 2017, Trump signed into law the Tax Cuts and Jobs Act of 2017. Among other things, the final version of this bill repealed the requirement for individuals and companies to get health care for themselves and their employees. It was this mandate which kept health care costs down under Obamacare by promoting cost sharing over a larger pool.

> Do *you* think Canada should move toward a free-enterprise-type health care system? Why or why not?

3.2 *Comparison with the Cuban system*

Cuba is a small island nation that has operated on a **socialist** model since the Cuban Revolution of 1959. After the revolution, a number of doctors left Cuba. The USA, concerned about the proximity (only 150 km from Florida) of such a different system, imposed an economic blockade on Cuba. Until its demise in 1991, the Soviet Union supported Cuba politically and economically. The US sanctions plus the loss of Soviet support caused economic hardship in Cuba, prompting Cuba to develop its own medical equipment and drugs (TeleSUR, 2014).

Cuba has an extensive public health care system that covers all citizens for all medical interventions and medications, and at no charge. It does not cover devices such as wheelchairs, crutches, or prescription eyeglasses; however, the government provides subsidies to help people purchase these (TeleSUR, 2014). All health-related facilities and services are run by the government (InterNations, 2015). Physicians, nurses, and other health care workers are *government employees*. Medical education is free. Doctors are respected, but not paid much (Campion & Morrissey, 2013). Cuba has one of the highest ratios of doctors per patients in the world: 7.52/1,000, about three times the ratio in Canada (CIA, 2018).

Cuba's small health budget led it to develop an approach to health care that focuses on **prevention** and **primary care**. All Cuban physicians must do their first residency (a practical training experience after finishing medical school) in family medicine.

Health care delivery is organized at the local level, with patients and their caregivers generally living in the same community (Campion & Morrissey, 2013). The country is divided into about 500 districts, each composed of about 45,000 residents and having 30 or so "doctor-and-nurse" offices. Physicians head about half of these offices, with the others led by nurses who work under the supervision of a local doctor. A "polyclinic" serves each area, acting as the organizational centre for the offices (Reed, 2018).

Every Cuban gets at least one health exam yearly, exams that local doctors or nurses often do at the patient's home (InterNations, 2015; Reed, 2018). House calls and discussions with family members are often used to improve compliance (i.e., patients following medical advice). Patients with chronic conditions receive visits more frequently. Patients can be referred to a district polyclinic for specialty evaluation, but they return to the community team for ongoing treatment (Campion & Morrissey, 2013).

Cuba boasts good health outcomes for such an economically strained nation. Infant mortality rate is 4.4 infant deaths per 1,000 live births, better than in Canada (4.5) and the USA (5.8). Life expectancy at birth is almost 79 years, not far behind Canada and the USA (82 and 80 years, respectively; CIA, 2018).

Remember from Chapter 1 that medical care is only part—and often not the most important part—of health. Cuba's improved health outcomes result mainly from improvements in **social determinants of health**, such as nutrition and education. Cuba's literacy rate is 99%, and health education is part of the mandatory school curriculum (Campion & Morrissey, 2013).

3.3 *Comparison with the French system*

Like Canada, France is a *welfare state* economy. Virtually everyone living in France is covered by the health care system. The system is quite comprehensive, covering services in the clinic or hospital, dental services, and pharmaceuticals (drugs and medicines). The system blends public and private services, with funding shared by government, employers, and individuals.

All salaries are charged a health contribution, with the employer and employee each paying part of this. Government-run health insurance pays the majority (70% to 100%) of the cost of each medical visit. Users pay a small fee for each service. Most users purchase supplementary insurance that pays for all of most of the user fee.

The government sets the fees for each medical procedure. For example, the flat fee for visiting a general practitioner is 23 euros (night, weekend, and home-visit rates are higher). The user is reimbursed for most of this, leaving her to pay between 6 and 0 euros, depending on the type of insurance she has purchased. One individual reports that she and her husband purchased top-of-the line insurance for 50 euros a month, less than 20% of what health insurance had cost them in the USA (Lundberg, 2014).

French residents must register with a health insurer, and designate one general practitioner as their primary doctor. The user can consult with other doctors—including specialists. However, typically the user only gets reimbursed for specialist consults at the full government rate if his primary doctor referred him. Specialists can work in their own practice, a group practice with other physicians, in a private hospital, or in a government hospital. Many specialists divide their time between clinics and hospitals, and some work in both the government and private sectors (Expatica, 2016).

The French system is considered one of the best in the world (Expatica, 2016; About France, 2018). It covers virtually everyone. Costs to users are low. Quality of care is high. Patients have a lot of choice. Overall, the system is relatively expensive, accounting for 11.0 % of GDP in 2016 (OECD, 2018). An aging population, increasing patient expectations, and expensive new medicines and procedures are driving up costs (About France, 2018). Most developed countries are experiencing similar strains, regardless of the type of health care system they use.

4 Problems with Health Care in Canada

4.1 Cost

As a country's population increases, the amount it spends on health care tends to increase. Total health spending in China, for example, is much greater than in Canada because China has many more people. So, if we wanted to track changes in health expenditure over time, we could use per capita spending as a metric. But the value of currency changes over time (because of, e.g., inflation) and differs from one country to another. A good way to account for all these factors—population, inflation, and currency differences—is to look at the health spending as a percentage of *gross domestic product (GDP)*.

Health care is expensive. The average country in the Organization of Economic and Cooperation and Development (OECD) spends about 9% of its annual gross domestic product (GDP)—the total value of all goods and services produced—on health care. Canada's per capita health bill is among the highest internationally: 11.5% of GDP in 2016, or $6,604 per person (CIHI, 2017a). Although Canada is above the OECD average in terms of per-person spending on health care, the *public-sector* share of total health expenditure is below the OECD average (CIHI, 2017a).

The USA, which has by far the costliest system in the world, spends over 17% of its GDP on health care (OECD, 2018). In the Commonwealth Fund's comparison of 13 high-income countries, the USA was the top consumer of prescription drugs and of sophisticated diagnostic-imaging technology, such as CT and MRI scans. Prices for medical procedures were also the highest in the USA. For example, the average price of coronary artery bypass surgery was $75,345 in the USA, nearly twice the cost of the surgery in Australia, the next most expensive country at $42,130 (Squires & Anderson, 2013).

Since 1975, health care spending in Canada has increased from about 7% to over 11% of GDP (Figure 14.2). This is a concern because money spent on health care isn't available to spend on other things, such as education, food, or housing. Rising health care spending is not just a Canadian phenomenon. On average, the 35 counties in the OECD spent 7.2% of their GDP on health in 2000; by 2016, this had risen to 9.0%. Growth of health spending has been much more dramatic in the USA: below 9% in 1980, 12.5% in 2000, and 17.2% in 2016 (OECD, 2018).

Across the OECD, health spending grew by about 5% per year from 2000 to 2009 (OECD, 2013d). Since the 2009 global economic crisis, growth of spending on health care by OECD countries has been modest. "In many countries, governments have also decided to cut their spending on prevention and public health, although these typically represent only a small share of their overall health budgets" (OECD, 2013d). As noted by the OECD,

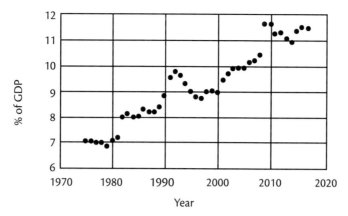

Figure 14.2. Trend in health expenditure in Canada from 1975 to 2017, as percentage of GDP. *Source:* Canadian Institute for Health Information. 2017a. *National Health Expenditure Trends, 1975 to 2017.* Data Table A-1. Ottawa: CIHI.

the number of hospital beds per capita has decreased over the past decade in most OECD countries. This reduction is part of a voluntary effort in most countries, partly driven by progress in medical technology, which has enabled a move to day surgery for a number of procedures and a reduced need for hospitalization. (OECD, 2018)

For example, in Canada, beds in public hospitals per 1,000 population decreased from 3.0 in 2006 to 2.6 in 2016 (OECD, 2018).

Other approaches to cost-cutting measures were taken by the British Columbia Liberal government of Christie Clark (2011–2017). "Government bargained tough new agreements with nurses and doctors and also drove better deals with medical laboratories throughout the province. It urged greater collaboration among health authorities in an effort to find efficiencies that would save cash." It changed the way hospitals were funded, from block funding to giving more money to those hospitals that handled more patients. It slowed the increase in drug costs by driving harder bargains with drug manufacturers, using generic drugs more often, and joined with other Western provinces to make bulk purchases of drugs (Mason, 2015).

4.1.1 *The role of physicians in cost*
Physicians are key figures in the health care delivery system. However, fees paid to physicians are *not* the major portion of direct health care costs. Hospitals are the biggest "line item" in the budget. In the mid-1970s, hospitals accounted for 45% of total health expenditures in Canada. This decreased to 28% in 2017. "Other institutions" (i.e., long term care facilities) made up another 11% of the total in

2017. Physician services represent about 15% of total cost, while pharmaceutical (drug) costs are about 16%. While all costs have gone up over the decades, drug costs have risen more rapidly than other health care costs (CIHI, 2017).

But physicians have a major effect on the total costs to the system, depending, for example, on what tests they order, what medications they prescribe, and whether they recommend a patient go to hospital or stay at home and receive outpatient care.

Physicians order and perform more tests and also employ more expensive care than they used to. According to the British Columbia Ministry of Health, between 2001 and 2011 the number of CT scans (a special type of diagnostic X-ray) doubled, and the number of MRI exams (another type of diagnostic imaging) increased by almost 170% in British Columbia (de Jong, 2012, p. 8). New surgical techniques and equipment contributed to the increased use of joint replacement procedures. In British Columbia, the number of hip replacements increased by 102% and the number of knee replacements by 180% over the past decade (de Jong, 2012, p. 8).

4.1.2 The two-tiered health care system

A tier is a layer, like the layers in a wedding cake. A *two-tiered* health care system means there are two different standards of care. The lower level is government-funded public health care. The upper level is private health care. Canada does not officially have a two-tier system, but it is moving in that direction.

In a two-tier system, wealthier Canadians or those covered by extended health care plans paid for by their employer would be able to afford additional services not covered by the government health insurance plan. This would make Canada more like the United States, and is directly against the Canadian principle of universality.

It has been argued that a parallel private health care system would reduce pressure on the public system, and that the public system would then be better able to serve lower-income Canadians. On the other hand, users of the private system would likely be less willingly to support government expenditures on public health care. This would result in further cutbacks in government funding of health care.

4.1.3 Chronic diseases

Over the last century, death from infectious disease has declined dramatically. Chronic diseases such as heart disease, cancer, diabetes, and mental illness have replaced infectious disease as major causes of disability and death. Improved treatment and management allow people with chronic health conditions to live longer—and to continue costing the health care system money.

People with chronic conditions represent approximately 38% of the British Columbia population, and they consume about 80% of the combined physician payment, PharmaCare, and acute (hospital) care costs. Projections suggest that the prevalence of chronic conditions could increase 58% over the next 25 years (de Jong, 2012, p. 8).

> What do *you* think?
> If you were in charge, what would you do about the costs of the Canadian health care delivery system?
> a) Would you raise taxes and put more money into health care?
> b) Would you cut costs? If so, how?

4.1.4 Aging population
Canadians are living longer, and older people constitute a growing percentage of our total population. Older people tend to have more chronic diseases and thus need more health care.

The senior population of British Columbia currently makes up 15% of the total population and is expected to double within the next 20 years, making it one of the fastest growing senior populations in Canada. The aging population is a significant driver of demand, because the need for health services rises dramatically with age. People over age 65 make up 15% of the British Columbia population but use 33% of physician services, 48% of acute care services, 49% of PharmaCare expenditures, 74% of home and community care services, and 93% of residential care services (de Jong, 2012, p. 7).

Some OECD counties, such as Japan and France, spend less on health care (as a percentage of GDP) than Canada, despite having a higher portion of their populations over age 65 (CIHI, 2017b).

4.2 Wait lists
Critics have complained that Canadians have to wait too long to see a family physician or specialist, to get a specialized test such as a CT scan or an MRI, or to have surgery for non-life-threatening conditions (such as hip replacement for chronic hip pain). This is a controversial issue, with as much rhetoric as data. The Supreme Court of Canada ruled in favour of a Quebec resident who argued he had been on a wait list for treatment for too long. The Court agreed, writing that Canadians are entitled by law to health care and that access to a waiting list did not constitute access to health care.

Governments seem sensitive to criticism about waiting times. Wait times have shortened for selected procedures: "cancer, cardiac, joint-replacement and sight-restoration operations have decreased since 2004–2005, mostly because of the investments made to reduce waits for those treatments" (CTVNews Staff, 2012). Wait times may still exist for other conditions (CTVNews Staff, 2012), although figures given by government don't agree with figures offered by proponents of private health care.

The problem persists. In a study of 11 developed nations, Canadians reported high levels of satisfaction with the **quality** of their health care, but the **longest wait times** at emergency departments and the **slowest access** to specialists (Vogel, 2017a). The problem seems to be with access to family physicians (primary care). Over 40% of Canadians surveyed said their last visit to the emergency department was for a condition that could have been treated in primary care, but their regular family physician was not available—especially on evenings and weekends. Canadians seem quite dependent on family physicians, averaging 7.6 doctor visits per year, 30% more than residents of the other countries surveyed. Paradoxically, Canada's physician supply is growing faster than the population, but patient reports of wait times haven't changed in 10 years (Vogel, 2017a).

Walk-in clinics, which are places where patients can go without an appointment, have become more popular. Critics complain these clinics take the easy cases (colds or flu, vaccinations, minor wounds, etc.), with the result that cases seen by "regular" doctors in "regular" clinics have become, on average, more difficult.

> Think about the last time *you* wanted to see your family physician.
> a) Were you able to see her on that day?
> b) If not, how many days did you have to wait for an appointment?

4.3 Emphasis on treatment rather than prevention

Prevention of disease should minimize human suffering, relieve overworked health care professionals, and save money. The need for a preventive approach to health care was pointed out by the 1974 federal health report *New Perspectives on the Health of Canadians* (LaLonde, 1974). Unfortunately, little action was taken to implement the recommendations of this report.

Almost 30 years later, the Romanow report offered the same opinion:

> Keeping people well, rather than treating them when they are sick, is common sense. And so it is equally common sense for our health care system to place a greater emphasis on preventing disease and on promoting healthy lifestyles. This is the best way to sustain our health care system over the longer term. It requires us all to realize that our health and wellness is not simply a responsibility of the state

but something we must work toward as individuals, families and communities, and as a nation. (Romanow, 2002, pp. 21–22)

The 2010 report by British Columbia's Provincial Health Officer (Kendall, 2010), *Investing in Prevention,* makes many of the same points.

4.4 Unequal distribution of health care resources

The Hall Commission established **accessibility** as a key feature of the Canadian model. In fact, access to high-quality medical care is *not* equal for all Canadians. For example, small rural communities in northern Canada, some urban low-income people, Indigenous people, and ethnic minorities may all be under-serviced by the health care system.

There has been much discussion of the unequal distribution between urban and rural areas. Only 9.4% of physicians (15.7% of family physicians and 2.4% of specialists) were located in rural areas in 2008. In contrast, 21.4% of the general population resided in rural areas. In Canada, there has been a rapid increase in the last 10 years in the number of students enrolled in medical school; however, only about 11% of these students are from rural areas, compared with the 22% of students one would expect based on Canada's population (Rourke, 2008).

Nevertheless, there are continuing issues of access to care. The bottom 33% of Canadian income earners are—as compared to the top 33% of income earners—50% less likely to see a specialist when needed, 50% more likely to find it difficult to get care on weekends or evenings, and 40% more likely to wait five days or more for an appointment with a physician. (Mikkonen & Raphael, 2010, p. 38)

4.5 Fragmentation of services

A few decades ago, the family physician diagnosed and treated most of his patients' complaints. This was especially true in smaller rural communities and when individuals were less geographically mobile than they are now. One often visited the same physician for decades. Consequently, the physician came to know the patient quite well.

Medical practice has certainly become much more complex. It is unrealistic to expect any individual to stay abreast of *all* the recent developments in medicine. Modern medical practice is based on an initial visit to the general practitioner, which is frequently followed by a referral or a series of referrals to specialists. These specialists report their findings back to the general practitioner who originally referred the patient.

In theory, this process can work well. However, good communication between medical practitioners is necessary. It is also expensive. Each visit to a doctor means a bill to the medical insurance plan. And fees for the services of specialists are higher than general practitioners' fees.

Romanow agrees:

> We must transform our health care "system" from one in which a multitude of participants, working in silos, focus primarily on managing illness, to one in which they work collaboratively to deliver a seamless, integrated array of services to Canadians, from prevention and promotion to primary care, to hospital, community, mental health home and end-of-life care. (Romanow, 2002, p. 19)

4.6 Unnecessary testing and treatment

More is not better. A 2017 report by the Canadian Institute for Health Information found that up to 30% of the medical interventions studied were done against best-practice guidelines. For example, doctors commonly prescribe older Canadians sedatives for insomnia, when advice to skip naps and minimize evening screen time might be more appropriate. As another example, a third of low-risk patients with minor head injuries got brain scans, even though the scans wouldn't improve outcomes. As a final example, Canadians with simple low-back pain often got X-rays or other images, even though their pain usually resolved without treatment (Vogel, 2017b). The picture in the USA is similar. The problem is not just that the interventions are unnecessary, waste resources, and compound wait times for those in genuine need. These interventions can *harm* patients: sedatives increase risk of falls and car crashes; X-rays increase risk of mutations and cancer; and telling people with low-back pain that the X-ray shows a "degenerated spine" may cause them to *avoid* exercise, while exercise is one of the most effective remedies for their condition.

4.7 Focus on rare diseases and high-tech solutions

Most of the major health problems today are related to established risk factors. The incidence of these health problems could be reduced substantially through programs of basic health care. Such a program might include early detection and treatment of disease, periodic screening for known risk factors for these health problems, and education aimed at providing individuals with information and motivation to become more involved in their own health maintenance, and with specific techniques to make positive changes in their personal health habits.

Basic medicine is probably where the biggest health gains can be made for the largest number of people at the most reasonable cost. However, there appears to be an under-emphasis of these points in current medical practice. Rather, modern medicine seems drawn to the new, the unusual, and the application of the most recent scientific advances.

Advances in medical technology have contributed in a significant positive way to medical practice. For example, the technique known as **arthroscopy** enables a surgeon to insert a small, flexible instrument through a small incision to examine or repair a joint. Arthroscopic surgery to repair a torn cartilage in the knee has become a routine operation. This operation gives significant improvements in recovery time, time in hospital, and costs to society.

Perhaps it is unrealistic to expect physicians to deal with the entire spectrum of medical care from the simple to the complex. Perhaps some of the less demanding but still important tasks could be delegated to less highly trained health care professionals, such as nurses, psychologists, nutritionists, exercise specialists, health educators, and counsellors. This would allow the physician the time to diagnose and treat more complicated conditions demanding special skills.

However, such a system would compound the problem of fragmentation of services discussed above. It also poses the question of who would administer and coordinate such a team-based approach to medicine. Traditionally, the general practitioner or family physician has filled this role. There is a real risk that if politicians or bureaucrats were in charge of managing a patient-care system, cost considerations might become more important than quality of care. Physicians would certainly object to any change they felt compromised the quality of the care the patient received, the patient's freedom to choose whom he wanted to provide this care, or the special nature of the patient-doctor relationship.

5 Conclusion

We are fortunate as Canadians to have open access to high-quality health care. There are, however, trends suggesting that the system delivering this health care is increasingly strained. Some fundamental changes in the way health care is delivered are indicated. These changes could protect the basic principles of our welfare state model. A holistic approach, linking the talents of many different types of health care professionals, is needed. This approach should incorporate maintenance of high-level wellness, prevention of disease, and early detection and treatment of disease. Clearly, coordinated political action would be required to accomplish these changes. The individual, however, can play an active role in this political process. We can also take more responsibility for using health care resources appropriately, and for practising good health habits to help maintain our own health.

Study Questions

1a. List and explain briefly the five key features of the Canadian health care system as outlined by the 1963 Hall Commission.

1b. Which of these principles are threatened by current trends? Explain.

2. What are the conditions for a person to legally practise as a physician in British Columbia?

3. Explain how the Canadian/British Columbia health care delivery system works, including the role of each of the following:
   - BCMSP
   - BCMSC
   - College of Physicians and Surgeons
   - BCMA
   - Fee for service
   - Fee schedule

4. Outline the demographics (e.g., age and sex) of Canadian physicians and Canadian nurses.

5. What are the main strengths of the Canadian health care system?

6. Compare and contrast the Canadian health care delivery system with the systems of the USA, Cuba, and France.

7. Explain the following:
   - Extra-billing
   - Co-payment
   - Insurance premiums

8. Identify at least four problems with the current Canadian health care system.

9. Regarding the Canadian health care delivery system:
   - How are costs changing?
   - What are the main components of cost?
   - What factors are driving changes in cost?

Glossary

BCMA—a lobby group for physicians; membership is voluntary; negotiates with MSCBC re fee schedule for medical services

BCMSP—the health insurance plan that covers virtually all residents of BC

College of Physicians and Surgeons—a professional society that licenses doctors to practise in BC; sets standards and regulates conduct of its members (can revoke licence to practise)

extra-billing—where a health care provider charges the patient more than the amount specified in the fee schedule; thus, the health insurance plan is billed

for the specified amount and the patient is billed for the "extra" amount
above this

fee-for-service—a payment system in which a service provider is paid a fee every
time she provides a service; examples of other payment systems are yearly
salary, hourly wage, or paying a set fee per client or patient per year

fee schedule—a list of all of the services the provincial health insurance plan
will pay for; each service is given a code number, name, and a dollar amount
that will be given to the service provider for performing this service

free enterprise—an economic model in which the price and distribution of goods
and services are determined by supply and demand; if something is in great
demand, it will command a high price, and only those able (or willing) to
pay this price will get it

general practitioner—a medical doctor who is not a specialist; often called a
"family physician" or "primary-care provider"

gross domestic product (GDP)—the total value of goods and services produced
(typically per year) in a country, province, or other jurisdiction

MSC—the arms-length government agency (like a Crown Corporation) that
administers the MSCBC

specialist—a medical doctor who has taken additional training in a special area,
such as cardiology (heart) or orthopedics (bones)

two-tiered—a tier is a layer, so this means "two-layered" and refers to health
care systems in which some people get better care than others; for example,
those who can afford to pay for private care get treated sooner, get a private
room rather than a bed in a ward, and so on

welfare state—an economic model in which governments assume responsibility for services that typically include health, education, transportation, and
communication

Additional Resources

British Columbia Medical Association
    www.bcma.org
College of Registered Nurses of British Columbia
    https://crnbc.ca/Pages/Default.aspx
Medical Services Plan of British Columbia
    www.health.gov.bc.ca/msp/

References

About-France.com. (2018). The French health care system. Retrieved January 9, 2018
    from https://about-france.com/health-care.htm

BBC News. (April 1, 2014). "Obamacare" deadline sparks surge in insurance sign-ups. Retrieved May 9, 2014 from http://www.bbc.com/news/world-us-canada-26823837

British Columbia Ministry of Health. (May 1, 2018). Medical Services Commission Payment Schedule. Retrieved June 2, 2018 from https://www2.gov.bc.ca/assets/gov/health/practitioner-pro/medical-services-plan/msc-payment-schedule-may-2018.pdf

Campion, E. W., Morrissey, S. (January 24, 2013). A different model – Medical care in Cuba. *New England Journal of Medicine.* 368:297-299.

Cecere, D. (September 17, 2009). New study finds 45,000 deaths annually linked to lack of health coverage. *The Harvard Gazette.* Retrieved June 4, 2018 from https://news.harvard.edu/gazette/story/2009/09/new-study-finds-45000-deaths-annually-linked-to-lack-of-health-coverage/

CIA (Central Intelligence Agency). (2018). The World Factbook. Retrieved June 4, 2018 from https://www.cia.gov/library/publications/the-world-factbook/fields/2226.html

CIHI (Canadian Institute for Health Information). (2010). *Regulated Nurses: Canadian Trends, 2005 to 2009.* Ottawa, Ontario: CIHI. Retrieved July 31, 2014 from http://publications.gc.ca/collections/collection_2011/icis-cihi/H115-48-2009-eng.pdf

CIHI. (September, 2015). *Physicians in Canada, 2014.* Retrieved June 2, 2018 from https://secure.cihi.ca/free_products/Summary-PhysiciansInCanadaReport2014_EN-web.pdf

CIHI. (2017a). *National Health Expenditure Trends, 1975 to 2017.* Ottawa: Ontario: CIHI. Retrieved June 1, 2018 from https://www.cihi.ca/en/national-health-expenditure-trends

CIHI. (2017b). *How Canada Compares Internationally: A Health Spending Perspective — International Chartbook, 2017.* Ottawa, ON: CIHI. Retrieved June 1, 2018 from https://www.cihi.ca/en/national-health-expenditure-trends

CIHI. (June 2017). *Regulated Nurses, 2016.* Ottawa, Ontario: CIHI. Retrieved June 2, 2018 from https://www.cihi.ca/en/regulated-nurses-2016

CMAJ. (2013). Canadian physician supply on uptick. *Canadian Medical Association Journal.* 185(1), E1–E2.

CTVNews Staff. (November 29, 2012). *Wait times persist for ER, primary care, report says.* Retrieved March 10, 2013 from http://www.ctvnews.ca/health/wait-times-persist-for-er-primary-care-report-says-1.1059343

de Jong, M. (BC Minister of Health). (February 2012). Ministry of Health 2012/13–2014/15 Service Plan. Retrieved October 5, 2012 from http://www.bcbudget.gov.bc.ca/2012/sp/pdf/ministry/hlth.pdf

Economist, The, (March 29, 2014). Obamacare: Uphill all the way. *The Economist.* Retrieved May 8, 2014 from http://www.economist.com/news/united-states/21599786-deadline-signing-up-nears-obamacare-looks-precarious-uphill-all-way

Expatica. (2016). A guide to the French healthcare system. Expatica France. sRetrieved January 9, 2018 from https://www.expatica.com/fr/healthcare/french-healthcare-france-health-care-system_101166.html

InterNations. (2015). Living in Cuba? Retrieved January 9, 2018 from https://www.internations.org/cuba-expats/guide/life-in-cuba-15677/healthcare-and-education-in-cuba-2

Kendall, P. R. W. (2010). Investing in Prevention: Improving Health and Creating Sustainability. The Provincial Health Officer's Special Report. September, 2010. British Columbia. Office of the Provincial Health Officer.

Lalonde, M. (1974). A New Perspective On The Health Of Canadians. Ottawa: Health and Welfare Canada.

Lundberg, C. (January 27, 2014). $200 minus $200. Slate. Retrieved January 9, 2018 from http://www.slate.com/articles/business/dispatches_from_the_welfare_...ialized_medicine_vs_u_s_health_care_having_a_baby_in_paris_is.html

Makarenko, J. (April 1, 2007). Romanow commission on the future of health care: findings and recommendations. Mapleleafweb. Retrieved April 14, 2008 from http://www.mapleleafweb.com/features/romanow-commission-future-health-care-findings-and-recommendations

Mason, G. (February 17, 2015). How BC balanced its books. The Globe and Mail. Retrieved June 1, 2018 from https://www.theglobeandmail.com/news/british-columbia/how-bc-balanced-its-books-by-controlling-health-care-costs/article23042031/

Medical Services Commission. Payment Schedule. Medical Services Commission, British Columbia Ministry of Health. Retrieved October 5, 2012 from http://www.health.gov.bc.ca/msp/infoprac/physbilling/payschedule/index.html

Mikkonen, J., Raphael, D. (2010). Social determinants of health: The Canadian facts. Toronto: York University School of Health Policy and Management. ISBN 978-0-9683484-1-3.

O'Brien-Pallas, L., Tomblin, Murphy G., & Shamian, J. (2008). Final report: Understanding the costs and outcomes of nurses' turnover in Canadian hospitals. Final Report. Canadian Nurses Association. University of Toronto: Nursing Health Services Research Unit. Retrieved March 10, 2013 from http://cna-aiic.ca/~/media/cna/page-content/pdf-en/roi_nurse_turnover_2009_e.pdf

OECD (Organisation for Economic Co-operation and Development). (2012). OECD health data 2012—Frequently requested data. Retrieved March 10, 2013 from http://www.oecd.org/els/health-systems/oecdhealthdata2012-frequentlyrequesteddata.htm

OECD. (2013c). Health Data How does the United States compare. Retrieved May 4, 2014 from www.oecd.org/health/healthdata

OECD. (2013d). Health spending continues to stagnate, says OECD. Retrieved May 4, 2014 from http://www.oecd.org/els/health-systems/health-spending-continues-to-stagnate-says-oecd.htm

OECD. (2018). Health Statistics. Retrieved Retrieved June 1, 2018 from http://stats.oecd.org/Index.aspx?DataSetCode=SHA

Reed, G. (2018). Cuba's primary health care revolutions: 30 years on. Bulletin: World Health Organization. Retrieved January 9, 2018 from http://www.who.int/bulletin/volumes/86/5/08-030508/en/

Romanow, R. J. (2002). *Building on values: The future of health care in Canada*. Saskatoon: Commission on the Future of Health Care in Canada. Retrieved June 25, 2004 from www.healthcarecommission.ca

Rourke, J. (January 29, 2008). Increasing the number of rural physicians. *Canadian Medical Association Journal.* Retrieved April 14, 2008 from http://www.cmaj.ca/cgi/content/full/178/3/322

Squires, D., Anderson, C. (October 2015). U.S health care from a global perspective. The Commonwealth Fund. Retrieved June 5, 2018 from http://www.commonwealthfund.org/publications/issue-briefs/2015/oct/us-health-care-from-a-global-perspective

TeleSUR. (July 23, 2014). Healthcare systems in Canada, US and Cuba. Retrieved January 9, 2018 from https://www.telesurtv.net/english/telesuragenda/Healthcare-Systems-in-Canada-US-and-Cuba-20140723-0078.html

Vogel, L. (2017a). Canadians still waiting for timely access to care. *Canadian Medical Association Journal.* 189(9): E375-E376. Retrieved January 9, 2018 from http://www.cmaj.ca/content/189/9/E375

Vogel, L. (2017b). Nearly a third of tests and treatments are unnecessary: CIHI. *Canadian Medical Association Journal.* 189(16): E620-E621. Retrieved January 9, 2018 from http://www.cmaj.ca/content/189/16/E620

Wilson, D. M. & Kieser, D. M. (March, 1996). Values and Canadian health care: An Alberta exploration. *Nursing Ethics.* 3(1): 9–15.

15 Environment

Learning Objectives

By the time you have finished this chapter you should be able to

- Explain the concept of "spaceship Earth"
- Describe how alteration of Earth's physical environment impacts human health
- Identify five major domains of environmental impact
- Discuss human population and how it stresses global water, air, land, and energy resources from an "integrated systems" perspective
- Examine your own lifestyle and identify behavioural changes that would minimize the damage you cause Earth's environment

1 Overview

In this chapter we focus on the physical environment in which we humans live. We emphasize the interdependency of our relationship with the surrounding land, air, and water.

Indigenous cultures, which typically live in smallish tribes (of hundreds or thousands of people) close to the land and sea, usually have cultural and spiritual traditions with strong appreciation of and respect for the environment. "Modern" human society has tended to be more alienated. A reawakening of the connection between humans and the environment occurred around the middle of the 20th century in North America, Europe, and other developed countries. A seminal event was Rachel Carson's 1962 book *Silent Spring*, which documented the decline of North American songbird populations due to the insecticide DDT.

The exploration of space, including developing life-support systems for humans in space capsules and photographic images of Earth as a "blue bubble" floating in space, spawned the concept of "spaceship Earth." This concept recognized that, although Earth seems large to us as individual humans, it is finite, with finite amounts of land, air, water, food, energy, and other resources to support humans and other life. When we flush the toilet or take out the garbage, our waste seems to disappear, but of course it doesn't. It goes someplace else, where it may make conditions less livable for those there. In other words, we live on a small planet where everything is connected to everything else.

2 Water

2.1 Human requirement for water

Water is the most essential of the nutrients. If you don't drink any water (or other fluids such as tea, beer, soda, or fruit juice, which are all mostly water), you will die in a week or so.

Sweat is mostly water (plus a small amount of sodium and other minerals). If the temperature of our surroundings is too high or if we increase our physical activity level, the body sweats. Even at rest in moderate temperatures, the body loses water from the skin and especially from the moist membranes of the nose, mouth, airways, and lungs. Our blood is composed of water plus red and white blood cells and small amounts of glucose, sodium, and other molecules. The kidney filters the blood, returning most of the water to the blood vessels, but a portion of the water spills into the bladder and is excreted as urine. The body loses water every hour of the day, and we need to replace this water with the fluids we consume.

People need at least one litre of water a day to survive. Requirements are increased by heat, physical exertion, lactation (a mother producing milk for her nursing infant), and diarrhea. In addition to the several litres of water we may *consume* daily, we Canadians each *use* an average of hundreds more litres of water to wash dishes, wash clothes, shower or bathe, water lawns and gardens, and fill swimming pools.

2.2 Public water sources

Public drinking water is drawn from rivers, lakes, reservoirs (artificial lakes that are created by damming rivers), springs (places where underground water comes to the surface), and wells (holes drilled down to reach underground water).

What is the source of the tap water in *your* home?

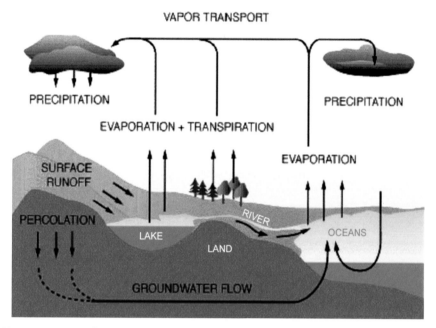

VAPOR TRANSPORT

PRECIPITATION

PRECIPITATION

EVAPORATION + TRANSPIRATION

EVAPORATION

SURFACE
RUNOFF

PERCOLATION

RIVER

OCEANS

LAKE

LAND

GROUNDWATER FLOW

Figure 15.1. In the water cycle, water circulates between atmospheric water vapour, precipitation such as rain and snow, surface water, and underground water.

Water evaporates from the surface of the earth: from the plants, the lakes, the oceans, and the ground itself. These water molecules go into the air, rise up, and collect in clouds. Eventually, water drops from the clouds as rain, snow, sleet, or hail. This water lands on the earth, where it soaks into the ground or runs downhill to collect in rivers, lakes, or oceans. This **water cycle** is illustrated in Figure 15.1.

Most parts of Canada have ample supplies of clean drinking water. This abundance has led many of us to take this water for granted. In Vancouver, for example, homeowners do not pay for the water they use. This isn't the same as saying the water is free. There are costs to build and maintain public water supply systems, costs that are factored into homeowners' property taxes. However, people are charged the same amount regardless of how much they use. It has been argued that it is less expensive for municipalities to allow this practice to continue than to install water meters and bill people for the amount they use. The result is that water appears to be free, and consequently people use water more extravagantly. Victoria, located in a region known for dry summers, meters homeowners' water and charges for the volume used. This is fairer, raises awareness of the cost (and value) of water, and promotes conservation.

2.3 *Water quality*

Sometimes public drinking water becomes contaminated—for example, with bacteria, often from human or animal feces, or with industrial chemicals, such as arsenic and mercury from the processes used to extract gold from the ore (rock) that is dug at gold mines. For the most part, though, tap water is no less healthy than bottled water. Some bottled water advertises that it is sourced from "pure glacial water" or "pure spring water." Some bottled water is drawn from exactly the same source as public drinking water.

> Do *you* drink bottled water or tap water? Why?

If you use a water bottle that you refill, there *is* a health issue. Repeated handling of the bottle, such as when you fill it or sip from it, can put pathogens such as bacteria into the bottle. At room temperature, these pathogens can multiply in the water. So it is a good idea to regularly—daily, if possible—empty, wash, and rinse water bottles, and allow them to dry completely before reusing.

There is a danger in the **commoditization** of water, which means viewing water as a commodity that is bought and sold rather than as a necessity for life to which all people should have a right. If the public perceives bottled water as *better* than tap water, then it will be more willing to pay for bottled water and less willing to pay for public water systems. Over time, decreased maintenance and expansion of public water systems would lead to a deterioration of public water. There is a similar issue regarding public versus private funding of health care (See Chapter 14: Health Care Delivery Systems).

> In addition to the issue of **commoditization,** there are other adverse environmental effects of drinking bottled water compared with tap water.
>
> Suggest two such effects.
>
> Hint: You will not find this answer directly in this text. You will need to think and apply concepts in this chapter to answer this question.

Agriculture accounts for 92% of humanity's **water footprint** (Shute, 2012). Meat production, especially beef, uses much more water per unit of nutritional value (for feed, drinking water, and maintenance) than production of vegetables, legumes, or cereals.

3 Air

A thick layer of gas forms an atmosphere that surrounds our planet. Without this atmosphere, we would die from lack of oxygen, be bombarded by deadly cosmic radiation, and experience daily extremes of temperature as the sun rose and set.

Humans breathe in and out an average of about 10 times a minute at rest and more frequently during heavy exertion. The lungs extract oxygen from the inspired air. Tiny hairs and the mucous coating on moist membranes in the nose, mouth, throat, and airways trap much of the dust and particulate matter, acting as a filter to protect the delicate tissues of the lungs.

We breathe out carbon dioxide as one of the waste products of our metabolism. Thus, we each "pollute" the air with our basic life processes. For millions of years, the burden of human pollution on Earth's atmosphere was relatively small. This has changed over the last century or so as global population has increased dramatically (Figure 5.2) and as human industrial activity has intensified. The air has become increasingly polluted with many different chemicals.

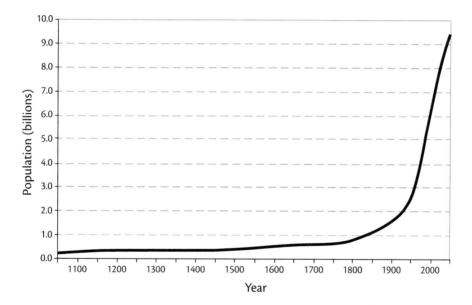

Figure 15.2. In 1800, Earth was home to less than one billion people. By 1900, this figure had doubled. In 2011, this number reached seven billion.

3.1 *Smog*

This compound (smoke plus fog) forms when sunlight reacts with nitrogen oxides and volatile organic compounds in the atmosphere. This results in a brownish haze. Smog occurs in all modern cities. It is more common in cities with lots of motor vehicles; in dry, warm, sunny areas; and in regions where hills or mountains reduce air circulation (think Los Angeles, or Vancouver after a week in the summer without rain).

3.2 *Acid rain*

This is produced when the gases **sulfur dioxide** and **nitrogen oxide** are washed out of the air and return to the earth as an acidic liquid. In Canada, the major sources of sulfur dioxide emissions are non-ferrous **metal smelters** (i.e., smelters for metals other than iron or steel), followed by **coal-fired power plants** (see the Energy section later in this chapter). Motor vehicles and, to a lesser extent, coal-fired power plants, are the major sources of nitrogen oxides (Environment Canada, 2012). Thousands of lakes in Canada and the northeastern USA have been affected by acid rain.

> Many species of fish, insects, aquatic plants and bacteria develop reproduction difficulties. Some even die. The decline in the population of any of these aquatic organisms affects the food chain. Dwindling populations of insects and small aquatic plants and animals are especially serious because the entire food chain is affected. (Environment Canada, 2012)

3.3 *Climate change*

Perhaps the most ominous air pollution issue humans currently face is climate change. **Weather** refers to the current state of the atmosphere (e.g., whether it is hot or cold, wet or dry, windy or still). **Climate** describes the typical variation in weather for a particular region, which is a function of that region's elevation, proximity to oceans and mountains, distance from the equator, and so on. For example, Calgary's prairie-type climate features hot summers and cold winters, with little rainfall throughout the year. Vancouver's oceanic or marine climate has more moderate temperatures and more rainfall, especially in winter. Conditions in any specific climatic zone vary from year to year, producing, for example, "the coldest year on record" or "above-average rainfall."

Over tens of thousands of years of history, the temperature of the Earth has fluctuated. There were times when tropical seas covered much of the planet. Other eras had ice ages and glacial periods. The last glacial period ended about 10,000 years ago. These temperature changes were caused by natural phenomena.

Virtually all atmospheric scientists agree that Earth is now experiencing a long-term change in climate, and this change is caused by human activity.

One symptom of climate change is **global warming**, caused by increased levels of *greenhouse gases* that trap some of the sun's energy in Earth's atmosphere, warming it like the air inside of a glass greenhouse or a closed car parked outside on a sunny day. **Carbon dioxide** is the major greenhouse gas. It is produced when gasoline is burned in motor vehicles, when oil is burned in thermal electrical generating plants, when forests are cleared to create land for crops or grazing animals, and when heavy oil or tar is dug from the huge deposits of sand in northern Canada. The bowels of cattle release **methane**, another greenhouse gas, and another negative impact of meat-eating on global health.

> Think about *your* lifestyle and the lifestyle of other people like you.
>   Assess the ways in which you produce, directly and indirectly, greenhouse gases.
>   Now, imagine that it was *critical* for you and your friends to cut in half the amount of greenhouse gas you each produce in a year. List at least six specific things you could do to meet this goal.

Environmental scientists estimate that greenhouse gas levels have increased the average temperature of the Earth by a couple of degrees centigrade over the last century or so. This may not seem like much, but it is, especially because it is quite a rapid change. Increasingly the debate has shifted from "Is global warming happening?" to "What are the consequences of global warming?" and "How can we deal with this?"

One likely consequence is melting of the ice sheets at the North and South Poles. This interferes with animal life (e.g., polar bear migration) and the livelihood of those who hunt these animals. Since ice normally *reflects* much of the sun's energy, the loss of polar ice accelerates the rate of global warming. Melting ice raises global ocean levels, which threatens to flood the many millions of people worldwide whose dwellings are within a couple of metres of current sea level.

Some parts of the globe will see hotter and drier conditions, while others will experience more rainfall. These changes will hurt crops, which could make it harder to feed the global population. Some parts of the world (e.g., Yemen and other countries in the Middle East; North Africa; northern Chile) are already very dry and have limited capacity to adapt to even drier conditions. For example, Chile has greatly expanded commercial agriculture in recent decades, growing grapes, avocados, and lemons for export. Much of this growth has been supported by irrigation from the many rivers that flow west from glaciers and snow packs in the tall Andes. As conditions become warmer and drier, more of the snow and ice is melting and less of it is forming (Salas et al., 2012). Some major rivers have already dried up completely. If this trend continues, where will the water to irrigate the crops come from?

4 Land
4.1 *Land as a place to live*
From a human point of view, land represents habitable space, a refuge from the remaining three-quarters of Earth's surface that is covered by water. Of

course, a multitude of species of other animals and plants are also terrestrial (land-living). Collectively, all living things create a **biosphere**, a complex web of life. In biological systems, diversity equates with stability; if one element of the system is harmed (e.g., if disease kills one species of plant), other elements compensate for this change.

4.2 Land to produce food

In addition to a place to live, the land provides food. From our origins as hunter-gatherers, humans learned how to grow crops and how to domesticate animals. These developments gave a measure of security to the human food supply; dried grain and salted, smoked, or dried meat and cheese keep for months to years. These agricultural advances allowed (and to a sense, required) humans to transition from nomadic to more settled lives, and led to the formation and growth of cities. City life promoted non-agricultural occupations (e.g., shoe-making, pottery, carpentry) and the commercial trading of goods and services.

In recent centuries, many humans have become increasingly distanced from the production of food. For example, I produce very little of my own food. Instead, I work as a teacher, and I use a portion of my salary to buy food produced by others. According to Statistics Canada (2006) in 1931, the first year the farm population was counted, 32% of the Canadian population lived on farms. By 2006, this had shrunk to 2.2%. Many fewer Canadians farm, and the average farm is much larger.

4.2.1 Small-scale farming

In traditional, small-scale, "peasant" agriculture, a variety of crops, such as beans, tomatoes, squash, and corn, are grown on small patches of land. This provides the variety of nutrients needed to feed the farmer's family. Nitrogen can be added to the soil by composting leaves and stems from last year's crop. Microbes in the soil accelerate the breakdown of this material and convert the minerals it contains into a form that is easier for the plant roots to absorb. Since one type of crop takes more of one type of mineral while other crops take different minerals, crops are rotated from one part of the land to another, which minimizes soil depletion. Certain crops, such as alfalfa or clover, are grown in order to **fix** the nitrogen in the soil, and then this crop is ploughed into the soil, enriching it with nitrogen. In addition, typically a part of the land is left **fallow** (unplanted) each year, which provides a rest for the soil to replenish its nutrients. Small farmers can handle pest control by planting specific pest-repellant plants (e.g., marigold flowers) and providing habitat for bug-eating birds and frogs.

4.2.2 *Large-scale farming*

In the last couple of centuries, commercial agriculture expanded greatly in scale. Farms and plantations of hundreds and thousands of hectares each were planted with a single crop, such as sugar cane, cotton, wheat, and corn (a hectare is a measure of land area). **Agribusiness** has capitalized on economies of scale. For example, seeds cost less per kilogram if you buy them for 1,000 hectares than for 10 hectares. When you have 1,000 hectares to cultivate, it is cheaper to buy a tractor and pay one person to drive it than it is to pay 10 people to cultivate it by hand. Around the 1950s, scientists discovered new high-yield varieties of grains, crops that produced more bushels of grain per hectare. At first, this **Green Revolution** seemed like a great thing: more food = less hunger. However, there are inherent problems with agribusiness:

- Large-scale high-technology agriculture works best with large inputs of synthetic fertilizers, petroleum-based pesticides and herbicides, and petroleum-fueled machinery. This makes it **energy intensive**.
- **Monoculture** (growing the same crop repeatedly on the same soil) depletes soil nutrients. For example, cotton uses a lot of the mineral boron. After several years of growing crop after crop of just cotton, the soil becomes boron deficient.
- Monoculture, by definition, reduces **biodiversity**. This makes the system more vulnerable to catastrophic damage from disease, insects, and weather extremes such as heat, drought, or flood.
- Agribusiness is **capital intensive**. You need lots of cash or big bank loans to fund start-up costs. Banks are reluctant to loan to low-income people without a credit history or collateral to secure the loan.
- The rich got richer. The poor got poorer, and were displaced from the land (because less human labour is needed with mechanized agriculture). They moved to cities, where many remained unemployed (lacking skills needed for city jobs) and lived in marginal shanty towns, often without electricity, running water, or sewers.
- The surge in agricultural productivity **flooded global markets**, driving down grain prices. Here in Canada, this led to the virtual demise of the independent family farm. In less developed countries, governments borrowed heavily to subsidize agribusiness but did not earn back enough to pay off the loans, which left these countries saddled with huge international debt and the associated cost of interest payments to service this **debt**.

4.2.3 A return to sanity?

Recently, there has been some useful reaction to the problems described above:

- The **100 Mile Diet** advocates consumption of locally produced food.
- Canadians appear more interested in shopping at **farmer's markets**.
- The Lawns to Loaves movement encourages homeowners to **replace their lawns** with trees and plants that produce food.
- Awareness of **local food security** has increased. It may be less expensive to buy tomatoes grown in Mexico and trucked to Canada, but this lower price is the result of a failure to fully account for costs, or **economic externalities**. For example, the grower in Mexico pays his workers much less than Canadian workers, and the workers have harsher and more unsafe working and living conditions. The workers get sick, which causes them medical expenses, expenses not included in the price of the tomatoes. The grower waters the tomatoes with water drawn from the Colorado River system, a system so overloaded by agricultural and residential expansion in the American Southwest that groundwater levels are dropping alarmingly. The cost of groundwater depletion is not included in the price of the tomatoes. The shipper's trucks exhaust carbon dioxide, particulates, and other pollutants into the air. The cost of air pollution is not included in the price of the tomatoes.

The most important take-home message from the preceding section (and this whole chapter) is that systems—bio-systems, ecosystems, socio-economic systems, and so on—are often **complex** and **highly integrated** (meaning lots of little pieces fit together and affect each other); that it is often **hard to predict** accurately the **consequences of manipulating the system**; and that such manipulations can have effects opposite to those intended.

> The next time *you* go shopping, notice what food items you purchase.
> Where were they each produced?
> What substitutions could you make to live on a 100 Mile Diet?

4.3 Land pollution

4.3.1 Dumping

Finally, we'll look at land pollution. The land can be contaminated in several different ways. The first is dumping of garbage or refuse (these words are sometimes used interchangeably; to me "garbage" contains organic material that can rot and could have been composted, while "refuse" is dry material, such as packaging, used automobile tires, and wood and glass from demolished houses). In rural areas with large acreages, landowners may create a dump in a less-conspicuous part of their property. As population density increases, people become unable to dump on their own small properties, and it's not cool to dump on someone else's property, or on public land such as a park or schoolyard. Thus, public garbage-collection systems tend to emerge. Typically, trucks collect garbage, which they bring to a transfer station, where bulldozers crush and push around mounds of garbage.

In addition to **municipal** collection and dumping, dumping also occurs at the **industrial** level. For example, an automobile manufacturer in New Jersey dumped industrial-sized containers of unwanted paint for years on wooded land it owned. An even more widely know example of this type of land pollution occurred at Love Canal, in upper New York state. This former industrial site was redeveloped as residential housing. It was not long before toxic waste the corporation had buried began leaking out of the ground and into the local water. Such sites are often very difficult and expensive to clean up, and the cost burden may fall on government, especially if the polluting company has since gone out of business.

Increasingly, municipal garbage and refuse are sorted, either by the resident before putting it out at the curbside for collection, or at the transfer station. For example, used refrigerators and other large appliances are stacked together and later recycled as scrap steel. Branches, leaves, and other garden debris are shredded and composted. Cardboard and paper are bundled and trucked to paper mills, where the paper fibres are extracted and used to make recycled paper. Eventually, the material that isn't recycled gets loaded on trucks and driven to **landfills**, where it is dumped.

Landfills "solve" the problem of disposing of unwanted stuff, but they present a couple of other problems. First, they take up space. For example, the City of Vancouver doesn't have enough available land for a landfill. Some Vancouver refuse goes to a regional disposal site in the municipality of Delta, while the rest is trucked to Cache Creek, hours north and east of the city. Second, material dumped in landfills doesn't all stay there. For example, boxes of discarded batteries decompose, and heavy metals that were inside the batteries, such as lead and cadmium, leak out into the ground. From there, these metals can slowly trickle or flow downhill and eventually enter water systems. Then plants or animals take up these heavy metals when they take in water.

Other countries (e.g., The Netherlands) have more advanced recycling programs than those in Canada. Increasingly, legislation makes the manufacturers of products such as electronics and appliances responsible for receiving these products at the end of their life cycle, to extract and reuse materials where possible, and otherwise to responsibly dispose of them.

> Think about the things *you* dispose of in an average week: scrap paper, beverage containers, packaging from consumer goods, food scraps, and so on.
>
> Now, apply the "reduce, reuse, recycle" concept to your disposal habits and list specific ways in which you could reduce the amount of material you add to municipal landfills (garbage dumps).

4.3.2 Runoff

A second way the land can become polluted is runoff. Farmers use chemicals to nourish their crops and to control weeds and insect pests. When it rains, some of the chemical residue washes off the plants and into the ground. Gravitational force pulls water downhill, and eventually the water, and the chemicals it contains, can re-enter the biosphere at places sometimes quite remote from their origin.

4.3.3 Fallout

Fallout involves material falling from the air and landing on the ground. Acid rain, mentioned in Section 3: Air, provides an example. Accidents at nuclear power plants—such as the ones at Chernobyl, Ukraine, and more recently, Fukushima, Japan—produce radioactive fallout. Radioactive atoms, such as iodine-131 or strontium-90, rise high into the air over the accident site, and then the wind can carry them thousands of kilometres. These radioactive particles eventually fall to earth, where they may land on crops and be eaten by dairy cows, which concentrate these elements in their tissues and in their milk, which would expose human milk-drinkers to the radiation.

> How does urban planning affect air, water, and land pollution?
>
> Be specific. For example, "zoning that encourages conversion of farm land to suburban housing means food has to be transported to urban and suburban residents from further away, which increases the burning of fossil fuels in cars, trucks, and trains, which in turn pollutes the air with more nitrogen dioxide and carbon dioxide."

5 Energy

Energy is defined as "the ability to do work, to move a force though a distance." In earlier chapters, we considered the energy we take in from food, the energy expended in physical activity, and the excess energy stored as body fat and resultant weight gain. In this section we look at non-food energy use by humans and its environmental impact.

Like air and water, energy seems so abundant and inexpensive we often take it for granted. To light a room, we flip a switch. To operate an appliance, we plug it into the wall. To drive a car, we turn a key, and only periodically fill the tank with more gasoline. To warm our home, we push a couple of buttons on the wall thermostat.

5.1 Electricity

As with water and food, modern energy needs are supplied (especially to urban dwellers, who represent an increasing portion of the global population) by an extensive distribution system. Electricity is a convenient medium for distributing energy, and it is "clean" at the point of consumption. A fire produces heat and light but also makes carbon dioxide, carbon monoxide, soot (dirty particles that collect on walls and inside chimneys) and other pollution. None of this happens when we flip an electric switch at home. But where does the electricity *come from*?

> Why do *you* think people tend to use more of something, such as water, when it's free, or at least very inexpensive? (For example, in British Columbia electricity costs about six cents to operate a 100-watt light bulb for 10 hours.)

There are three common ways to generate electricity commercially: hydro, nuclear, and thermal.

5.1.1 Hydroelectricity

Hydroelectricity uses the force of falling water—usually water captured in a reservoir by building a dam across a river—to turn giant turbines (Figure 15.3). Turbines look sort of like boat propellers, except instead of the propeller turning and its blades pushing the water, the water pushes the blades of the turbine. The main environmental impacts of hydroelectric projects are that they flood large areas of land, rendering it useless for terrestrial habitation, agriculture, and forestry. Dams also change the amount, temperature, oxygen content, sediment level, and nutrient level of the water that flows into the river downstream from the dam.

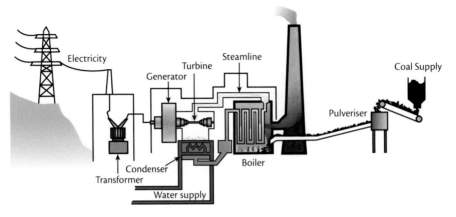

Thermal Power Plant

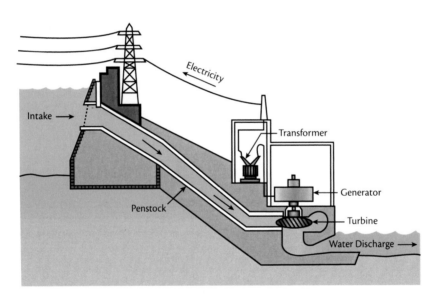

Hydroelectric Power plant

Figure 15.3. Both thermal and hydro power plants use a rotating turbine to generate electricity.

5.1.2 Nuclear reactors

These also produce electricity by causing turbines to rotate. In this case, steam provides the turning force. The steam comes from water that is heated by a (hopefully) controlled decomposition of radioactive material, such as uranium or plutonium, in the reactor core. The main environmental risks of nuclear power concern radiation: acute high doses cause rapid death; lower exposures can cause birth defects, infertility, and cancer. The 2011 failure of a nuclear reactor in Fukushima, Japan, following an earthquake and tsunami (tidal wave) raised public awareness of the dangers of catastrophic radioactive leaks. Radiation can also escape during uranium mining and processing. Workers in these industries have elevated risk of lung cancer.

A less well-recognized problem is the disposal of used radioactive material from normal reactor operation. The radioactive material decomposes to a level where it is not commercially viable, and is replaced. However, the spent reactor material is not completely decomposed, and it continues to emit radioactivity for thousands of years. To date, disposal methods have included sealing the radioactive materials in (we hope) secure containers and burying them deep underground. Will there be a rail or truck accident during transport? Will an earthquake disrupt a burial site? It is impossible to guarantee safety for thousands of years.

5.1.3 *Thermal power plants*

These work like nuclear plants in that they heat water and use steam to turn turbines, and the turning turbines generate electricity (Figure 15.3). In thermal plants, the energy to heat water comes from burning coal, natural gas, or petroleum (oil). These are all **fossil fuels**. Trees and plants take carbon dioxide from air and use energy from sunlight to create carbon bonds that store energy. This energy is released when the plants are burned or when they are eaten and digested by animals. Hundreds of millions of years ago, plants died and were buried in the earth. Over time, their carbon energy became more and more concentrated and formed the materials we call coal, natural gas, and petroleum.

There are four main environmental problems with thermal power plants:

- The extraction and burning of fossil fuels produce **greenhouse gases**, which contribute to global warming.
- If they burn fossil fuel with high sulfur content, they emit **sulfur oxides**, which contribute to acid rain.
- Transportation of the fossil fuel to the power plant poses the risk of a **spill**. Spilled coal is easy to clean up. Spilled natural gas may explode and cause serious damage locally. Petroleum (oil) is the most problematic. It is transported by bulk in pipelines, which go across rivers and other vulnerable ecosystems. When an oil pipeline develops a leak, it may be hours or days before the leak is detected and fixed, during which large quantities of oil are spilled onto the ground or into the water.

- Fossil fuels are **non-renewable**. It took millions of years to form them, and we are using them up very much more rapidly than the rate at which new fossil fuels are being formed.

5.2 *Alternative energy*

Other options for commercial generation of electricity to date represent a small fraction of total global human energy use. However, the environmental and economic problems with the three main methods described above have increased interest in **alternative energy** sources. These include

- **Solar power:** A huge amount of energy reaches Earth from the Sun every hour. This can be captured with solar panels mounted on the ground, on buildings, and perhaps even on cars and airplanes. Solar panels allow energy to be captured locally. Solar energy can be used to charge electric batteries to power lights or appliances, and to heat water for bathing and washing.

- **Wind power:** The windmill is an old idea; the force of the wind turns propeller blades, and gears convert this turning action into movement that will grind grain, raise water from wells, or do other work. In recent decades, wind turbines have been used to generate electricity. Typically, these turbines are large and mounted about 100 m above the ground. There is a growing suspicion that vibrations produced by the wind turbines may harm human health.

    Wind turbines also pose a threat to migrating bats and birds. For example, "the Spanish Ornithological Society in Madrid estimates that Spain's 18,000 wind turbines may be killing 6 million to 18 million birds and bats annually" (Subramanian, 2012). As huge as this number sounds, wind turbines seem to kill many fewer birds overall than other hazards such as communication towers, power lines, buildings, automobiles, agricultural pesticides, and cats. However, turbines threaten species that are *already* struggling, such as bats and eagles. Also, turbines are killing some at-risk species that tend not to fall victim to the other hazards mentioned above.

- **Wave action:** The up-and-down action of waves and the back-and-forth motion of tides represent mechanical energy. Clever devices have been invented that can be anchored offshore to convert this mechanical energy to electrical energy. This field appears to be still in the early stages of development.

6 Population

It's hard to pick a "worst environmental problem." As we are discovering, things are connected. At the root of many environmental problems is global population shifts. In this section, we will explore some of these trends and their implications for the physical and social environment.

6.1 *Population stresses on resources*

People consume oxygen, water, and food. They occupy space. They produce carbon dioxide and other waste products. They use petroleum, wood, metal, and other materials. People stress Earth's environment ... but some individuals stress it much more than others. This is the concept of **carbon footprint**. Imagine yourself standing barefoot on damp sand. When you step away, you can see that you have left a footprint in the sand. Basic human life functions consume oxygen and produce carbon dioxide. Other activities, such as heating our homes in winter, expand our carbon footprint. Meat-eaters have a bigger carbon footprint than vegetarians because grazing land absorbs less carbon than forest does, the animals use food energy, and the animals emit greenhouse gases from their lungs and digestive systems. If you own 10 shirts, you are responsible for more carbon than if you own four shirts. Driving a motor vehicle expands your carbon footprint compared with taking the bus or train, or carpooling. Air travel spreads your carbon footprint even more.

There are two basic population factors that stress the environment:

- How many people are on the planet?
- How conservative or extravagant is each person's lifestyle?

A number of free carbon footprint calculators are available on the Internet, for example, at the following websites:

- https://treecanada.ca/reforestation-carbon-offsetting/carbon-offsetting/carbon-calculator/ (sponsored by Tree Canada, a registered charity that plants and nurtures trees)
- www.nature.org/greenliving/carboncalculator/index.htm (sponsored by The Nature Conservancy, a large non-profit society that seems to be based in the USA)
- www.carbonfootprint.com/calculator.aspx (sponsored by Carbon Footprint Ltd, an environmental consulting company in the UK

I used the Nature Conservancy calculator to compare the footprints of two hypothetical couples, each living in Washington state (Canadian provinces are not included in this calculator).

Couple A lives in a one-bedroom apartment in a building with more than five units. They use efficient home lighting, heating, and appliances. They do not own a vehicle and have not taken any airplane trips in the past year. They recycle paper, bottles, and so on but do not compost kitchen scraps. They eat meat most days but not at every meal, and eat organic food sometimes. The calculator estimates their total annual greenhouse gas emissions at the equivalent of 11 tons of CO_2 (carbon dioxide)—right at the world average impact for two people, and much less than the 53 tons of an average US couple.

Couple B lives in a two-bedroom house. They do not use efficient home lighting, heating, or appliances. They own one small vehicle, which they drive 24,000 km (15,000 mi.) per year. In the past year, they took one long and one short airplane flight. They don't recycle or compost. They eat meat at most meals and rarely eat organic food. The calculator scores them at 40 tons of CO_2 annually—almost four times as much as Couple A.

> Why does living in an apartment have a smaller carbon footprint than living in a house?
>
> Why does living in an apartment in a building with more than five units have a lower carbon footprint than living in the same apartment in a building with fewer units?

6.2 Population dynamics

People are born, live, and die. The number of people on the planet at the end of each year equals the number who were alive at the beginning of the year plus those who were born that year, minus those who died that year. Thus, **fertility rate** (number of births per population, usually per 100,000) and **mortality rate** (number of deaths per population, again usually per 100,000) are key factors in the population equation.

Globally, in the 1970–1975 period, **life expectancy** at birth averaged 56 and 60 years for males and females, respectively. Those born forty years later (2010–2015) can expect to live 13 years longer (United Nations Population Fund, 2017).

World population has almost doubled in the last 50 years. In 1970, global population was 3.7 billion. In 2000 it reached 6.1 billion, and by 2012 it was 7 billion (United Nations, 2013). In 2018, it exceeded 7.6 billion (Worlometers, 2018).

The world population grew by 1.2% annually in the 2010–2015 period. This average masks large regional differences. North America and Europe grew at only 0.8% and 0.1%, respectively. Latin America and Asia each experienced growth of 1.1%, while the growth rate in Africa was 2.6% (United Nations Population Fund, 2017).

6.3 *How development affects mortality and fertility*

An interesting phenomenon has occurred in various parts of the world as they have transitioned from **agricultural** to **industrial** society, and then transitioned further into post-industrial **information economies** in countries such as Canada. In agricultural societies, most of the population live in small villages and practise mostly subsistence agriculture. People grow most of their own food and sell or trade some cash crops for shoes, sugar, salt, and the other things they do not produce themselves. The peasant's main asset is her labour, and that of her family. The benefits of children as a source of labour outweigh the costs of children. Not surprisingly then, birth rates tend to be high. The standard of living is low: housing is crowded and may be dirty, hot, cold, damp, or drafty. Children are under-nourished. Drinking water may be contaminated with pathogens. Complete vaccination against infectious disease is uncommon. Consequently, **child mortality rates** are also high (Table 15.1).

Table 15.1
Child Mortality Rates (Deaths Under Age Five per 1,000 Live Births)

Location	1990	2011
World	87	51
Sub-Saharan Africa	178	109
South Asia	119	62
Middle East and North Africa	72	36
Eastern Asia and the Pacific	85	20
Latin America and the Caribbean	53	19
Central and Eastern Europe and Commonwealth of Independent States	48	21

Source: United Nations Population Division, 2017.

When the society develops somewhat, the picture changes. Improvements in public health (sanitation, nutrition, vaccination) reduce mortality rates, especially infant mortality. More people live to childbearing age. Large families are still the norm. Thus, for a couple of generations the population "explodes." The population profile of such a country is pyramidal (see Figure 15.4), with young people constituting a large portion of the population.

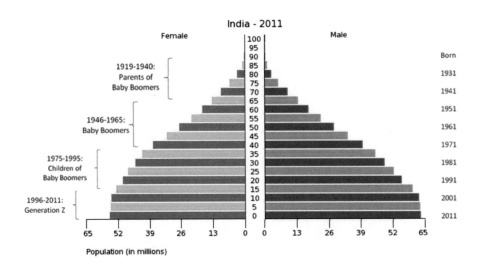

Figure 15.4. India's population profile resembles a pyramid, with a wide base and a narrow top. This pattern, typical of developing countries, means a large fraction of the population is young.

As the society transitions further from its agricultural roots, other changes occur. More children attend school and stay in school longer. People move to towns and cities, where they work for wages and buy their food rather than grow it themselves. They probably rent an apartment or home rather than owning a shack in the countryside. They have access to electrical appliances, such as radios and refrigerators, which enhance their perceived quality of life. They rely more on government and less on their children for social security. The economic benefits of having large families go down. The costs go up: rent, food, school supplies, and with further economic development, the "right" clothes and hairstyles, automobiles, ballet lessons, cell phones, and so on.

In addition, society tends to become more pluralistic (i.e., more than one set of political and religious beliefs are tolerated) and liberal. Contraception becomes more available. Other options for women become more numerous: advanced education, political office, and work outside the home in traditional and non-traditional careers. Women marry at a later age and delay starting a family. Some women choose to live independently from men or to have no children. Collectively, the result is that the fertility rate goes down. This balances the lower mortality rate experienced a couple of generations earlier. The population stabilizes at a new, higher level. The population profile at this stage looks more rectangular (Figure 15.5).

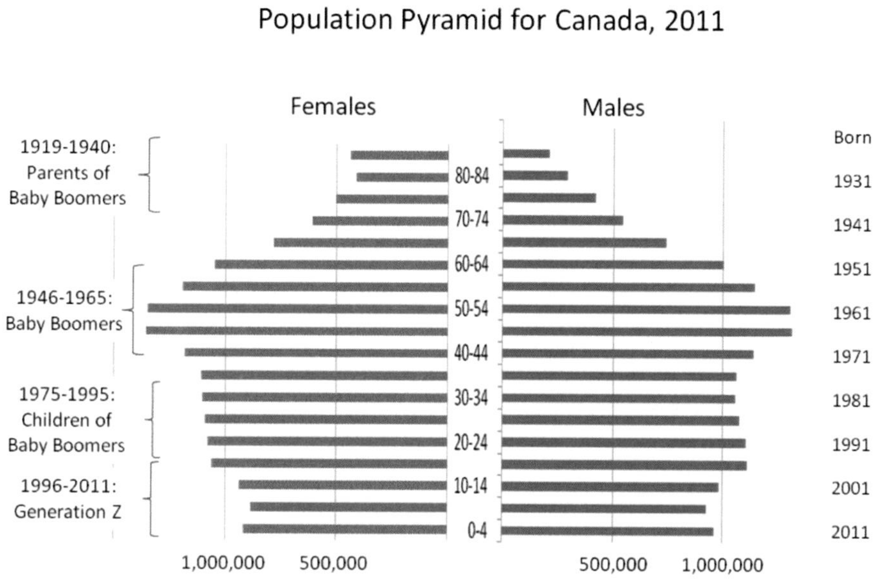

Population Pyramid for Canada, 2011

Figure 15.5. Canada's population profile, 2011.

Like other developed countries with proportionally fewer young people and more old people, Canada's population profile looks less like a triangle and more like a rectangle. A "baby boom" occurred in the years following the end of World War II. These baby boomers, now in their sixties and seventies, create a bulge in the population profile.

There are three main take-home messages in this **demographic transition**:

- It takes a couple of generations for the effect to become fully realized, during which time the population increases rapidly.
- The changes in fertility occur *spontaneously*, independent of any political messaging to have fewer children.
- An approach that emphasizes comprehensive social, political, and economic development will likely have more powerful and more rapid effects on population control than more narrowly focused **family planning** programs.

> Imagine that *you* were the new leader of a developing country.
>
> You have huge popular support and lots of money to use (maybe you have a personal fortune, or maybe your country has valuable resources such as oil or diamonds).
>
> Your main priority is to slow your country's population growth rate.
>
> Outline your strategy.

7 Conclusion

In this chapter we have taken a big-picture look at some major environmental issues facing the world today. Instead of details of atmospheric science or environmental toxicology, we leave with four simple messages:

- We are enmeshed with, not separate from, our environment.
- We are in this together.
- You can make a difference.
- We don't have to go back to living in caves. Many small changes, such as turning off lights when you leave a room, can add up to big results.

Study Questions

1. Explain in your own words the concept of "spaceship Earth."
2. Which one of the essential nutrients is most essential? Why?
3. Why is the water cycle labelled a cycle?
4. Each Canadian uses on average hundreds of litres of water per day. However, the human stomach will only hold a couple of litres when it is full. Explain this apparent contradiction.
5. What does the City of Victoria do to promote water conservation that the City of Vancouver does not do?
6. What can you do to avoid getting sick if you use a water bottle you refill?
7a. Which is the major greenhouse gas?
7b. What generates this gas?
8. Describe the likely adverse effects of climate change.
9. Discuss the adverse social, economic, and environmental problems with agribusiness (large-scale commercial farming).
10. In your own words, explain the concept of "economic externalities."
11. What are three major ways in which land can be contaminated?
12a. What are the three ways that electricity is most commonly generated commercially?
12b. Explain briefly the adverse environmental consequences of each method.
13a. Explain in your own words the concept of "carbon footprint."
13b. Imagine your peers (i.e., other people like you). What are they currently doing that helps minimize adverse effects on the environment?
13c. List 10 *other* simple things they could do to further reduce their environmental impact.
14. According to the author, what is the most fundamental of the six environmental issues discussed?
15a. Explain how (and why) fertility and mortality rates change with the transition from agricultural to industrial society.

15b. What are the three main take-home messages in this transition phenomenon?

16. What four simple messages are given in the Conclusion of this chapter?

Glossary

acid rain—precipitation that is more acidic than normal water because the precipitation combines with atmospheric pollutants

greenhouse gases—gases such as carbon dioxide that act to trap more of the sun's energy within Earth's atmosphere, causing global temperature to rise

smog—a "smoky fog," or brownish haze, formed by the reaction of sunlight with nitrogen oxides and volatile organic compounds in the atmosphere

References

Beun-Chown, J. (2007). Canada's healthiest city. *Canadian Living.* Retrieved January 12, 2013 from http://www.canadianliving.com/health/prevention/canadas_healthiest_city.php

Environment Canada. (2012). *Acid rain.* Retrieved February 8, 2013 from http://www.ec.gc.ca/eau-water/default.asp?lang=En&n=FDF30C16-1

Harris, M. (n.d.). *Health tap.* Retrieved January 21, 2013 from https://www.healthtap.com/topics/human-cell-regeneration

Macrae, F. (February 28, 2012). You CAN live forever … as long as you are a flatworm, scientists say. *Daily Mail Online.* Retrieved January 21, 2013 from http://www.dailymail.co.uk/sciencetech/article-2107236/You-CAN-live-forever--long-flatworm-say-scientists.html

Salas, S., Jiminez, E., Montna, E., Garay-Fluhmann, R., Gauthier, D., Diaż, H. P. (2012). *Vulnerabilidad al cambio climatico.* Instituto Interamericano para la investigacion del Cambio Global in collaboration with Universidad de La Serena, Chile and University of Regina, Canada. ISBN 978-956-351-091-1.

Shute, N. (September, 2012). Precious water. *National Geographic.* p. 28.

Statistics Canada. (2006). *Canada's farm population: Agriculture-population linkage data for the 2006 census.* Retrieved February 7, 2013 from http://www.statcan.gc.ca/ca-ra2006/agpop/article-eng.htm

Statistics Canada. (2012). *Life expectancy, at birth and at age 65, by sex and by province and territory.* Retrieved January 12, 2013 from http://www.statcan.gc.ca/tables-tableaux/sum-som/l01/cst01/health72a-eng.htm

Subramanian, M. (June 20, 2012). The trouble with turbines: An ill wind. *Nature.* 486(7403) Retrieved May 10, 2014 from http://www.nature.com/news/the-trouble-with-turbines-an-ill-wind-1.10849

UNICEF. (2012). *Committing to child survival: A promise renewed.* Progress Report 2012. Division of Policy and Strategy. Retrieved July 31, 2014 from http://www.unicef.org/lac/Committing_to_Child_Survival_APR_9_Sept_2013.pdf

United Nations. (2013). *Demographic yearbook 2012*. ST/ESA/STAT/SER.R/42. Department of Economic and Social Affairs. New York. ISBN 978-92-1-051106-3.

United Nations Population Division. (2017). *World Population Prospects 2017*. Retrieved June 5, 2018 from https://esa.un.org/unpd/wpp/Download/Standard/Mortality

Wang, H. et al. (December 15, 2012). Age-specific and sex-specific mortality in 187 countries, 1970–2010: A systematic analysis for the Global Burden of Disease Study 2010. *The Lancet*. 380(9859), 2071–2094.

Worlometers. (2018). World Population Clock. Retrieved June 5, 2018 from http://www.worldometers.info/world-population/

Index

1-inch heels 159
100 Mile Diet 378
2015 Canadian Community Health
　Survey 137–138

A
Abdominal obesity 160–162
abortion rates 265, 286, 295, 297
abortions in clinics 288
Abstinence 270–271
accelerometer 110
acid rain 374, 380, 391
aerobic fitness 13, 64, 109, 112–113, 120,
　127, 184
Aerobic Fitness 118
age-standardized incidence rate (ASIR)
　84
age-standardized mortality rates 84
agriculture 135, 145, 154–155, 372,
　375–377, 381, 387, 391
AHCA Repeal and replacement 353
AIDS. *See* HIV/AIDS
alcohol 6, 8, 12, 13, 22, 23, 40, 65, 67, 92,
　103, 138, 139, 175, 199, 202, 205, 224,
　231, 233, 257, 259, 293, 313, 314, 317,
　317–320, 320, 323, 325, 326, 328, 329,
　331, 333–339
Americans and health insurance
　350–353
American teen pregnancy rates 295
amino acids 133, 153

anal intercourse 227, 243, 258, 259
anecdotal evidence 19, 29
anemia 142, 153, 277, 304
anorexia nervosa 170, 171, 179, 180, 181
antibiotic 49, 150
antibodies 42, 43, 54, 55, 240, 241, 250,
　251, 261
antibody 54, 101, 241, 247
antimicrobial agents 49
antioxidant 65, 133, 143, 144, 149, 304
antiretroviral drugs 241, 247, 263
anxiety disorders 187–189
arteriosclerosis 61, 62, 78
artery 20, 60, 61, 64–66, 74, 75, 78, 79,
　356
association vs. causation 27–28
atherosclerosis 59, 60, 61, 68, 77, 78, 183,
　224
autonomic nervous system 183, 193, 206

B
bacteria 25, 41, 45, 48, 49, 54, 55, 146,
　149, 150, 227, 372, 374
BC and free HIV/AIDS blood tests 250
BCMA 341, 346–348, 364
benign 87, 94, 104, 105, 333
"Berlin patient," the 247
Bill C-36 229, 236, 237
binge drinking 318, 319
binge eating disorder 172
Bipolar disorder 187, 208
blind experimental design 22–23, 187

blood/brain barrier 302
BMI (*See* body mass index)
body composition 114, 159, 160, 162, 177, 181
body mass index 68, 147, 159, 164, 179, 181
body weight 3, 15, 25, 34, 64, 68, 70, 114, 143, 157–160, 164, 165, 168, 171, 173, 174, 179, 184, 186
botulism. *See* food poisoning
breastfeeding, as contraceptive 267, 285
breast self-examination 92, 94, 106
British Columbia Medical Association 346, 347, 365
bulimia nervosa 171, 180

C
caffeine 66, 202, 301, 304, 305, 317, 325
calcium 60, 98, 131, 133, 134, 137, 143, 144, 148, 153, 155
Canada and prescription opioids 320
Canada Food Guide 135
Canadian Society for Exercise Physiology 109, 110, 118, 128
cancer 86–108
　breast cancer 24, 84, 86, 89–92, 94–96, 101, 104, 106–108
　lung cancer 6, 23, 24, 27, 28, 38, 84, 88–91, 106, 233, 305–307, 314, 315, 383
　multi-stage screening for 93–94
　prevention 102–103
　prostate cancer 84, 86, 95–97, 101, 104, 106
　skin cancer 84, 99, 107
　treatment 100
cannabis 205, 231, 293, 303, 312–317, 325, 331, 332, 333, 335, 337–339
Cannabis Act 332
cannabis usage rates 313
capacity 111
carbohydrate 76, 133, 140, 141, 155, 175
carbon dioxide 59, 314, 373, 378, 380, 381, 383, 385, 386, 391
carbon footprint 385, 386, 390
carcinogen 86, 89, 103, 154, 318
cardiovascular disease 20, 25, 59, 61–66, 68–70, 72, 73, 77–81, 89, 114, 115, 134,

140, 160, 195, 306, 309, 318
　prevalence 61–62
　risk factors 62–69
Carson, Rachel 369
cervix 98, 105, 218, 235, 252, 273, 276, 281, 290, 291, 297
　cervical cancer 86, 98, 99, 107, 252–254
　cervical cap for contraception 273
chain of infection 39, 44, 54, 256
childbirth 15, 265, 277, 290–291, 294, 299
chlamydia 98, 255, 256, 257, 258, 260
cholera 25, 40, 45, 251
cholesterol 25, 60, 63, 64, 65, 66, 68, 72, 74, 78, 79, 80, 92, 120, 139, 141, 147
cilia damage and repair 305–307
circumcision 219, 220, 234, 236, 237
climate change 151, 374, 390
clitoris 218, 221, 223, 226, 234, 235
cocaine 302, 303, 305, 311, 312, 313, 314, 320, 326, 332, 335, 339
cocaine 302, 311, 329, 339
communicable 39, 44, 45, 48, 51, 53–55, 239
communicable disease. *See* infectious disease
complex carbohydrates 141
condom 48, 54, 218, 227, 243, 249, 252, 258–260, 267–269, 273, 274–276, 287, 297
condom 259, 296
contraception. *See* fertility management
contraceptive patch and lawsuits for injury and deaths 280
control group 20–24, 36, 91, 204
coronary artery. *See* coronary artery disease
coronary artery disease 20, 60, 78
　coronary artery bypass 74, 78, 356
crack. *See* cocaine
cross-training 125–126
Cuban model: prevention and primary care; social determinants of health 354–355
cultivation of relationships 197–198
cunnilingus 226, 227, 235

D

Dalkon Shield 281
Danish experiment, the 232
decriminalization 302, 331, 335
defence mechanisms 183, 185, 205, 206, 231
dementia 2, 3, 319
demographics of HIV-infection 244–247
dependence 29, 303, 312, 317, 323, 325, 336, 337, 339
Depo-Provera 303
depression 186, 187, 190, 192, 199, 205–207
diabetes 3, 9, 11, 12, 39, 59, 63, 64, 68–72, 75–81, 113, 116, 124, 129, 134, 141, 147, 155, 160, 180, 306, 329, 358
    prevalence 71
    risk factors 72
    treatment 75–76
diaphragm, contraceptive method 218, 268, 269, 273, 276, 281
diarrhea 2, 41, 47, 48, 97, 370
dieting 158, 170, 174, 175, 178, 186
digestion 133, 137, 153, 154, 193, 206
discipline 16
double-blind 22, 23, 36
double-blind, experimental design 22, 36
drugs 301–340
    Four Pillars 326, 327, 330
    models of abuse 325–326
    psychoactive drug 301, 304, 305, 313, 327, 334–336
    routes of administration 302–303
    treatment 327–329
    why people take drugs 322–325
dual-energy X-ray absorptiometry (DXA) 163

E

eating disorders 157, 170–172, 178, 180, 181
e-cigarettes and regulation 311
e-cigarette vapour or "aerosol" 310–311
economic externalities 378, 390
effects of pornography 211, 230–232

Eisner, David 31, 38
elevated cortisol 194
endemic 52, 55, 244
ENDS and gateway effect 310
ENDS, defined 309
environment 369–392
epidemiology 19, 24, 26, 37, 38, 183, 239, 245, 260
estrogen 8, 86, 91, 92, 101, 143, 217, 278
ethanol. *See* alcohol
eustress 195, 196, 206
evaluating health claims 19–38, 62, 114, 115, 136, 159, 232, 279
evidence 19–38
exercise 109–130
    benefits of exercise 113–115
experiment 20–24
experimental group 20–23, 36, 37, 91, 204
extra billing 347
extra-billing 341, 347, 364

F

Fallopian tube. *See* oviduct
farming. *See* agriculture
fat intake 20, 139, 146
fee-for-service 348, 350, 365
fee-for-service payments 348
fee schedule 346, 364, 365
fellatio 226, 227, 235
female GPs 344
fentanyl 302, 321, 322
fertility management 265–300
    barrier methods 273–276
    effectiveness 266–268
fibre 65, 76, 98, 103, 131, 138, 141, 142, 144, 146, 176
first-degree relative 95
fitness 109–130
    aerobic 13, 64, 109, 110, 112, 113, 118–120, 123, 127, 133, 174, 184
    flexibility 123–124
    health-related 113–116
    muscular 120–122
    performance-related 113
five-year survival rate 88–89
flexibility 109, 112, 123, 127

flu. *See* influenza
foreskin 218, 220, 235
four food groups 134, 135, 170
Four Pillars 326, 327, 330
Framingham Heart Study 38, 62, 115
free enterprise 365
free radicals 60
French model: welfare state economy, salaries and contributions, fees, health insurers 355
funding (health care) 343–344

G

general adaptation syndrome 183, 193, 194, 206, 222, 304
genetically modified foods 131, 155
genital anatomy 216–220
    female 216–218
    male 218–220
glans 218, 221, 235
global HIV infections 245–247
global warming 374, 375, 383
gonorrhea 45, 255, 256, 257, 258, 260
good health habits 47–49
Government budget for health care 343–344
gratitude journaling 204
greenhouse gas 374, 375, 386, 390

H

Hall Commission 342, 347, 361, 364
harm reduction 329
hash, hashish. *See* cannabis
HCV hepatitis C virus 251
HDL. *See* lipoprotein
health 1–18
    holistic model 1, 6, 6–8, 231, 341
    medical model 4–5
    risk factor 6, 64–66, 68, 71, 72, 80, 90, 96, 98, 102, 111, 142, 160, 190, 254
    social determinants 10–12
    wellness model 14–14
health and GDP 356
health care 341–368
    American system 350–353
    Canadian system 342–350
cost 356–359
funding 343–349
nurses 346
physicians 357–358
health insurance premiums 344–345
heart attack 30, 61, 74, 77, 79, 117, 188, 318
hectare 377
height-weight tables 158–159
hepatitis 45, 86, 239, 242, 250, 251, 260, 303, 321, 330
herd immunity 51–52
heroin. *See* opiates
herpes simplex 48, 219, 239, 253, 260, 262–264
high blood pressure. *See* hypertension
high-density lipoprotein. *See* lipoprotein
high environmental temperature 117
high-fructose corn syrup (HFCS) 140–141
HIV/AIDS 3, 237, 240, 241, 241–252, 258, 261–263, 298, 337
    epidemiology 243–249
    prevention 248–250
    transmission 241–243
    treatment 247
homeostasis 192, 193, 206, 207
homosexuality 227–228
hormone replacement therapy 92
HPV. *See* human papilloma virus
HPV immunization 253
HSV. *See* herpes simplex
HSV-1 and HSV-2 infection 253–255
human papilloma virus 98, 219
hydrostatic weighing 162, 163
hypertension 11, 25, 38, 66–68, 72, 77, 79, 147, 160, 329
hypothesis 20, 36, 37

I

immune system 40–43, 86, 87, 98, 101, 150, 152, 184, 194, 240, 241, 247, 254, 261
immunity 42, 43, 51, 52, 54–56, 240, 251, 256
immunization 15, 43, 50, 51, 55, 253

impact factor 31, 36
Implanon 279
incidence 39–40
incubation period. *See* latent period
Indigenous Services 190
infant mortality 2, 3, 15, 16, 152, 351, 387
infant mortality rate 2, 3, 15, 16
infection 39–58
    natural defences 53, 54
infectious disease 2, 9, 39–40, 45, 48, 49,
    52–55, 248, 251, 358, 387
infirmity 14, 16, 127
inflammatory biomarkers 204
influenza 40, 43, 44, 46, 47, 54–56, 88,
    116, 125
injury, activity-related 114, 116, 117, 120,
    122, 124–127
    prevention 124–125
    treatment 125–126
Insite: fatal overdoses, interventions,
    detox, drug related crime, Hep C and
    HIV 322, 330, 331, 337, 338, 340
Insite safe injection facility 330–331
intimate relationships 211–238
intrauterine device. *See* IUD
iron, dietary 131, 133, 137, 138, 142–144,
    147, 148, 153
IUD 267, 269, 281–283, 296
IUD most effective form of birth control
    281–282

J
J-shaped 318

K
Kinsey Reports 227
Kutchinsky, B. 232, 236

L
labia 218, 221, 223, 235
labour. *See* childbirth
latent period 23, 36, 37, 40, 54, 55, 89, 90,
    105, 247, 259–261
legalized cannabis 332–334
leisure time physical activity 110
leptin 68, 164, 165

lesion 60, 61, 79, 256
life expectancy 2, 3, 7–10, 15, 84, 114,
    129, 145, 247, 304, 351, 386
lifetime prevalence 84, 171, 172
lipoprotein 64, 66, 114, 147
low-density lipoprotein. *See* lipoprotein

M
malaria 40, 44, 45, 53
malignant 86–88, 97, 99, 104, 105
marijuana. *See* cannabis
marriage 211–214, 216, 224, 225, 227, 229,
    235, 236, 253, 259, 294
Maslow, Abraham 184, 205, 207, 209
Masters & Johnson 221
masturbation 225, 226
measles 20, 40, 50, 51, 53, 55–57, 152, 260
medical interventions and best practice
    362
medical model 4, 5, 16, 18
Medical Services Commission 347, 366,
    367
Medical Services Plan of BC (MSP) 288,
    347, 348, 349
menstrual cycle 216, 235, 271, 272
mental health 183–210
    treatment 191–192
metastasis 86–88, 105
meth. *See* amphetamines
method of taking drugs 302–303
miscarriage 285, 290, 297, 307, 319
model 3–14
mood and anxiety disorders 186–187
mood disorders 9, 190, 207
mortality 2, 3, 5, 6, 13, 15–18, 27, 28, 39,
    46, 54, 56, 59, 63, 68, 71, 73–75, 78,
    79, 83, 84, 90–92, 94, 95, 98, 99, 104,
    108, 111, 113, 115–117, 128, 129, 145, 152,
    160–163, 170, 171, 181, 212–214, 234,
    237, 239, 245, 262, 338, 351, 352, 354,
    386–388, 390, 392
most prevalent STI 252
multi-stage screening 93, 104, 105
mutation 49, 91, 101, 105

N

narcotics. *See* opiates
National Lung Screening Trial 91
national prohibition. *See* prohibition
neurotransmitter 187, 207, 305
nicotine 60, 64, 68, 202, 305, 307–310, 323, 335–337, 340
    nicotine replacement therapy 309
normal sexual behaviour 211, 211–212
norovirus. *See* stomach flu
nuclear reactor 382–383
Nunavut 9
nutrition 131–156
    developing world 151–152
    dietary recommendations 138
    modern North American diet 137–138
nutritional supplements 137, 138, 155

O

Obamacare 352, 353, 366
obese 12, 63, 68, 69, 72, 76, 157–159, 164, 165, 167, 168, 172, 177, 178, 180, 181
obesity 17, 68, 79, 80, 96, 158, 160, 164, 167, 181
    causes 164–167
    prevalence 164
    social issues 167–169
obsessions and rituals 189
obsessive-compulsive disorder 189, 209
OECD defined 356
omega-3 fatty acid 65, 138, 140, 144
omega-6 fatty acid 140, 144
opiates 320–322
opioid overdose crisis 321
oral sex 226, 226–227, 235, 249, 258
organic food 148–149, 153, 386
orgasm 95, 218, 221, 222–224, 227, 228, 235
osteoporosis 115, 127, 143, 154, 171, 277
other STIs & anti-microbial agents 255–258
overfat 158, 164, 178, 179, 181
overweight 17, 30, 63, 68, 69, 71, 72, 75–77, 138, 157–161, 164, 166, 168, 178, 179, 181
oviduct 216, 218

P

panic attack 188, 205, 207
panic disorder 188, 205, 207
Pap test 98, 99, 105, 282
pathogen 40, 42–45, 52, 54, 55, 240, 251, 252, 260, 261
peer review 30–31
penis 45, 218, 221, 223, 226, 235, 243, 249, 271, 273, 276
pertussis (whooping cough) 51
physical activity 3, 11, 16, 48, 67, 70, 76, 92, 98, 109–130, 133, 135, 166, 169, 172–174, 178, 180, 192, 204, 208, 232, 293, 370, 381
placenta 43, 241, 290, 292, 297
polio 50, 52, 56
pollution 193, 199, 373, 374, 378–380, 381
    air pollution 374, 378
    land pollution 378–380
pooling risk 353
population 385–389
    definition of 386
    dynamics 386–387
    pyramid 387–389
    stresses on resources 385–386
population health 1, 2, 16
porn addiction 231
pornography 211, 230, 231, 232, 234, 235, 236, 237. *See also* sex, commercial
portal of entry; of exit. *See* chain of infection
potential years of life lost (PYLL) 84
pregnancy 72, 91, 98, 144, 154, 165, 216, 218, 225, 259, 265, 268–271, 277, 279, 283–285, 287–290, 293–300, 307, 312, 316
    having a healthy pregnancy 293–294
    teenage pregnancy 294–295
prevalence 3, 9, 17, 20, 61, 62, 66, 71, 72, 77, 79, 84, 90, 94, 136, 141, 155, 157, 164, 166, 168, 171, 172, 178, 181, 186, 190, 228, 237, 239, 252, 255, 260–263, 297, 298, 312, 320, 327, 353, 359
prevention 6, 17, 18, 59, 62, 69, 73, 74, 78–89, 92, 102–108, 114, 123, 134, 143,

177, 180, 183, 191, 208, 220, 239, 240,
251, 269, 301, 327, 333, 354, 356, 360,
362, 363, 391
  of illness 6
  of suicide 191
  secondary prevention 59, 74, 78, 79,
    89, 92, 104, 105, 134
processed food 138
producing reward 204
progesterone 8, 278
progestin. See progesterone
prohibition 331, 333–335, 347
prolonged sitting 111
prospective, studies 116, 128
prostate 83, 84, 86, 95–97, 101, 102, 104,
  106, 108, 218, 284
  cancer 84, 86, 95–97, 101, 104, 106
  gland 95, 218
prostitution. See sex, commercial
protein 54, 55, 64, 76, 79, 96, 98, 121, 131,
  135, 138, 139, 143–145, 147, 151, 152, 155,
  194
psychoactive drug. See drugs
public health agencies 131, 134
purging 171, 179
PYLL. See potential years of life lost

R
radioactive atoms 380
radioactive fallout. See fallout
relative risk 50–51
respiratory infection 2
risk-benefit ratio 51
risk factor 6, 64–66, 68, 71, 72, 79, 80,
  90, 96, 98, 102, 111, 142, 160, 190, 254
Romanow report 360, 361, 362, 367, 368
routine circumcision 220

S
salmonella. See food poisoning
salt. See sodium
sample size 22
saturated fat 64, 79, 139, 144, 146
schizophrenia 185, 209
screening 6, 83, 91, 93–97, 99, 104, 105,
  106–108, 126, 230, 252, 255, 256, 362

screen time 109–111, 127, 128, 362
scrotum 218, 221, 223, 284
self-actualization 184
Selye, Dr. Hans 192–195, 206, 210
set point theory 165, 179
sex 211–238
  anal 227
  assault. See rape
  commercial sex 228–230
  human sexual response 221–224
  oral sex 226–227
  sexual health promotion 232–233
  sex with children 225
sexuality 16, 211, 212, 237, 270, 283
sexually transmissible infections
  239–264
sex workers 228–230
signs, of disease 4, 23, 37, 105, 127, 259
  signs and symptoms 14, 91, 117, 125,
    240, 247
skinfold thickness 161–163
sleep 48, 64, 66, 68, 118, 160, 183,
  186–188, 197, 199, 200, 200–204, 206,
  208, 209, 308, 312, 313, 323
smallpox 260
smog 373
smoking 6, 12, 20, 23, 25, 27–29, 33, 64,
  68, 73, 75, 77, 88, 90, 98, 102, 233, 293,
  303, 305, 307–311, 313–317, 322, 324,
  332, 335–337
  cannabis 314, 315–317
  prevalence 307
  quitting 308–309
  reasons people smoke 307–308
social anxiety disorder 188–189
sodium 63, 67, 138, 142, 144, 145, 155,
  293, 370
solar power 384
spaceship Earth 369, 370, 390
specificity 28
sperm 7, 8, 85, 218, 234, 235, 271, 273,
  279, 282–285
Spiegelhalter, David 51
  Spiegelhalter 51, 56
Stevenson, V. 229, 237
stress 192–200

stressor 116, 193–196, 206, 207, 223

stroke 61, 66, 68, 71, 79

suicide 6, 9, 11, 13, 171, 172, 183, 186, 187, 189–191, 205, 208, 210, 319
    epidemiology 189–190
    prevention 191
    risk factors 190–191

symptoms, of disease 4, 14, 23, 37, 40, 91, 105, 117, 125, 127, 240, 247, 259

syndrome 7, 26, 123, 183, 193, 194, 206, 207, 209, 222, 240, 261, 293, 304, 316, 319
    acquired immune deficiency syndrome (AIDS) 26, 261
    general adaptation syndrome 183, 193, 194, 206, 222, 304

syndrome, definition 193

syphilis 255, 256, 258, 260, 262

syphilis resurgence and poverty 257

Systemic inequality, HIV and AIDS 246–247

T

tanning beds 100, 107

testicle 8, 218, 224, 235, 256

testing for diseases 93–94
    testing vs screening 93–94

tetanus 45, 294

The Pill. *See* oral contraceptives

thermal power plants 383–384

time management 197

tolerance 41, 232, 312, 325, 329, 336

total calories consumed 137

toxin 45, 48, 65, 131, 140, 149, 293

traffic injury 2, 331

trans-fats 139, 140, 144, 155

treatment for HPV-infection 252

tubal ligation. *See* tubal sterilization

tubal sterilization 283

tuberculosis 2–4, 15, 18, 40, 337

tumour 86–89, 91, 92, 97, 100, 101, 104, 105, 163, 305

two-tiered health care system 358

U

umbilical cord 290, 291, 297

undue exploitation of sex 230

unprotected sex 232, 257

unsafe abortions 286, 294

urethra 41, 218, 221, 235, 256

USA Patient Protection and Affordable Health Care Act 352–353

uterus 43, 91, 98, 102, 105, 216, 218, 221, 234, 235, 277, 281, 282, 284, 290–292, 297

V

vaccination. *See* immunization

vaccine 5, 43, 46, 47, 50–52, 56, 248, 251, 253, 255, 262, 263

vagina 41, 45, 98, 105, 216, 218, 221, 223, 224, 226, 227, 235, 243, 249, 256, 271, 273, 276, 278, 281, 291, 297

vaginal ring 278, 281

valid data 110

vas deferens 218, 221, 235, 284, 297

vasectomy 267–269, 284, 285, 296, 297

vector 44, 45, 53, 55

vegan. *See* vegetarian

vegetarian 131, 140, 145, 146, 148, 153, 154

viral gastroenteritis. *See* stomach flu

virus 26, 43–48, 55, 88, 98, 219, 239–243, 247, 248, 251, 253, 254, 260–264

W

waist girth, circumference 161–162

wait lists, for health service 359–360

walk-in clinics 360

water 370–372
    cycle 371
    drinking 372
    quality 372

weakened immune system 98, 194

weight control 172–177

welfare state 342, 350, 355, 363, 365

wellness 1, 13, 14, 15, 16, 18, 184, 204, 205, 212, 231, 308, 360, 363

wellness model 14

whole body electrical impedance 163

whole foods 138

wind power 384

withdrawal 267, 271, 296, 312, 326

drugs 308, 309, 312, 321, 325, 326, 328,
336
intercourse 271, 274
World Health Organization (WHO) 1,
2, 14, 16–18, 49, 52, 56, 57, 139, 150, 152,
155, 161, 181, 237, 253, 262, 263, 281,
286, 299, 311, 346, 367

This book's text is set in Warnock, a contemporary typeface grounded in the classic proportions of oldstyle Roman type. The headings are set in Cronos, which derives its appearance from the calligraphically inspired type of the Italian Renaissance. Both typefaces were designed by Robert Slimbach.

This book was printed by Hignell Book Printing on Ph neutral paper that is processed chlorine free.